The Impact of Addictive Substances and Behaviours on Individual and Societal Well-being

D1465248

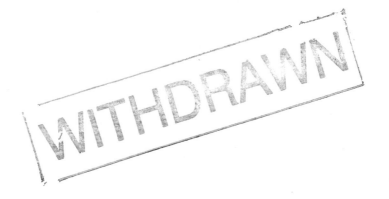

Governance of Addictive Substances and Behaviours Series

Series Editors:
Peter Anderson and Antoni Gual

Titles in the series

Governance of Addictions: European Public Policies

Tamyko Ysa, Joan Colom, Adrià Albareda, Anna Ramon, Marina Carrión, and Lidia Segura

The Impact of Addictive Substances and Behaviours on Individual and Societal Well-being

Edited by

Peter Anderson

Jürgen Rehm and

Robin Room

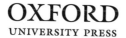

OXFORD
UNIVERSITY PRESS

OXFORD
UNIVERSITY PRESS

Great Clarendon Street, Oxford, OX2 6DP,
United Kingdom

Oxford University Press is a department of the University of Oxford.
It furthers the University's objective of excellence in research, scholarship,
and education by publishing worldwide. Oxford is a registered trade mark of
Oxford University Press in the UK and in certain other countries

First Edition published in 2015

Impression: 1

Published in the United States of America by Oxford University Press
198 Madison Avenue, New York, NY 10016, United States of America

British Library Cataloguing in Publication Data

Data available

Library of Congress Control Number: 2014953420

ISBN 978–0–19–871400–2

Printed in Great Britain by
Clays Ltd, St Ives plc

Foreword

This book, *The Impact of Addictive Substances and Behaviours on Individual and Societal Well-being*, is the second in a planned series of six books arising out of ALICE RAP (Addictions and Lifestyles in Contemporary Europe—Reframing Addiction's Project), a 5-year, €10 million endeavour co-financed by the Social Sciences and Humanities division of FP7 within the European Commission and led by the Foundation for Biomedical Research based in Barcelona and the Institute of Health and Society at Newcastle University (<http://www.alicerap.eu/>). The first book described current European approaches to governing addictive substances and behaviours (Ysa et al., 2014). Subsequent books will address the determinants of harm from addictive substances and behaviours, how concepts of addictive substances and behaviours have changed across time and place, the impact of market forces on addictive substances and behaviours, and how we can work towards a new governance of addictive substances and behaviours.

ALICE RAP studies the place of addictions and lifestyles in present-day Europe and aims to inform how we can better redesign their governance. By addictions, we mean the regular and sustained heavy use of drugs, such as alcohol, nicotine, and cocaine and regular and sustained heavy engagement in actions such as gambling or internet gaming.

Three things in particular strike one on reading this book. First, the extent of the harm done by addictive substances is phenomenal. In 2010, for the world as a whole, out of sixty-seven risk factors for a combined measure of ill-health and premature death (measured as disability-adjusted life years, DALYs), tobacco use was the second most important risk factor, alcohol the fifth, and illicit drug use the eighteenth (high blood pressure was the first, household air pollution from solid fuels the third, and a diet low in fruits the fourth; Lim et al., 2012). Secondly, harm is not just about health but about all aspects of life. Addictive substances can impair quality of life through their impact on work, education, civic engagement, social connections, and personal security; they can impair material living conditions through their impact on income and wealth, jobs and earnings, and housing; and, they can impair the sustainability of well-being over time by diminishing economic, human, and social capital. Thirdly, harm does not result just from the addictive drug itself, but also the societal response to the drug, which can cause more harm than the drug itself through stigma, social exclusion, and actions of the criminal justice system.

What is also clear from this book is that money features highly when considering addictive substances. Too much money through the greed of those who produce and market addictive substances is a driver of harm. Too little money amongst those who use drugs is a driver of harm—for the same level of drug use, poorer people are more likely to die from drug-related causes than richer people. And, too much money is wasted—the untaxed retail value of cannabis alone in the European Union is between €18 and €30 billion per year, with profits accruing to organized criminal networks and unregulated markets.

This book shows that as far as human experience with drugs is concerned, there is nothing new. Psychoactive drug use is a pan-human phenomenon, widespread in the archaeological record, at least for the last 12,000 years. Beyond this, during the evolution of the human lineage there were biological fitness benefits associated with regulated consumption of psychoactive drugs, which are primarily plant toxins. Humans were thus active agents in drug-seeking behaviour, and its neurophysiological basis could have evolved because of beneficial effects of neurotoxins. But, in present-day society, with the globalization of markets, heavy use is common, and going beyond a certain boundary leads to stigmatization, particularly for poorer and marginalized groups of society. We can understand the concept of addiction as a particular way of explaining why so much harm can result from something so attractive. The problem, though, is that the addiction concept tends to dichotomize harm, when this is not the case—harm being on a continuum—and it narrows societal attention to the individual level of those engaged in the behaviour, neglecting the fact that the environment in which someone lives is a major determinant of drug use and harm.

Hippocrates (1978), writing 2,500 years ago, advised anyone coming to a new city to enquire whether it was likely to be a healthy or unhealthy place to live, depending on its geography and the behaviour of its inhabitants ('whether they are fond of excessive drinking'). He continued 'as a general rule, the constitutions and the habits of a people follow the nature of the land where they live'. When redesigning the governance of addictions, we need to take this into account. The bad news is that, as the first book in this series pointed out, there is no group of countries in Europe whose policies on addictive substances could be described as optimal in promoting quality of life, material living conditions, and sustainability of well-being over time (Ysa et al., 2014). The good news is that we can all do better.

Peter Anderson

International coordinator of the ALICE RAP project; chief series editor, Governance of Addictive Substances and Behaviours; Professor of Substance Use, Policy and Practice, Newcastle University, UK; Professor of Alcohol and Health, Maastricht University, the Netherlands

References

Hippocrates (1978). *Hippocratic Writings*. Edited with an introduction by G.E.R. Lloyd. Harmondsworth: Penguin.

Lim, S.S., Vos, T., Flaxman, A.D., et al. (2012). A comparative risk assessment of burden of disease and injury attributable to 67 risk factors and risk factor clusters in 21 regions, 1990–2010: a systematic analysis for the Global Burden of Disease Study 2010. *Lancet*, **380**, 2224–2260.

Ysa, T., Colom, J. Albareda, A., Ramon, A., Carrión, M., & Segura, L. (2014). *Governance of Addictions: European Public Policies*. Oxford: Oxford University Press.

Acknowledgements

The editors thank all the people involved in the ALICE RAP project for their support, comments, and contributions along the years. We would especially like to thank Toni Gual and all the team from the Hospital Clínic of Barcelona for being excellent facilitators and providing the necessary support to reach the desired goals. The research leading to much of this book has received funding from the European Community's Seventh Framework Programme (FP7/2 007–2013), under grant agreement no. 266,813—Addictions and Lifestyle in Contemporary Europe—Reframing Addictions Project (ALICE RAP). Participant organisations in ALICE RAP can be seen at <http://www.alicerap.eu/about-alice-rap/partners.html>.

Contents

List of contributors xi

1 Introduction to addictive behaviours 1
Peter Anderson, Jürgen Rehm, and Robin Room

2 Passive vulnerability or active agency? An ecological
and evolutionary perspective on human drug use 13
Roger J. Sullivan and Edward H. Hagen

3 What are addictive substances and behaviours and how far do they
extend? 37
Laura A. Schmidt

4 Well-being as a framework for understanding addictive
substances 53
Laura Stoll and Peter Anderson

5 The effects of addictive substances and addictive behaviours on
physical and mental health 77
Kevin D. Shield and Jürgen Rehm

6 Drug and alcohol policy for European youth: current evidence
and recommendations for integrated policies and research
strategies 119
*Patricia J. Conrod, Angelina Brotherhood, Harry Sumnall,
Fabrizio Faggiano, and Reinout Wiers*

7 Addictive substances and behaviours and social justice 143
Jacek Moskalewicz and Justyna I. Klingemann

8 Impact of the economic recession on addiction-prone
behaviours 161
Aleksandra Dubanowicz and Paul Lemmens

9 Social costs of addiction in Europe 181
Kevin D. Shield, Maximilien X. Rehm, and Jürgen Rehm

10 Addictive substances and socioeconomic development 189
*Robin Room, Sujatha Sankaran, Laura A. Schmidt, Pia Mäkelä,
and Jürgen Rehm*

11 Addictive substances and behaviours and corruption, transparency,
and governance 215
David Miller and Claire Harkins

12 Conclusions 239
Jürgen Rehm, Robin Room, and Peter Anderson

Index 247

List of contributors

Peter Anderson
MD PhD MPH, Professor of Substance Use, Policy and Practice, Institute of Health and Society, Newcastle University, UK; Professor of Alcohol and Health, Faculty of Health, Medicine and Life Sciences, Maastricht University, the Netherlands

Angelina Brotherhood
Public Health Researcher, Centre for Public Health, Liverpool John Moores University, UK; Doctoral Candidate, Department of Sociology, University of Vienna, Austria

Patricia J. Conrod
PhD, Research Professor, Department of Psychiatry, Université de Montréal, Canada; Senior Clinical Lecturer, Addictions Department, King's Health Partners, Institute of Psychiatry, King's College London, UK

Aleksandra Dubanowicz
MSc Global Health, BSc European Public Health, Maastricht University, The Netherlands

Fabrizio Faggiano
MD, Associate Professor of Public Health, Department of Translational Medicine, Avogadro University of Eastern Piedmont, Novara, Italy

Edward H. Hagen
PhD Associate Professor of Anthropology, Washington State University, Vancouver, WA, USA

Claire Harkins
PhD candidate and research associate, University of Bath, UK

Justyna I. Klingemann
PhD, sociologist, Assistant Professor at the Department of Studies on Alcohol and Drug Dependence, Institute of Psychiatry and Neurology, Warsaw, Poland

Paul Lemmens
PhD, Associate Professor, Department of Health Promotion, Faculty of Health, Medicine and Life Sciences, Maastricht University, the Netherlands

Pia Mäkelä
Senior researcher and head of Alcohol and Drugs, National Institute for Health and Welfare, Helsinki, Finland

David Miller
Professor of Sociology, Department for Social and Policy Sciences, University of Bath, UK; Director, Public Interest Investigations, UK; Member, Centre for Tobacco and Alcohol Studies, Centre for Public Health Excellence, UK

Jacek Moskalewicz
PhD, Head, Department of Studies
on Alcoholism and Drug
Dependence, Institute of Psychiatry
and Neurology, Warsaw, Poland

Jürgen Rehm
PhD, Professor, head of an
epidemiological research unit,
Technische Universität Dresden,
Germany; Chair, Professor,
University of Toronto, Canada;
Director, Social and
Epidemiological Research
Department, Centre for Addiction
and Mental Health, Toronto,
Canada

Maximilien X. Rehm
Student, Faculty of Arts
and Sciences/Politics and
Governance, Ryerson University,
Toronto, Canada

Robin Room
PhD, Professor, Melbourne School
of Population and Global Health,
University of Melbourne, Australia;
Professor, Centre for Social
Research on Alcohol and Drugs,
Stockholm University; Director,
Centre for Alcohol Policy Research
at Turning Point, Fitzroy, Victoria,
Australia

Sujatha Sankaran
MD, Assistant Clinical Professor,
Division of Hospital Medicine,
Department of Medicine, University
of California San Francisco, USA

Laura A. Schmidt
PhD, MSW, MPH, Professor, Philip
R. Lee Institute for Health Policy
Studies and Department of
Anthropology, History and Social
Medicine, School of Medicine,
University of California at
San Francisco, USA

Kevin D. Shield
MHSc, PhD student, World Health
Organization/Pan-American Health
Organization Collaborating Centre in
Addiction and Mental Health, Centre
for Addiction and Mental Health,
Toronto, Canada; PhD student,
Institute of Medical Science,
University of Toronto, Toronto,
Canada

Laura Stoll
Researcher, Wellbeing Economics
and Policy, London, UK

Roger J. Sullivan
PhD, Associate Professor of
Anthropology, California State
University, Sacramento, CA, USA

Harry Sumnall
PhD, Professor of Substance Use,
Centre for Public Health, Liverpool
John Moores University, UK

Reinout Wiers
PhD, Professor of Developmental
Psychopathology, Addiction
Development and Psychopathology
(ADAPT) Lab, Department of
Psychology, Universiteit van
Amsterdam, the Netherlands

Chapter 1

Introduction to addictive behaviours

Peter Anderson, Jürgen Rehm, and Robin Room

1.1 Addictive behaviours as a conceptual frame

This book focuses on a set of behaviours which are commonly described as 'addictive'. As will be discussed, the behaviours that are considered 'addictive' have varied by time and place, although they have always included the use of at least some psychoactive substances. The common characteristics identified by the descriptor 'addictive' are: that the behaviour has attractive effects for the person engaged in it; that the effects are attractive enough that some who try it go on to repeated and heavy patterns of the behaviour; and that the behaviour often has negative health and social consequences for the person engaged in it, and often also for others.

To focus on the addictive dimension of behaviours is to emphasize thinking and action at the level of the interaction between the substance or behaviour and the individual consumer. The concept of addiction was first popularized as an explanation in terms of an individual's loss of self-control over his or her own behaviour (alcohol consumption), despite negative consequences or an apparent desire to desist (Levine, 1978). For the individual, the attraction and reinforcement of the behaviour become so great that often neither disincentives nor willpower can curb it.

In this book we expand the perspective on the dynamics of addictive behaviours beyond the individual consumer, and beyond substances. Firstly, addictive behaviours often cause harm to or carry costs for others, which may not be taken into account in an individual's decisions about the behaviour. The heavy gambler is often using up collectively owned resources—the family's joint finances and assets—in pursuit of his or her personal pleasure in or devotion to gambling (Borch, 2012). A heavy drinker's behaviour often causes harms to family members, friends, and strangers (Laslett et al., 2011). And second-hand smoke threatens the health of people who happen to be close enough to smokers (US Department of Health and Human Services, 2006). Besides harms to specific others, the behaviour may also result in harm at a collective level, for instance in loss of productivity for the consumer's workplace or the disturbance of peace and order for a community (see Chapter 9). The term 'externalities' used in economics conveys the reality that behavioural choices about consumption are often made considering only the interest of the consumer without taking into account the interests of others.

Secondly, most of the behaviours considered as addictive are potentially commodifiable and subject to market forces. Because of their attractions for use, and particularly for repeated and heavy use, commercialized addictive products or behaviours are potentially especially profitable. History is replete with examples of extreme levels of addictive behaviours, with large societal harms and costs, when commercial interests have had free rein to promote and sell addictive products and behaviours in a laissez-faire system of market governance.

Thirdly, history also records many instances of substantial societal reaction to addictive behaviours as a consequence of these harms and costs. The radical response, to prohibit commercial sale and promotion altogether, has been quite widespread. Most commercialized gambling was outlawed in many countries in the later nineteenth century and the first half of the twentieth (e.g. Dixon, 1991; Campbell and Smith, 2003). All alcohol sales were prohibited at some time in the period between 1910 and 1935 in at least 13 self-governing states, including four in Europe (Schrad, 2010). The non-medical sale and use of over 250 psychoactive substances is currently globally prohibited under international drug control treaties (Room and Reuter, 2012). Between the extremes of laissez-faire and prohibition, governments and societies have pursued various strategies of regulation and normative control of addictive behaviours, and particularly of the commercial promotion of such behaviours. A burgeoning public health-oriented literature considers these strategies and the evidence on whether and how they are effective in limiting addictive behaviours (e.g. Babor et al., 2010a,b; Ysa et al., 2014).

An important corollary of the societal importance of addictive behaviours and their consequences is that legislative and normative responses often seek to limit the behaviour by derogating and stigmatizing consumers and their behaviour. To be called a 'drunk' in English, a '*clochard*' in French, or a '*Säufer*' in German is not a compliment. As will be discussed in later chapters, these social processes of derogation become sources of secondary harms to consumers and those associated with them, and this needs to be taken into account in policy-making.

1.2 **Addictive behaviours in Europe in the last fifty years**

The last fifty years have been characterized by important changes in people's lives and lifestyles and in European society, social structures, and values. The changing nature of work and of private life, the evolution of the patterns of consumption, values, attitudes, and beliefs of modern societies have all changed the place and challenges of addictions in current European society. Addictions are an extensive feature of modern societies, bringing considerable concerns. As their number seems to have increased over the last decades, they have become a focus of social, economic, and political attention, sometimes polarizing societies and politics. In addition to the widely acknowledged problem of addiction to various substances, there is a growing problem of new addictions such as gambling, eating disorders, and use of the internet. A considerable proportion of all expenditure in European health systems flows into the treatment of various addictions, and even more into the treatment of their mental and physical health consequences. In addition, there are the costs of prevention and the associated crime, which increasingly have global dimensions. Thus the governance (the way in which a society or organization steers itself with respect to addictions) and stewardship of addictions need to balance individual freedom and social responsibility while taking into account social, economic, and ethical considerations.

1.3 **Framing the book**

This book addresses the impact of addictive substances and behaviours on individual and societal well-being. The book arises out of the ALICE RAP project, a 5-year scientific endeavour to analyse and take stock of the challenges of addictions and lifestyles to the cohesion, organization, and functioning of present-day European society (<http://www.alicerap.eu/>). This book is the second in a series of six on the governance of addictive substances and behaviours. The first book described current European approaches to the governance of addictive substances and behaviours (Ysa et al., 2014). Subsequent books will address the determinants of harm from addictive substances and behaviours, how concepts of addictive substances and behaviours have changed across time and place, the impact of market forces on addictive substances and behaviours, and progress towards a new governance of addictive substances and behaviours. The frame of the ALICE RAP project, and thus of this book, is public health and well-being, and included within this is a consideration of harm, whether at individual, interpersonal, or social and societal levels. Charting the adverse consequences of addictive behaviours, considered both in terms of direct harms and of their negative impact on well-being, is a major focus of this book.

What we mean by addictive substances and behaviours are primarily substances such as alcohol, nicotine, and illegal drugs (e.g. cannabis, cocaine, and opiates) and behaviours such as gambling. In this book we touch on all of these, but largely focus on alcohol, nicotine, and illegal drugs. This simply reflects the much greater literature on drugs than on behaviours.

Addictive substances and behaviours interact with a wide range of dimensions and domains of individual and societal well-being (see Chapter 4). In terms of quality of life, these include health, work–life balance, education and skills, civic engagement and governance, social connections, personal security, and subjective well-being itself. In terms of material living conditions, these include jobs and earnings, and housing. Addictive substances and behaviours also interact with the sustainability of well-being over time, by impacting upon trajectories of human, social, and economic capital. The interactions across all these dimensions are two-way. Take jobs and earnings as an example. On the one hand, heavy use of drugs (alcohol, tobacco, and illicit drugs) impairs an individual's employability and performance at work; on the other hand, highly demanding unrewarding jobs increase the risk of heavy drug use. So, while this book addresses the impact of addictive substances and behaviours on individual and societal well-being, it also addresses the dimensions and domains of societal well-being as drivers of both heavy drug use and the harm done by drug use—which in turn cause more harm to individual and societal well-being. Take social exclusion as an example. As already noted, heavy drug users are often stigmatized and socially excluded (see Chapter 7). Social exclusion can exacerbate drug use, and at any given level of drug use the socially excluded suffer more harm (see Chapter 10). Drug users can also be sent to prison, which disenfranchises them and removes them from the labour market, severely diminishing their future employment and earning prospects. So, the relation between drug use and adverse consequences is not a simple process; it is compounded by society's reaction to drugs, which can sometimes cause more harm than the drugs themselves.

1.4 **Overview of the book**

In Chapter 2, Sullivan and Hagen remind us that the aetiological theory of human drug use has historically been dominated by the notion that drug use is initiated and sustained by biological and behavioural rewards and reinforcement. They note that the operationalization of drug reward theory has invoked other aetiological concepts, including the nature of novelty in human encounters with drugs, and human behavioural and biological vulnerability to drugs. They go on to point out that if one stands back and considers drugs from anthropological, ethnohistorical, and evolutionary perspectives, the notion is actually very different. With respect to many drugs, human evolution has entailed a long and dynamic relationship that has been active and functional, rather than passive and vulnerable; and that fundamental ecological dynamics, rather than rewards, have been the primary 'cause' of human drug use.

Sullivan and Hagen note that the use of psychoactive drugs primarily involves plant toxins which, while triggering avoidance mechanisms in most individuals have been an important part of animal diets for hundreds of millions of years. Yet psychoactive drug use is a pan-human phenomenon, involving similar substances and concentrations across a diverse array of cultures, and is widespread in the archaeological record, at least for much of the Holocene era (the last 11,700 years). To explain this, Sullivan and Hagen suggest that during the evolution of the human lineage there were biological fitness benefits associated with regulated consumption of these substances. These fitness benefits could include pharmacophagy (the consumption of pharmacologically active substances), the exploitation of plant toxins against parasites, and the use of ingested compounds that chemically resemble endogenous signalling molecules at times when internal signalling functions could become compromised due to deficiencies in other dietary precursors in marginal environments. Thus, Sullivan and Hagen argue that, in principle, drug-seeking behaviour, and its neurophysiological basis, could have evolved because of the beneficial effects of neurotoxins. Although there is no doubt that such neurotoxins can constitute serious health hazards, these hazards, which often only appear at high doses or later in life, may have been offset by immediate benefits, resulting in a net increase in biological fitness.

Sullivan and Hagen do not discuss alcohol, but other evidence of the presence of ethanol within ripe fruit suggests low-level but chronic dietary exposure for all fruit-eating animals (Dudley, 2004). Volatilized alcohols from fruit could potentially serve in olfactory localization of transient nutritional resources, whereas ethanol consumed during the course of frugivory (fruit consumption) may act as an appetitive stimulant. As a consequence, natural selection may have acted on all frugivorous animals, including human ancestors, to associate ethanol consumption with nutritional reward. Studies of the evolution of the functions of ancestral alcohol dehydrogenases in primates has found that while the enzymes from the most ancient primate ancestors of humans were largely *inactive* against ethanol they could metabolize *other* alcohols, including the terpene alcohols abundant in the leaves of plants (Benner, 2013). Primate ancestors living 16–21 million years ago could not effectively metabolize consumed ethanol. However, by 6–12 million years before the present, the last common ancestor of humans with gorillas and chimpanzees had evolved a digestion fully able to metabolize consumed ethanol at the levels found in fermenting fruits. Later effects of alcohol use on human evolution are discussed in McGovern (2009), who identifies alcohol as crucial in humans making the transition to becoming farmers.

In Chapter 3, Laura Schmidt follows the recent trend in professional psychiatry towards expansion of the addiction concept to include new substances, such as sugar, and new habitual behaviours, such as gambling, internet gaming, and pornography use, into a pan-addiction model that would provide a single explanatory framework encompassing both substance and behavioural addictions. Schmidt argues that the widening scope of addictive disorders is a response to tangible changes unfolding in the information age, as globalized markets make a greater abundance of pleasurable substances and experiences available to consumers on a 24-hour, 7-day a week basis than ever before. She notes that discussions around expanding diagnoses of addiction also reflect psychiatry's own territorial and financial interests in responding to the growing demand for ways to help individuals achieve hedonic balance in a social context that increasingly fails to support it.

In Chapter 4, Laura Stoll and Peter Anderson describe how measures of societal well-being are increasingly being used as a holistic way of measuring societal progress rather than the single measure of national economic productivity (i.e. gross domestic product, GDP). They describe the Organisation for Economic Co-operation and Development's (OECD) Framework for Measuring Wellbeing and Progress, including quality of life, material living conditions, and sustainability over time. Stoll and Anderson give three examples of the interactions of well-being with addictive substances. First, they argue that quality of life and material living conditions are potentially adversely affected by addictive substances. In their second example, classifying cannabis as an illegal substance is argued to impair quality of life, material living conditions, and sustainability of well-being over time. Thirdly, while people have a diminished quality of life and material living conditions upon entering opioid substitution treatment, this is often, but not always, improved by treatment. Finally, based on the work of Ysa et al. (2014), Stoll and Anderson point out that there is no group of countries in Europe whose policies on addictive substances could be described as optimal in promoting quality of life, material living conditions, and sustainability of well-being over time.

In Chapter 5, Kevin Shield and Jürgen Rehm summarize the findings on risk factors for disability or death from the most recent global burden of disease study. For the world as a whole, tobacco use was the second largest contributor to the burden of disease in 2010 [measured as disability-adjusted life years (DALYs), a summary measure of ill-health and premature death], alcohol was the fifth largest contributor, and illicit and non-medical drug use was the eighteenth largest contributor. (High blood pressure was the first, household air pollution from solid fuels the third, and a diet low in fruits the fourth; Lim et al., 2012.) Reflecting variations in how much use there is, and also in the magnitude of competing risk factors, there is substantial variation in the rankings by global region, with the ranking of tobacco, alcohol, and drugs in Europe at least as high as the global average. The rankings and estimated magnitude of DALYs also vary over time. When corrected for population structure, for example, the global burden of alcohol use actually decreased from 1636 DALYs per 100,000 people in 1990 to 1444 DALYs per 100,000 people in 2010. However, although alcohol's burden of disease per 100,000 people has slightly decreased, the percentage of all DALYs attributable to alcohol use has increased from 2.9% in 1990 to 3.9% in 2010, an increase of a third. This increase basically reflects that deaths attributable to alcohol and the other health burdens it caused did not decrease to the same degree as the decrease of burden of disease in general. Other factors contributing are the change in population age structure and the fact that alcohol use is mainly increasing in low-income countries as they became wealthier and their overall health indicators improve (alcohol use is strongly correlated with the GDP of a country adjusted for purchase power parity; see Chapter 10).

The next two chapters shift attention from the harms directly attributable to addiction behaviours to the evidence on commonly used preventive approaches, considering first such strategies as education and second the indirect effects of deterrence strategies. In Chapter 6, Patricia Conrod and colleagues find that although binge-drinking and illicit drug use are common among European youth, there is little evidence to support the majority of approaches currently adopted and delivered by many European countries to address substance-related harm in young people. Although some individual prevention programmes have shown beneficial effects on addictive behaviour outcomes, Conrod and colleagues argue that it is not currently possible to generalize beyond implementation of specific interventions to recommend any broad policy approaches based upon the underpinning principles of these programmes.

In Chapter 7, Jacek Moskalewicz and Justyna Klingemann give a devastating account of the social stigma associated with addictive substances. Throughout history, stigma has been extended to cover large segments of society, the lower classes and ethnic minorities, in order to discredit their claims for more social justice and to legitimize the superior position of the dominant classes. Moskalewicz and Klingemann describe how social stigma reinforced by the criminal justice system is used to justify the imposition of harsh control measures on individuals and social classes which are not considered as deserving social justice due to their moral inferiority manifested by their apparently excess use of psychoactive substances. Moskalewicz and Klingemann note that the disease concept of addiction has failed to remove stigma, as, in public perception, a moral condemnation of addictions is reinforced by a medical stigma of chronic disease with poor prospects for recovery. Addiction treatment has very low social status—for both its patients and its providers—and thus attracts only low investment, resulting in poor treatment outcomes, further stigmatization, and progressive marginalization.

In Chapter 8, Aleksandra Dubanowicz and Paul Lemmens describe the impacts of economic downturns, with their associated cuts in public spending, increases in unemployment, and decreases in income, on addictive substances. While finding that the use of alcohol and tobacco in general declines in times of economic crisis, mainly due to decreased affordability, patterns of use alter and become more harmful, so that, for example, deaths from alcohol use disorders may increase in times of economic crisis (Stuckler et al., 2009). Dubanowicz and Lemmens find mixed evidence for illicit drug use—in some studies economic downturns are associated with reductions in illegal drug use, while in others the opposite is true. The main mechanisms identified are effects of declining disposable income and changes in the structure of everyday life due to unemployment and loss of social roles. Dubanowicz and Lemmens find that the negative impacts of recessions are worsened by the introduction of welfare cuts by hard-pressed governments.

In Chapter 9, Kevin Shield and colleagues demonstrate that addictive substances and behaviours result in enormous social costs for Europe. Although they focus on people who fit the criteria of dependence, using data from their original sources and updating to 2010, alcohol and tobacco together are found to cost the European Union some €300 billion in terms of costs relating to health, crime, and lost productivity. Many of these costs are avoidable. However, to access such savings, societies have to do something effective to reduce the use of alcohol and tobacco.

In Chapter 10, Robin Room, and co-authors describe the interplay between various socioeconomic dimensions and addictive substances—alcohol, tobacco, and other psychoactive drugs. Room and colleagues note that poorer users tend to suffer greater health and injury consequences for a given level of substance use than richer users. Poorer users are also usually subject to greater stigmatization and marginalization than less poor users. Using the example of alcohol, Room and colleagues find that economic development fuels a growing market for alcohol, compounded by commercial forces pushing for open and greater markets—yet problems arising from this growing market are a drag on economic development itself.

In Chapter 11, David Miller and Claire Harkins describe how corporate actions influence policy decisions and the way in which they are implemented and enforced (or not). They highlight the murky waters of corruption, and especially institutional corruption and the responses to it, including lack of transparency. Miller and Harkins argue that policy responses to enhance well-being should, in addition to comforting those afflicted by addictions, also focus on those economic and policy levers that can have very significant effects downstream in terms of both individual behaviours and the wider societal impact.

1.5 **Bringing it all together**

There are things about psychoactive substances which humans have always found positive, though the positives may be trivialized in one place and time and dramatized in another. It is also clear that the negative consequences of psychoactive substances have long been recognized, and that the impulse to control the supply of drugs goes back a long way in history.

What is also clear is that while the market and market forces have been fruitful instruments of capital accumulation (whether or not this is viewed as good or bad; Sloterdijk, 2014), if they are left to flourish undisturbed the result can easily be heavy substance use, which is frequently problematic for individuals and societies. In an era when economic and political ideology discourages government intervention in markets, governments frequently resort instead to approaches aiming to single out and punish the individual heavy substance user. Unfortunately, such societal reactions to reduce such problematic use often produce their own problems. They are also usually differentially applied to produce social injustice and inequality, compounded by the perverse negative interference of criminal justice systems.

We can understand the concept of addiction as a particular way of explaining why so much harm can result from something so attractive. The concept of addiction is rooted in personal experiences, but these experiences need to be understood in terms that reach beyond the individual to include the market, governments, and civil society, with the outcomes also driven by the demands of many different stakeholders. From a pragmatic public health perspective, the primary sources of harm are sustained heavy use, with some contribution from sporadic heavy use. Unfortunately, the addiction concept and its baggage can often just get in the way of this, by narrowing societal attention to the level of the individual engaged in the behaviour.

How can public health be preserved or increased in such circumstances? In Chapter 12 we stress favourable environments and health-promoting societal contexts (Davies et al., 2014). Such contexts are characterized by cultures in which healthy behaviours are the norm, and in which the institutional, social, and physical environment supports such norms. Achievement of this ambition will require a positive, holistic, eclectic, and collaborative effort, involving a broad range of stakeholders. To move towards achieving this goal, the value of health and incentives for healthy behaviour should be emphasized (Anderson et al., 2011), healthy choices in behaviour should become the default (Bloomberg, 2011), and factors that create a culture and environment which promote unhealthy behaviour should be minimized.

References

Anderson, P., Harrison, O., Cooper, C., & Jané-Llopis, E. (2011). Incentives for health. *Journal of Health Communication*, **16**(Suppl. 2), 107–133.

Babor, T., Caetano, R., Casswell, S., et al. (2010a). *Alcohol: No Ordinary Commodity— Research and Public Policy*, 2nd edn. Oxford: Oxford University Press.

Babor, T., Caulkins, J., Edwards, G., et al. (2010b). *Drug Policy and the Public Good*. Oxford: Oxford University Press.

Benner, S. (2013). Paleogenetics and the history of alcohol in primates. *AAAS 2013 Annual Meeting Abstracts*. URL: <https://aaas.confex.com/aaas/2013/webprogram/Paper8851. html>.

Bloomberg, M. (2011). Mayor Bloomberg's remarks at the United Nations General Assembly high level meeting on non-communicable diseases. URL: <http://mikebloomberg. com/index.cfm?objectid=88C81DF6-C29C-7CA2-FCBB0555D5B99541>.

Borch, A. (2012). The Real of problem gambling households. *Journal of Gambling Issues*, issue 27. URL: <http://jgi.camh.net/doi/pdf/10.4309/jgi.2012.27.6>.

Campbell, C.S. & Smith, G.J. (2003). Gambling in Canada—from vice to disease to responsibility: a negotiated history. *Canadian Bulletin of Medical History*, **20**, 121–149.

Davies, S.C., Winpenny, E., Ball, S., Fowler, T., Rubin, J., & Nolte, E. (2014). A new wave in public health improvement. *Lancet*, doi: 10.1016/S0140-6736(13)62341-7.

Dixon, D. (1991). *From Prohibition to Regulation: Bookmaking, Anti-Gambling and the Law*. Oxford: Clarendon Press.

Dudley, R. (2004). Ethanol, fruit ripening, and the historical origins of human alcoholism in primate frugivory. *Integrative and Comparative Biology*, **44**, 315–323.

Laslett, A.-M., Room, R., Ferris, J., Wilkinson, C., Livingston, M., & Mugavin, J. (2011). Surveying the range and magnitude of alcohol's harm to others in Australia. *Addiction*, **106**, 1603–1611.

Levine, H.G. (1978). The discovery of addiction: changing conceptions of habitual drunkenness in America. *Journal of Studies on Alcohol*, **15**, 493–506.

Lim, S.S., Vos, T., Flaxman, A.D., et al. (2012). A comparative risk assessment of burden of disease and injury attributable to 67 risk factors and risk factor clusters in 21 regions,

1990–2010: a systematic analysis for the Global Burden of Disease Study 2010. *Lancet*, **380**, 2224–2260.

McGovern, P. (2009). *Uncorking the Past: The Quest for Wine, Beer, and Other Alcoholic Beverages*. Berkeley, CA: University of California Press.

Room, R. & Reuter, P. (2012). How well do international drug conventions protect public health? *Lancet*, **379**, 84–91.

Schrad, M.L. (2010). *The Political Power of Bad Ideas: Networks, Institutions and the Global Prohibition Wave*. Oxford: Oxford University Press.

Sloterdijk, P. (2014). *In the World Interior of Capital*. Cambridge: Polity Press.

Stuckler, D., Basu, S., Suhrcke, M., Coutts, A., & McKee, M. (2009). The public health effect of economic crises and alternative policy responses in Europe: an empirical analysis. *Lancet*, **374**, 315–323.

US Department of Health and Human Services (2006). *The Health Consequences of Involuntary Exposure to Tobacco Smoke: A Report of the Surgeon General*. Atlanta, GA: U.S. Department of Health and Human Services, Centers for Disease Control and Prevention, Coordinating Center for Health Promotion, National Center for Chronic Disease Prevention and Health Promotion, Office on Smoking and Health.

Ysa, T., Colom, J. Albareda, A., Ramon, A., Carrión, M., & Segura, L. (2014). *Governance of Addictions: European Public Policies*. Oxford: Oxford University Press.

Chapter 2

Passive vulnerability or active agency? An ecological and evolutionary perspective on human drug use

Roger J. Sullivan and Edward H. Hagen

2.1 An introduction to the ecological perspective of drug use

Drug policy is strongly influenced by aetiological theories of human drug use. Historically, such theories have been dominated by two key concepts—human drug use is initiated and sustained by *reward* and *reinforcement* at both biological and behavioural levels. The operationalization of these ideas has invoked several other historical concepts, including the nature of *novelty* in the human encounter with drugs, and human *vulnerability* to drugs in moral, behavioural, and biological dimensions. This chapter will explore a contrasting viewpoint that follows from anthropological ethnohistory and evolutionary theory. We will draw from several of our previous publications to demonstrate that human evolution and history has entailed a long and dynamic relationship with 'drugs' that has been active and functional, rather than passive and vulnerable; and that fundamental ecological dynamics, not reward and reinforcement, have been the primary 'cause' of human drug use (Sullivan and Hagen, 2002; Sullivan et al., 2008; Hagen et al., 2009, 2013; Roulette et al., 2014). We will close by proposing that an *active* rather than a *passive* human drug-use dynamic has implications for drug policy and clinical practice.

2.2 The paradox of drug reward

According to Sullivan et al. (2008)

 The use of psychoactive substances is one of the most perplexing human [behaviours. Some substances cause immeasurable harm to individuals and societies (e.g. heroin), or impose a tremendous social burden in the form of preventable chronic illnesses (e.g. tobacco), while others appear to be mostly harmless and are widely enjoyed by people around the world (e.g. coffee and chocolate). Historically [and conceptually], a broad range of psychosocial, behavioural, and neurobiological theories seeking to understand drug phenomena are [unified] by the notions of reward and reinforcement (Thorndike, 1911). According to these theories, recreational drugs reward and/ or reinforce consumption, often via hedonic effects (Koob and Le Moal, 2005; Nestler, 2005).

All 'commonly used psychoactive drugs are secondary metabolites of plants or fungi (e.g. alkaloids) or their close chemical analogues' (Sullivan et al., 2008) (Table 2.1). (Ethanol is the only commonly used drug that is not a plant toxin and therefore falls outside the boundaries of the current discussion; see Dudley (2002).)

Table 2.1 Relationships between commonly used plant toxins and the human nervous system.

Receptor	Neurotransmitter	Plant toxin	Plant	Drug
Nicotinic	Acetylcholine	Nicotine[a]	*Nicotiana, Duboisia*	Tobacco, pituri
Muscarinic	Acetylcholine	Arecoline[a]	*Areca catechu*	Betel nut
Adrenergic	Norepinephrine	Cocaine[c]	*Erythroxylum*	Coca
	Epinephrine	Ephedrine[c], cathinone[a,c]	*Catha edulis*	Khat
Serotonin	Serotonin	Mescaline	*Lophophora*	Peyote
Dopamine	Dopamine	Cocaine[c]	*Erythroxylum*	Coca
		Cathinone[a,c]	*Catha edulis*	Khat
Adenosine	Adenosine	Caffeine[b]	*Coffea, Cola nitida*	Coffee, cola nut
		Caffeine[b], theophylline[b], theobromine[b]	*Camellia sinensis*	Tea
		Theobromine[b]	*Theobromine cacao*	Chocolate
Opioid	Endorphins	Codeine[a], morphine[a]	*Papaver somniferum*	Opium
Cannabinod	Anandamide	Δ9-THC[a]	*Cannabis sativa*	Cannabis

THC, tetrahydrocannabinol.

[a]Receptor agonist.

[b]Receptor antagonist.

[c]Re-uptake inhibitor.

Adapted from Sullivan, R. J. et al., Revealing the paradox of drug reward in human evolution, Proceedings of the Royal Society Biological Sciences, Volume 275, Number 1640, pp.1231–1241, Supplementary Online Materials, Copyright © 2008, reproduced under the Creative Commons Attribution 3.0 Unported (CC BY 3.0).

Evolutionary biologists studying plant–herbivore interactions have [convincingly] argued that many plant secondary metabolites, including nicotine, morphine, cocaine [and THC] are potent neurotoxins that evolved [because they punished and deterred] consumption by herbivores (Karban and Baldwin, 1997). On the other hand, neurobiology's reward model sees interactions between drugs and the nervous system as rewarding and reinforcing. Hence, in their current forms, [neurobiology's] reward model, and evolutionary [biology's] punishment model, appear to be incompatible. We term this incompatibility the *paradox of drug reward*. (Sullivan et al. 2008)

2.3 **The hijack hypothesis (reward model)**

The mesolimbic dopamine system (MDS) plays a key, though still not fully understood, role in the ability of laboratory rats and monkeys to learn an association between a stimulus, such as a tone, and a natural reward, such as sugar water, and to approach and consume the reward. However, both neurobiological and psychological perspectives have tended not to consider the degree to which experimentation and the modelling of reward and reinforcement reflect the natural world. The importance of acknowledging ecologically valid versus artificial/abstract contexts of reward phenomena was revealed by the classic studies of Garcia and Ervin (1968) and Petrinovich and Bolles (1954) which

> showed that murine experimental outcomes that contradict conventional classical and instrumental conditioning theory, [respectively], are explicable only when interpreted from [ecological and] evolutionary perspectives. Garcia and Ervin (1968) showed that rats will avoid novel foods paired with an aversive association after a single trial, but only if the aversive experience is nausea. Petrinovich and Bolles (1954) demonstrated that rats find it easier to learn relationships that are consistent with their natural ecology, and will make such associations independent[ly] of experimentally induced motivational states such as hunger and thirst. The common element in [both] these studies, experimental conditions that are ecologically ['normal'] to the laboratory animal, is missing from [earlier] studies that have been hugely influential on theory of drug reward such as Olds and Milner's (1954) classic research of electrical brain stimulation in the rat. (Sullivan et al. 2008).

The 'naturalness' of the contexts of drug use is additionally important in that drugs of abuse have neurobiological and behavioural effects that closely resemble the effects of sugar and other natural rewards, activating the MDS and producing approach and consummatory behaviour, positive feelings, and the learning of cues that predict drug availability. The neuromedical approach to drug use would seem to demand, however, that drugs differ fundamentally from natural rewards such as sugar. Otherwise, the consumption of drugs would be no different from consumption of food: it is difficult to make a distinction on a chemical basis alone. Drugs and sugar are both small organic molecules that act as ligands for various receptors. Numerous, highly cited articles that review the neurobiology of drug use rely on similar metaphors to distinguish natural rewards from drugs: Natural rewards 'activate' the MDS, whereas drugs 'hijack', 'usurp', 'co-op', or artificially stimulate it (e.g. Wise, 2000; Kelley and Berridge, 2002; Schultz, 2011; Sulzer, 2011). Schultz, for instance, opens a recent review by asking 'How do addictive drugs hijack the brain's reward system?' and then goes on to consider how 'normal, physiological reward processes may be affected by addictive drugs' (Schultz, 2011, p. 603). Kelley and Berridge (2002, p. 3306) similarly open their review by stating that:

> Addictive drugs act on brain reward systems, although the brain evolved to respond not to drugs but to natural rewards, such as food and sex. Appropriate responses to natural rewards were evolutionarily important for survival, reproduction, and fitness. In a quirk of evolutionary fate, humans discovered how to stimulate this system artificially with drugs.

On the evolutionary novelty of drug use, Wise (2000, p. 27) is more explicit:

> Addiction is quite a recent phenomenon, largely dependent upon the controlled use of fire (smoking), hypodermic syringes (intravenous injection), and the cork and bottle (storage and transportation of alcohol). Thus, while brain dopamine is activated by most drugs of abuse, the drugs have undergone mostly human selection for their ability to activate the system; the system has not undergone natural selection because of its sensitivity to the drugs.

We refer to these arguments collectively as the 'hijack hypothesis'. While recognizing that 'hijack' is a metaphor invoked by drug researchers to help explain the effects of drugs of abuse on the brain, drug abuse researchers apparently do consider that it provides a fundamental distinction between addictive substances and food. This distinction is based on the following evolutionary (Darwinian) propositions. First, the MDS evolved to enhance access to some substances, like sugar, that increased fitness; these are termed 'natural rewards'. Second, it did not evolve to respond to known drugs of abuse because these did not increase fitness and because repeated consumption of such substances is an evolutionary novelty. In this evolutionary sense, the 'hijack hypothesis' is useful for our purposes here, as opposed to referring to 'reward hypotheses' generally, in that it is an implicit acknowledgement by drug researchers that the aetiology of drug-use phenomena must accommodate the natural antecedents of drug reward phenomena.

2.4 **Historical and archaeological evidence of ubiquitous substance use in antiquity**

Whereas the hijack perspective sees drug use as novel, an anthropological–historical perspective describes a long human relationship with drugs. Archaeological evidence and historical accounts of substances used by indigenous peoples at European contact (Fig. 2.1) provide some insight into the use of psychoactive substances in prehistory. It is important to consider that as the origin of these practices is unknown, their actual antiquity is on an open-ended time-scale.

In the case of *Areca catechu* (betel nut), today the fourth most used drug in the world after nicotine, ethanol, and caffeine (Marshall, 1987), archaeological evidence suggests that it may have been chewed in Timor as early as 13,000 years ago (Glover, 1971, 1977) and in Thailand 10,700 years ago (Gorman, 1970; Yen, 1977). At the time of European contact, Aborigines were exploiting the indigenous plant pituri (*Duboisia hopwoodii*) for its nicotine content in western Queensland, and an indigenous *Nicotiana* in central Australia (*Nicotiana gossei*) (Watson, 1983). As Aborigines had lived in Australia for at least 40,000 years before the arrival of European colonists (see Bellwood, 1985), the antiquity of the exploitation of these native plants may be considerable. Tobacco species (*Nicotiana tabacum* and *N. rustica*) were spread throughout most of the Americas by the time of European conquest, and were 'one of the oldest of the New World cultigens' (Schultes, 1979, p. 152). Similarly, the use of khat (*Catha edulis*) in Ethiopia and northeast Africa was already an 'ancient' practice before the arrival of European colonists (Weir, 1985). According to Plowman (1984), coca (*Erythroxylum coca*) was being domesticated in the western Andes by 7000 years ago, and archaeological artefacts date the use of coca in Ecuador to at least 5000 years ago (Balick and Cox, 1997).

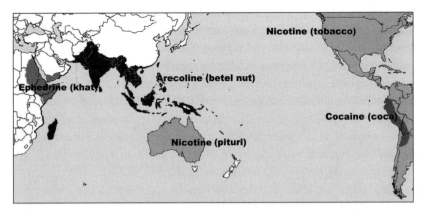

Fig. 2.1 Examples of commonly used plant toxins in the pre-colonial world.
Reproduced with permission from Sullivan, R.J. and Hagen, E.H., Psychotropic substance-seeking: evolutionary pathology or adaptation? Addiction, Volume 97, Issue 4, pp. 389–400, Copyright © 2002 John Wiley & Sons, Ltd.

2.4.1 **Route of administration**

At the time of first European contact, as today, betel nut, khat, tobacco, and coca were chewed in the buccal cheek cavity. The buccal mucosa is a blood-rich tissue that allows the passage of substances directly into the blood stream, avoiding the elimination that occurs via the intestine and liver when a drug is introduced orally (first-pass metabolism). This process is facilitated, with the exception of khat, by mixing the substance with an alkali (lime or wood ash), that converts it into the free base (pituri: Watson, 1983; tobacco: McKim, 1991; betel nut: Johnston et al., 1975; Wink, 1998c; coca: Balick and Cox, 1997; Wink, 1998c). That people in the past used alkalis to free base psychotropic substances is evident in the alkali-bearing vessels found in the archaeological record (Fox, 1970; Balick and Cox, 1997). This combination of physiological and cultural processes produces a pure drug introduced into the body by a direct route. Although a universally used method, the buccal route was only one of several direct routes of administration used in antiquity. For example, the smoking of tobacco and the nasal and rectal administration of psychedelics were common in the Americas (McKim, 1991).

2.4.2 **Pharmacology and potency**

The nicotine-bearing plants used by indigenous peoples at the time of European colonization tended to be more potent than the commercial *N. tabacum* used today (which contains up to approximately 1.5% nicotine; Goodman et al., 1985). The *N. rustica* used by indigenous Americans contains up to 8% nicotine, and the pituri of Australian Aborigines has between 3.5 and 5% nicotine (Watson, 1983).

Despite being one of the most commonly used drugs globally, betel nut is virtually unknown in the west and is rarely mentioned in texts describing commonly used drugs. Chewing a betel nut in combination with the conventional pepper leaf and lime exerts potent parasympathetic effects in the intolerant user, including salivation, sweating, tremor, nausea, bronchoconstriction, and vasodilation (Chu, 1993, 1995). The betel nut's most abundant constituent alkaloid is arecoline (Farnworth, 1976), a non-selective muscarinic agonist that crosses the blood–brain barrier and increases levels of acetylcholine in the brains of animals by 150–250% (Shannon et al., 1994, p. 279).

Khat's active constituents include cathine (norpseudoephedrine) and ephedrine (Luqman and Danowski, 1976), both central stimulants structurally similar to noradrenaline. Cathine is a sympathomimetic that increases the release of serotonin, noradrenaline, and dopamine and inhibits their re-uptake (Schmeller and Wink, 1998). Ephedrine inhibits the re-uptake of noradrenaline (Wink, 1998b), and is a drug of frequent abuse elsewhere (Mattoo et al., 1997). The spectrum of khat's pharmacological action is estimated to be between amphetamines and caffeine (see Luqman and Danowski, 1976).

Cocaine, the active alkaloid in *E. coca*, is a central stimulant exerting its pharmacological action by preventing the re-uptake of noradrenaline and dopamine (Wink, 1998b). The approximately 15 million regular coca chewers in South America consume around 50 g of fresh leaves per day each, equivalent to 0.4 g of cocaine (Mann, 1992; Wink, 1998c).

2.4.3 Drugs as food

It is pertinent to consider what 'drugs' represented for people in the ancestral environment. The ways in which indigenous peoples perceive traditionally used psychoactive and/or 'medicinal' plants are different from the pharmaceutical concepts understood in the industrial west. Today, when we think of 'drugs' we visualize processed commodities such as packaged cigarettes, pills, or powders. These processed products had no counterpart in the environments of indigenous peoples, or in the ancestral environment: 'drugs' were plants, and thus were eaten as food (Etkin, 1994; Balick and Cox, 1997). While researching the effects of betel chewing on people with schizophrenia in Micronesia (Sullivan et al., 2000), the first author found that betel nut was not perceived as a drug in the western sense. Rather, it is chewed in the manner of a food, is conceived as imparting energy and sustenance in the manner of a food, and comes from a palm that is tended and grown around dwellings in the manner of a food-bearing plant. Moreover, when chewers were questioned about their perceptions of the effects of chewing, the response was invariably that the nut was chewed for energy or to prevent fatigue rather than for its psychotropic effects.

Similar accounts of a blurred distinction between drugs and food can be found in the ethnomedical and anthropological literatures. Marshall (1981) relates that in Yap and Chuuk, tobacco is considered akin to a strength-imparting food or drink, and is governed by similar taboos and restrictions. Etkin and Ross (1982) found that of the 107 plant species used for gastrointestinal disorders by the Hausa of Nigeria, 50% (53) are also used in dietary contexts where they are regarded solely for their nutritive value. Moerman (1994) found that a large number of plant species used by native North Americans were used as both foods and medicines. Of the 2646 utilized species, 1222 were used exclusively as medicines, 745 were used exclusively as foods, and 679 were used as both foods and medicines. Thus, roughly half of all food plants (48%) were also medicinal. He concluded that 'people have, over the millennia, sought out as foods those species that were likely to contain disproportionate quantities of secondary chemicals, many of which are poisonous' (Moerman, 1994, p. 178).

Describing drugs as foods does not necessarily constitute a metaphor, as many ubiquitously used substances have considerable nutritional value. For example, Balick and Cox (1997) note that the calcium, phosphorus, iron, and vitamins A, B_2, and E in 100 g of Bolivian coca leaf exceed the daily recommended US dietary allowance. Khat contains vitamin C (150 mg/100 g of fresh leaves) and trace amounts of thiamine, niacin, riboflavin, and carotene, as well as iron and amino acids (Luqman and Danowski, 1976). Moreover, as many alkaloids are based chemically on tryptophan or tyrosine (Waterman, 1998), and these essential amino acids may become available after oral consumption.

Although the evidence presented above is not proof of ubiquitous substance use in the ancestral environment, it is sufficient to give pause to some of the assumptions of the hijack (reward) hypothesis and suggests that further research is warranted.

2.5 Ecology: the punishment model of drug origins

In parallel with the above account detailing a long human relationship with plant toxins, considerable biological evidence points to a deep-time co-evolutionary relationship between plants and animals in general. There is a 300–400 million year history of antagonistic interrelationships between terrestrial plants which photosynthesize chemical forms of energy for their own reproduction and the bacterial, fungal, nematode, invertebrate, and vertebrate herbivores that exploit plant tissues and energy stores for food and other nutrients, often severely damaging a plant's ability to reproduce. To limit such damage, most plant species have evolved aggressive defence strategies to punish herbivores that feed on them. These strategies include mechanical defences, such as thorns, as well as chemical defences such as toxins that interfere with herbivore growth, development, fecundity, and other aspects of functioning (Karban and Baldwin, 1997).

2.5.1 Plant chemical defences against herbivores

One broad category of chemical defences includes compounds with relatively non-specific effects on a wide range of molecular targets in the herbivore. Tannins and other phenolics, for instance, can form multiple hydrogen and ionic bonds with numerous proteins, changing their conformation and impairing their function (Wink, 2003). Another broad category of defensive compounds interferes with specific aspects of herbivore physiology. Of central interest to us are those compounds that have evolved to interfere with signalling in the central nervous system (CNS) and peripheral nervous system. Psychoactive plant-based drugs fall into this category. It is striking that different plant compounds interfere with nearly every step in neuronal signalling, including: (1) neurotransmitter synthesis, storage, release, binding, and re-uptake; (2) receptor activation and function; and (3) key enzymes involved in signal transduction (Wink, 2000). In many cases, plant compounds achieve these effects because they have evolved to resemble endogenous neurotransmitters. Many plant drugs are alkaloids—secondary metabolites containing nitrogen. Several alkaloids form a quaternary nitrogen configuration under physiological conditions, a structural motif that is present in most neurotransmitters (Wink, 2006) (Table 2.1).

The punishment model has successfully explained the function of many plant secondary metabolites (Wink, 1998a). Even so, the precise evolved functions of most plant secondary compounds are still unknown, and among the popular plant drugs only nicotine, which we discuss next, has been conclusively shown to serve plant defence.

2.5.2 Nicotine

The defensive functions of nicotine are particularly well documented. We use nicotine examples throughout this chapter because, unlike other plant drugs, nicotine has been extensively studied from both ecological and neurobiological perspectives and is one of the world's most popular plant drugs. Furthermore, smoking is estimated to account for 12% of global adult mortality (Ezzati and Lopez, 2004), which makes tobacco consumption one of the most urgent, unsolved problems in international public health.

Nicotiana attenuata, a wild North American tobacco plant used by Native Americans, is an important model species for the analysis of plant–herbivore interactions involving nicotine. It is attacked by over 20 different herbivores, ranging from mammalian browsers to intracellular-feeding insects. These attacks induce defensive responses, including the production of nicotine; because synthesis of nicotine is costly for the plant it is allocated to tissues that are particularly important for plant fitness and/or are likely to be eaten by herbivores (Baldwin, 2001). Data on the ecological function of psychoactive compounds in most other plant drugs, such as THC, cocaine, morphine, codeine, and caffeine, are still emerging. However, studies to date also indicate defensive functions for these substances, such as deterrence of herbivore feeding and microbe or animal toxicity (e.g. Wink, 1998a). It is therefore likely that an ecological role similar to that of nicotine will be established for these psychoactive drugs too.

2.5.3 Co-evolved herbivore countermeasures

In response to the evolution of chemical defences in plants, herbivores have co-evolved a number of countermeasures (Karban and Agrawal, 2002; Petzinger and Geyer, 2006), including: (1) compounds that prevent or attenuate the induction of plant chemical defences; (2) detoxification mechanisms, including enzymes and symbiotic relationships with microbes to detoxify or extract nutrients from plant defence compounds, and cellular membrane carrier proteins for toxin transport; and (3) chemosensors and aversive learning mechanisms that permit selective feeding on less toxic tissues.

Plant toxins, in addition to their direct effects on herbivores, often have pronounced effects on organisms directly or indirectly feeding on the herbivore (the third and higher trophic levels). These phenomena are termed *tritrophic*, or *multitrophic*, interactions (Price et al., 1980; Ode, 2006). Nicotine is one of the toxins shown to have an impact on multiple trophic levels (Thurston and Fox, 1972; Bentz and Barbosa, 1990). Numerous invertebrates and vertebrates even actively sequester dietary toxins for their own chemical defence against predators (e.g. Daly et al., 2002). This and other types of exploitation of plant secondary compounds is called *pharmacophagy* (Boppre, 1984) (see Figs 2.2 and 2.3).

From the perspective of the herbivore, there are costs but also potential benefits from the consumption of tobacco nicotine (Fig. 2.2). Bentz and Barbosa (1990) 'demonstrated that the food-utilization efficiency of unparasitized tobacco hornworm larvae (*Manduca sexta*) was significantly reduced by ingestion of nicotine. Yet, larvae that consumed food containing nicotine were themselves protected from parasitism by the wasp *Cotesia congregate*' (Sullivan et al. 2008). Wasp-parasitized nicotine-treated larvae had significantly greater efficiency in conversion of ingested and digested food than did parasitized larvae without dietary nicotine. In another study, Singer et al. (2009) found that

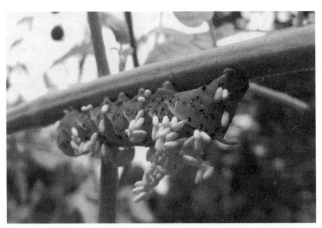

Fig. 2.2 Tomato hornworm caterpillar (*Manduca quinquemaculata*) parasitized by wasp larvae.

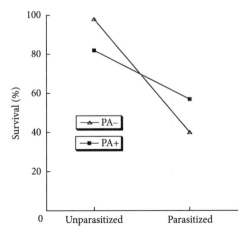

Fig. 2.3 Percentage survival to adulthood of unparasitized and parasitized *Grammia incorrupta* caterpillars given a synthetic food lacking toxins (PA−) or containing toxins (PA+) (0.1% monocrotaline).

Reproduced from Singer, M. S. et al., Self-Medication as Adaptive Plasticity: Increased Ingestion of Plant Toxins by Parasitized Caterpillars, PLoS ONE Volume 4, Issue 3, Copyright © 2009. licensed under the Creative Commons License version 2.5

Grammia incorrupta caterpillars fed artificial food containing a toxin (0.1% monocrotaline) were more resistant to parasitic flies (*Exorista mell*a) then those fed food without the toxin (Fig. 2.3). On the other hand, caterpillars fed the toxin-free diet did better when unparasitized.

These examples demonstrate both 'the cost of toxin consumption even to co-adapted species (e.g. tobacco hornworm/*Nicotiana*), and how a targeted plant predator may counter-exploit the toxins deployed against it' (Sullivan et al., 2008). Note that the ability of the animals to exploit plant toxins as a beneficial 'adaptation' does not equate to positive or 'good' attributes of the toxin. In the examples given here the plant toxin remains poisonous to the caterpillar, and the cost–benefit ratio of the effects of toxicity becomes positive only when the caterpillar is itself parasitized: the neurotoxin is exploited *because* it is 'bad' (toxic).

2.5.4 **Summary of the ecological perspective**

In the story of life since the rise of complex terrestrial organisms more than 400 million years ago, one of the main plot lines has been the constant battle between plants, which dominate the biosphere, and diverse legions of herbivores. Plant secondary compounds have been potent, effective weapons for punishing and deterring herbivore enemies.

The foregoing 'punishment' model is an ultimate-level explanation of drug origins—it construes broad categories of plant compounds as defences which arose during antagonistic co-evolution between plants and herbivores. Mayr (1961) introduced a distinction between such *ultimate* biological explanations, which invoke evolved responses to particular ecological conditions, and *proximate* biological explanations, which invoke physiological mechanisms (we will use the term 'mechanism' to refer to proximate mechanisms). The punishment model is at marked variance with the proximate, neurophysiological hijack model introduced above, and more usually employed by neurobiologists investigating human recreational drug use.

2.6 Towards resolving the paradox

We now explore three avenues for resolving the paradox of drug reward: evolutionary novelty, non-defensive functions of secondary compounds, and counter-exploitation.

2.6.1 Is drug exposure an evolutionary novelty?

Wise (2000) and Nesse and Berridge (1997), among others, have proposed that current patterns of drug exposure are an evolutionary novelty, and therefore drugs, at least in their pure form, were probably not a selective pressure on human neurophysiology. If true, our brains might not be adapted to recognize psychoactive drugs as toxic, and reward circuits might inadvertently be triggered when such drugs are consumed.

Although particular drugs are probably evolutionarily novel, we note that psychoactive drug use: (1) primarily involves plant toxins, compounds that have been an important part of animal diets for hundreds of millions of years; (2) does trigger toxin avoidance mechanisms in most individuals, including aversive reactions to evolutionarily novel compounds such as nicotine, even in pure form; (3) is a pan-human phenomenon, involving similar substances and concentrations across a diverse array of cultures; and (4) is widespread in the archaeological record, at least for much of the Holocene (Sullivan and Hagen, 2002; Sullivan et al., 2008). Moreover, humans, like other animals, have evolved several layers of protection against plant toxins, including receptors for detecting and enzymes for metabolizing plant neurotoxins and other xenobiotics. Evidence of conserved function, stabilizing selection, and population-specific selection of at least some human bitter taste receptors (Soranzo et al., 2005; but see Wang et al., 2004) and xenobiotic-metabolizing cytochrome P450 genes indicates a long evolutionary exposure to plant toxins as a class, albeit at reduced levels relative to other primates (Sullivan et al., 2008). Aversion and aversive learning and the blood–brain barrier, which provide protection against many plant toxins, are additional evidence that mammalian evolution has been shaped by exposure to plant defensive compounds.

Nesse and Berridge (1997) have argued that novel routes of drug administration bypass adaptive information-processing systems to act directly on the mechanisms controlling emotion and behaviour. This might be true for some drugs (e.g. injected heroin) but not for others (e.g. chewed coca or tobacco leaves). Even so, the injection of pure drugs can still cause aversive reactions in most individuals (for data on subcutaneous injection of pure nicotine in humans see Foulds et al., 1997).

Tobacco, marijuana, areca palm, opium poppy, coca, coffee, tea, and cacao are domesticated plants. This means that in the last several thousand years their profile of secondary compounds is likely to have been tailored by artificial selection to fit human preferences. Hence, the precise recipes of these drug cocktails are evolutionarily novel. Nevertheless, at least when it comes to nicotine, the level of drug in commercially marketed products is similar to that in the tobacco and other nicotine-containing plants (wild and domestic) long used by indigenous peoples (Sullivan and Hagen, 2002). Domestication also implies significant interaction between humans and the wild progenitor species, presumably to obtain access to the same psychoactive substances. We therefore conclude that, despite these complications, exposure to potent psychoactive plant toxins as a class is probably not an evolutionary novelty for humans.

2.7 Counter-exploitation of plant neurotoxins

As an alternative to the hijack/reward model, or the notion that drug use follows the novel availability of domesticates, we propose that attraction to toxic plant compounds might have actively evolved because of benefits accruing from their consumption. We have argued for the existence of superbly well-functioning neurobiological mechanisms for defence against toxins, and that interactions between appetite and aversion clearly play a central role in patterns of drug use. In light of this conclusion, the inability of the latter defence mechanisms to completely prevent any use of tobacco, cocaine, opiates, and other psychoactive drugs raises the possibility that during the evolution of the human lineage there were biological fitness benefits associated with regulated consumption of these substances.

2.7.1 Pharmacophagy: exploiting plant 'research and development' against parasites

Terrestrial plants account for about 50% of net primary production, and represent over 99% of the primary producer biomass (Field et al., 1998). Excluding a large class of decomposers (organisms that consume dead plant and animal tissue), a substantial fraction of the world's viruses, bacteria, fungi, nematodes, and arthropods feed off living plants. Hence, an enormous amount of pharmaceutical 'research and development' against these parasites has been, and continues to be, conducted by naturally evolving plant species. The same major categories of parasites also attack humans and other animals.

To inhibit and kill their own parasites, some animals might have evolved to counter-exploit the products of hundreds of millions of years of 'research' by plants (Villalba and Provenza, 2007). As we noted earlier, there is evidence that a number of herbivores evolved to subsist on a mixed diet of palatable and toxic plants, in effect trading off diet quality (and thus growth) for what is termed *enemy-reduced* or *enemy-free* space (Singer and Stireman, 2003). Even more intriguing is evidence that some herbivores contingently vary the toxicity of their diet in response to infection. In one study, for example, unparasitized *Platyprepia virginalis* caterpillars were more likely to survive on a diet of lupin (low toxicity), whereas caterpillars parasitized by a tachnid parasitoid (*Thelaira americana*) were more likely to survive on poison hemlock. When offered a choice of both plants in field tests, parasitized caterpillars were more likely to choose hemlock and unparasitized caterpillars were more likely to choose lupin (Karban and Baldwin, 1997). (For a more recent review of this field see Ode, 2006.)

Primates, too, appear to engage in pharmacophagy (Johns, 1990; Huffman, 1997). In humans 'it has been proposed that toxins in fava beans and cassava might be effective against *Plasmodium falciparum* infections' (Sullivan et al. 2008), explaining the geographic patterns of use of these plants and genetic polymorphisms (Jackson, 1990, 1996); and 'the ubiquitous use of spices could be an adaptation to exploit plant toxins to combat bacterial infections of food (Billing and Sherman, 1998)'. Sullivan and Hagen (2002) hypothesized 'that hominins may have exploited plant toxins to overcome nutritional and energetic constraints on CNS signaling' (Sullivan et al. 2008).

2.7.2 **Nicotine and other popular plant drugs fight parasites**

Intriguingly, some recreational drugs are remarkably effective treatments for mammalian pathogens. For example, nicotine, arecoline (betel nut), and THC, three of the world's most popular plant drugs, are potent anthelmintics: nicotine, arecoline, and their close chemical relatives have been widely used to deworm livestock (Hammond et al., 1997; WHO, 1981; Iqbal et al., 2006) and cannabis is toxic to plant-parasitic nematodes (Grewal, 1989; McPartland and Glass, 2001). These compounds are also frequently mentioned as anthelmintics in the enthnomedical literature (Fabricant and Farnsworth, 2001; McPartland and Glass, 2001).

Thus, speculatively, the widespread recreational use of tobacco, betel nut, and cannabis could be a form of human pharmacophagy, an evolved response to chronic infections of helminths or other parasites with nicotinic or muscarinic receptors in ancestral human populations. We doubt, however, that there was selection for use of these plant drug specifically; instead, there could have been selection to seek out and use plants rich in cholinergic agents—there are a number of cholinergic plant toxins (Wink and Schimmer, 1999) and other toxins of various types.

2.7.3 **Other potential benefits**

Neurotoxins have other effects that may be beneficial under certain conditions: cannabis and opiates are powerful analgesics and caffeine and nicotine can act as cognitive enhancers (Rezvani and Levin, 2001; Lieberman, 2003). These effects are related to the fact that plant drugs chemically mimic endogenous signalling molecules (Table 2.1).

The question is, if it is possible to enhance performance by ingesting compounds that chemically resemble endogenous signalling molecules, why didn't natural selection simply increase production of the endogenous signalling molecules? There are a variety of potential answers involving evolutionary constraints, tradeoffs, and the like. Sullivan and Hagen (2002) suggested that although levels of endogenous signalling molecules are probably close to optimal in healthy individuals under normal circumstances, internal signalling functions would occasionally become compromised, perhaps due to deficiencies in dietary precursors in marginal environments, excess utilization of signalling molecules (e.g. as a consequence of chronic high stress), or disease. In such cases, limited doses of some plant secondary compounds might have been able to partially compensate for impaired functionality. It is also possible, in humans at least, that cultural evolution could identify benefits from plant compounds that offset the costs of exposure. This is obviously the case in modern medicine, which often exploits plant-derived compounds for clinical applications: one-third of the current top twenty drugs on the market are derived from plants (Howitz and Sinclair, 2008).

Cholinergic brain systems play important roles in attention and memory, for example, and have also been implicated in Alzheimer's disease, schizophrenia, and other mental illnesses. Nicotine and other nicotinic agonists correspondingly improve performance on attention and memory tasks, and clinical studies have shown nicotine to be an effective treatment for some of the cognitive deficits associated with the aforementioned diseases (Rezvani and Levin, 2001).

Thus, in principle, drug-seeking behaviour, and its neurophysiological basis, could have evolved because of beneficial effects of neurotoxins. We do not doubt that these neurotoxins constitute serious health hazards. Rather, these health hazards, which often appear only at high doses or later in life, may have been offset by immediate benefits, resulting in a net increase in biological fitness.

2.8 **Policy, treatment, and research**

We have made a case for prioritizing the consideration of ecological and evolutionary perspectives in understanding human (and mammalian) drug use phenomena. Extending the ecological principles that predict behaviour between animals and toxin-bearing plants (drugs) in nature to humans may provide novel insights for drug-use theory, treatment, and policy. We are scientists/evolutionary theorists trying to understand the ultimate causes of human drug use. We do not do policy work, are not trained in policy practice, and have not invested in studying possibilities for the application of our work to clinical practice or policy. However, it is clear that our ideas, if they have merit, have implications for policy, and here we will briefly outline some initial possibilities.

One of the key differences between the conventional hijack hypothesis and the ecologically orientated hypothesis is that the former describes an actor that is passive in the face of the biological effects of drugs while in the latter the actor is an active agent. Seeing the drug user as an active agent who is possibly following ecologically evolved behavioural strategies is suggestive of alternative avenues of drug behaviour research for both human and animal models (Sullivan et al., 2008). For example, we can:

1 Make a casual distinction between the ecology of initial seeking, and addiction, i.e. the causes of use by a neophyte are distinct from the physiological and behavioural processes associated with chronic drug use.

2 Utilize information about natural patterns of seeking and use, for example what are the ecologically salient factors affecting initial patterns of use in humans and animals?

3 Utilize independent variables that are ecologically meaningful, or plausible, to the experimental subject, i.e. that reflect a plausible aspect of the animal's natural ecology and evolutionary phylogeny. For example, the key elements of Garcia and Ervin's (1968) classic study—food paired with nausea—are 'ecologically plausible' to the rat. In contrast, the electrical brain stimulation used in Olds and Milner's (1954) famous study has no natural parallel in the ecology or phylogeny of the rat.

4 Focus on the primary neurobiological target of the neurotoxin rather than 'downstream' interactions with dopamine and/or the nucleus accumbens.

For example, the neurotoxin nicotine has evolved to bind with cholinergic receptors, not dopaminergic receptors; what are the primary physiological (and behavioural) correlates of cholinergic receptor binding, and how do they relate to points 1, 2, and 3?

5 Consider the possibility of an adaptive process. Animals that are ecologically exposed to neurotoxins often develop strategies and adaptations to counter-exploit the neurotoxin.

At a very simple level, if humans are not inherently vulnerable to drugs in the biological sense there is no need to 'protect' people by restricting their access to drugs. This means primarily that top-down policies designed to control human drug use on a large scale (e.g. the US federal 'war on drugs') are doomed to failure, because substance use is not 'caused' by biological frailty in humankind collectively, although it may be an important factor in individual people. This insight would suggest moving away from aetiological models explaining a normative vulnerability of humans to drug use and towards a greater understanding of individual variation in biological and behavioural vulnerability to problem drug use, both in terms of research and treatment resources.

This point also speaks to the theme that availability and potency are primary causes of human drug use. In particular, substances that are highly potent are often emphasized across-the-board, from neurobiological research to federal policy, as being a principal driver in problem drug use. We compiled data from the 2004 annual federal survey of drug use in the United States to show that regular heroin users are an extremely small proportion of the population (0.2%) and even the proportions of regular users of cocaine, 'crack', and amphetamines are markedly smaller (2.4, 0.5, and 0.6% of the population, respectively) than the proportions for users of tobacco and cannabis (34 and 11%, respectively, 'used in the last year') (Fig. 2.4). These data suggest that the exception—the use of potent euphoric drugs by small proportions of human populations—has been used to prove the 'rule' of hedonic drug reward in humankind (and mammals). Stiff legal penalties might partially explain the exceptionally low frequency of consumption of potent euphoric drugs (DuPont and Voth, 1995), but they obviously cannot explain the high frequency of consumption of non-euphoric drugs.

These data support our contention that 'solving' problem drug use by focusing on apparent normative human vulnerability is incorrect; instead, as the majority of people do not in fact use 'hard drugs' the focus needs to shift to the relatively small proportion of individuals that do use them.

Both passive (vulnerability) and active (evolutionary and ecological) perspectives of drug use may be illuminated by concentrating on problem users,

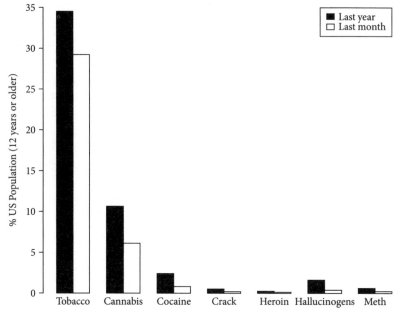

Fig. 2.4 Drug use in the United States (2004).
Source: data from the US National Survey on Drug Use and Health 2004, Substance Abuse and Mental Health Services Administration, 2004, available from http://www.icpsr.umich.edu/icpsrweb/SAMHDA/studies/4373

rather than global populationse. Continued investment in research into *individual* biological variation as it relates to drug use represents the passive perspective, i.e. are individual 'vulnerabilities' to drug use unique to each user rather than normative? The active perspective may also contribute to research into individual differences, but could have a particular impact on clinical practice. Current clinical practice, influenced by approaches that prioritize reward-based models, tends to view problem drug use ('abuse') as a clinical *end point*. A typical approach is to focus resources on ending the substance use and/or insulating the patient from exposure to drugs, and is entirely consistent with the passive viewpoint of human drug use. An active perspective, on the other hand, could consider the patient's drug-using behaviours and their contexts as a clinical *starting point*; what is going on in the *ecology* of the patient's life—the ecological contexts and dynamics—that may influence the patient's drug use? This approach is novel and would be dependent on future research to ascertain what constitutes 'ecology' in modern lifestyles. We found, for example, that reducing parasite load in central African 'pygmy' men who were heavy smokers reduced their exposure to nicotine (Roulette et al., 2014). Is the higher parasite burden in the developing world contributing in some small way to the explosion of tobacco use in these populations? Our speculation highlights one of the key advantages that emerge from utilizing evolutionary theory and perspectives; the generation of novel hypotheses to explain familiar phenomena. Even if this particular speculation turns out to be incorrect, we urge the adoption of evolutionary and ecological insights to open up new directions of research and to further understanding of the biology and behaviour of human drug use.

Acknowledgements

Text extracts from Sullivan, R. J. et al., Revealing the paradox of drug reward in human evolution, Proceedings of the Royal Society B: Biological Sciences, Volume 275, Number 1640, pp. 1231–1241, Copyright © 2008, reproduced under the Creative Commons Attribution 3.0 Unported (CC BY 3.0).

Text extracts from Sullivan, R. J. and Hagen, E.H., Psychotropic substance-seeking: evolutionary pathology or adaptation? *Addiction*, Volume 97, Issue 4, pp. 389–400, Copyright © 2002, reproduced with permission of John Wiley & Sons, Ltd.

References

Baldwin, I.T. (2001). An ecologically motivated analysis of plant–herbivore interactions in native tobacco. *Plant Physiology*, **127**, 1449–1458.

Balick, M.J. & Cox, P.A. (1997). *Plants, People, and Culture: The Science of Ethnobotany.* New York: Scientific American Library.

Bellwood, P. (1985). *Prehistory of the Indo-Malaysian Archipelago.* Sydney: Academic Press.

Bentz, J. & Barbosa, P. (1990). Effects of dietary nicotine (0.1%) and parasitism by *Cotesia congregata* on the growth and food consumption and utilization of the tobacco hornworm, *Manduca sexta. Entomologia Experimentalis et Applicata*, **57**, 1–8.

Billing, J. & Sherman, P.W. (1998). Antimicrobial functions of spices: why some like it hot. *Quarterly Review of Biology*, **73**, 3–49.

Boppré, M. (1984). Redefining 'pharmacophagy'. *Journal of Chemical Ecology*, **10**, 1151–1154.

Chu, N.S. (1993). Cardiovascular responses to betel chewing. *Journal of the Formosa Medical Association*, **92**, 835–837.

Chu, N.S. (1995). Betel chewing increases the skin temperature—effects of atropine and propranolol. *Neuroscience Letters*, **194**, 130–132.

Daly, J.W., Kaneko, T., Wilham, J., et al. (2002). Bioactive alkaloids of frog skin: combinatorial bioprospecting reveals that pumiliotoxins have an arthropod source. *Proceedings of the National Academy of Sciences of the United States of America*, **99**, 13996–14001.

Dudley, R. (2002). Fermenting fruit and the historical ecology of ethanol ingestion: is alcoholism in modern humans an evolutionary hangover? *Addiction*, **97**, 381–388.

DuPont, R.L. & Voth, E.A. (1995). Drug legalization, harm reduction, and drug policy. *Annals of Internal Medicine*, **123**, 461–465.

Etkin, N. (1994). *Eating on the Wild Side.* Tucson, AZ: University of Arizona Press.

Etkin, N.L. & Ross, P.J. (1982). Food as medicine and medicine as food: an adaptive framework for the interpretation of plant utilization among the Hausa of northern Nigeria. *Social Science and Medicine*, **16**, 1559–1573.

Ezzati, M. & Lopez, A.D. (2004). Smoking and oral tobacco use. In: *Comparative Quantification of Health Risks: Global and Regional Burden of Disease Attributable to Selected Major Risk Factors* (ed. M. Ezzati, A.D. Lopez, A. Rogers, & C.J.L. Murray), pp. 883–957. Geneva: WHO.

Fabricant, D.S. & Farnsworth, N.R. (2001). The value of plants used in traditional medicine for drug discovery. *Environmental Health Perspectives*, **109**(Suppl. 1), 69–75.

Farnworth, E.R. (1976). Betel nut—its composition, chemistry and uses. *Science in New Guinea*, **4**, 85–90.

Field, C.B., Behrenfeld, M.J., Randerson, J.T., & Falkowski, P. (1998). Primary production of the biosphere: integrating terrestrial and oceanic components. *Science*, **281**, 237–240.

Foulds, J., Stapleton, J.A., Bell, N., Swettenham, J., Jarvis, M.J., & Russell, M.A.H. (1997). Mood and physiological effects of subcutaneous nicotine in smokers and never-smokers. *Drug and Alcohol Dependence*, **44**, 105–115.

Fox, R.B. (1970). *The Tabon Caves*. Manila: National Museum.

Garcia, J. & Ervin, F.R. (1968). Gustatory–visceral and telereceptor–cutaneous conditioning: adaptation in internal and external milieus. *Communications in Behavioral Biology*, **1**, 389–415.

Glover, I.C. (1971). Prehistoric research in Timor. In: *Aboriginal Man and Environment in Australia* (ed. D.J. Mulvaney & J. Golson), pp. 158–181. Canberra: Australian National University Press.

Glover, I.C. (1977). Prehistoric plant remains from Southeast Asia, with special reference to rice. In: *South Asian Archaeology 1977* (ed. M. Taddei), pp. 7–37. Naples: Istituto Universitario Orientale.

Goodman, L.S., Gilman, A., Rall, T.W., & Murad, F. (1985). *Goodman and Gilman's The Pharmacological Basis of Therapeutics*. New York: Macmillan.

Gorman, C.F. (1970). Excavations at Spirit Cave, North Thailand: some interim interpretations. *Asian Perspectives*, **13**, 79–108.

Grewal, P.S. (1989). Nematicidal effects of some plant-extracts to *Aphelenchoides composticola* (Nematoda) infesting mushroom, *Agaricus bisporus*. *Revue de Nématologie*, **12**, 317–322.

Hagen, E.H., Roulette, C.J., & Sullivan, R.J. (2013). Explaining human recreational use of 'pesticides': the neurotoxin regulation model of substance use vs. the hijack model and implications for age and sex differences in drug consumption. *Frontiers in Psychiatry*, **4**, 142.

Hagen, E.H., Sullivan, R.J., Schmidt, R., Morris, G., Kempter, R., & Hammerstein, P. (2009). Ecology and neurobiology of toxin avoidance and the paradox of drug reward. *Neuroscience*, **160**, 69–84.

Hammond, J.A., Fielding, D., & Bishop, S.C. (1997). Prospects for plant anthelmintics in tropical veterinary medicine. *Veterinary Research Communications*, **21**, 213–228.

Howitz, K.T. & Sinclair, D.A. (2008). Xenohormesis: sensing the chemical cues of other species. *Cell*, **133**, 387–391.

Huffman, M.A. (1997). Current evidence for self-medication in primates: a multidisciplinary perspective. *American Journal of Physical Anthropology*, **104**(Suppl. 25), 171–200.

Iqbal, Z., Lateef, M., Jabbar, A., Ghayur, M.N., & Gilani, A.H. (2006). In vitro and in vivo anthelmintic activity of *Nicotiana tabacum* L. leaves against gastrointestinal nematodes of sheep. *Phytotherapy Research*, **20**, 46–48.

Jackson, F.L.C. (1990). Two evolutionary models for the interactions of dietary organic cyanogens, hemoglobins, and falciparum malaria. *American Journal of Human Biology*, **2**, 521–532.

Jackson, F.L.C. (1996). The coevolutionary relationship of humans and domesticated plants. *Yearbook of Physical Anthropology*, **39**, 161–176.

Johns, T. (1990). *With Bitter Herbs They Shall Eat It: Chemical Ecology and the Origins of Human Diet and Medicine*. Tucson, AZ: University of Arizona Press.

Johnston, G.A.R., Krogsgaard-Larsen, P., & Stephenson, A. (1975). Betel nut constituents as inhibitors of gamma-aminobutyric acid uptake. *Nature*, **258**, 627–628.

Karban, R. & Agrawal, A.A. (2002). Herbivore offense. *Annual Review of Ecology and Systematics*, **33**, 641–664.

Karban, R. & Baldwin, I.T. (1997). *Induced Responses to Herbivory*. Chicago, IL: University of Chicago Press.

Kelley, A.E. & Berridge, K.C. (2002). The neuroscience of natural rewards: relevance to addictive drugs. *Journal of Neuroscience*, **22**, 3306–3311.

Koob, G.F. & Le Moal, M. (2005). Plasticity of reward neurocircuitry and the 'dark side' of drug addiction. *Nature Neuroscience*, **8**, 1442–1444.

Lieberman, H.R. (2003). Nutrition, brain function and cognitive performance. *Appetite*, **40**, 245–254.

Luqman, W. & Danowski, T.S. (1976). The use of khat (*Catha edulis*) in Yemen: social and medical observations. *Annals of Internal Medicine*, **85**, 246–249.

McKim, W.A. (1991). *Drugs and Behavior: An Introduction to Behavioral Pharmacology*. New Jersey: Prentice Hall.

McPartland, J.M. & Glass, M. (2001). Nematicidal effects of hemp (Cannabis sativa) may not be mediated by cannabinoid receptors. *New Zealand Journal of Crop and Horticultural Science*, **29**, 301–307.

Mann, J. (1992). *Murder, Magic and Medicine*. London: Oxford University Press.

Marshall, M. (1981). Tobacco use in Micronesia: a preliminary discussion. *Journal of Studies on Alcohol*, **42**, 885–893.

Marshall, M. (1987). An overview of drugs in Oceania. *Drugs in Western Pacific Societies: Relations of Substance*, pp. 13–50. Lanham, MD: University Press of America.

Mattoo, S.K., Basu, D., Sharma, A., Balaji, M., & Malhotra, A. (1997). Abuse of codeine-containing cough syrups: a report from India. *Addiction*, **92**, 1783–1787.

Mayr, E. (1961). Cause and effect in biology. *Science*, **134**, 1501–1506.

Moerman, D.E. (1994). North American food and drug plants. In: *Eating on the Wild Side* (ed. N.L. Etkin), pp. 166–181. Tucson, AZ: University of Arizona Press.

Nesse, R.M. & Berridge, K.C. (1997). Psychoactive drug use in evolutionary perspective. *Science*, **278**, 63–66.

Nestler, E.J. (2005). Is there a common molecular pathway for addiction? *Nature Neuroscience*, **8**, 1445–1449.

Ode, P.J. (2006). Plant chemistry and natural enemy fitness: effects on herbivore and natural enemy interactions. *Annual Review of Entomology*, **51**, 163–185.

Olds, J. & Milner, P. (1954). Positive reinforcement produced by electrical stimulation of septal area and other regions of rat brain. *Journal of Comparative Physiology and Psychology*, **47**, 419–427.

Petrinovich, L. & Bolles, R. (1954). Deprivation states and behavioral attributes. *Journal of Comparative Physiology and Psychology*, **47**, 450–453.

Petzinger, E. & Geyer, J. (2006). Drug transporters in pharmacokinetics. *Naunyn-Schmiedeberg's Archives of Pharmacology*, **372**, 465–475.

Plowman, T. (1984). The origin, evolution, and diffusion of coca, *Erythroxylum* spp., in South and Central America. In: *Pre-Columbian Plant Migration* (ed. D. Stone), Papers of the Peabody Museum of Archaeology and Ethnology 76, pp. 129–163. Cambridge, MA: Harvard University Press.

Price, P.W., Bouton, C.E., Gross, P., McPheron, B.A., Thompson, J.N., & Weis, A.E. (1980). Interactions among three trophic levels: influence of plants on interactions between insect herbivores and natural enemies. *Annual Review of Ecology and Systematics*, **11**: 41–65.

Rezvani, A.H. & Levin, E.D. (2001). Cognitive effects of nicotine. *Biological Psychiatry*, **49**: 258–267.

Roulette, C.J., Mann, H., Kemp, B., et al. (2014). Tobacco vs. helminths in Congo basin hunter-gatherers: self medication in humans? *Evolution and Human Behavior*, **35**, 397–407.

Schmeller, T. & Wink, M. (1998). Utilization of alkaloids in modern medicine. In: *Alkaloids: Biochemistry, Ecology, and Medicinal Applications* (ed. M.F. Roberts & M. Wink), pp. 435–459. New York: Plenum Press.

Schultes, R.E. (1979). Solanaceous hallucinogens and their role in the development of New World cultures. In: *The Biology and Taxonomy of the Solanaceae* (ed. J.G. Hawkes, R.N. Lester, & A.D. Skelding), pp. 137–160. London: Academic Press.

Schultz, W. (2011). Potential vulnerabilities of neuronal reward, risk, and decision mechanisms to addictive drugs. *Neuron*, **69**, 603–617.

Shannon, H.E., Bymaster, F.P., Calligaro, D.O., et al. (1994). Xanomeline: a novel muscarinic receptor agonist with functional selectivity for M2 receptors. *Journal of Pharmacology and Experimental Therapeutics*, **269**, 271–281.

Singer, M.S., Mace, K.C., & Bernays, E.A. (2009). Self-medication as adaptive plasticity: increased ingestion of plant toxins by parasitized caterpillars. *PLoS ONE*, **4**(3): e4796. doi: 10.1371/journal.pone.0004796.

Singer, M.S. & Stireman, J.O. (2003). Does anti-parasitoid defense explain host-plant selection by a polyphagous caterpillar? *Oikos*, **100**, 554–562.

Soranzo, N., Bufe, B., Sabeti, P.C., et al. (2005). Positive selection on a high sensitivity allele of the human bitter-taste receptor TAS2R16. *Current Biology*, **15**, 1257–1265.

Sullivan, R.J., Allen, J.S., Otto, C., Tiobech, S., & Nero, K. (2000). The effects of chewing betel nut (*Areca catechu*) on the symptoms of people with schizophrenia in Palau, Micronesia. *British Journal of Psychiatry*, **177**, 174–178.

Sullivan, R.J. & Hagen, E.H. (2002). Psychotropic substance-seeking: evolutionary pathology or adaptation? *Addiction*, **97**, 389–400.

Sullivan, R.J., Hagen, E.H., & Hammerstein, P. (2008). Revealing the paradox of drug reward in human evolution. *Proceedings of the Royal Society B: Biological Sciences*, **275**, 1231–1241.

Sulzer, D. (2011). How addictive drugs disrupt presynaptic dopamine neurotransmission. *Neuron*, **69**, 628–649.

Thorndike, E.L. (1911). *Animal Intelligence: Experimental Studies*. New York: Hafner.

Thurston, R. & Fox, P.M. (1972). Inhibition by nicotine of emergence of *Apanteles congregatus* from its host, the tobacco hornworm. *Annals of the Entomological Society of America*, **65**, 547–550.

Villalba, J.J. & Provenza, F.D. (2007). Self-medication and homeostatic behaviour in herbivores: learning about the benefits of nature's pharmacy. *Animals*, **1**, 1360–1370.

Wang, X., Thomas, S.D., & Zhang, J. (2004). Relaxation of selective constraint and loss of function in the evolution of human bitter taste receptor genes. *Human Molecular Genetics*, **13**, 2671–2678.

Waterman, P.G. (1998). Chemical taxonomy of alkaloids. In: *Alkaloids: Biochemistry, Ecology, and Medicinal Applications* (ed. M.F. Roberts & M. Wink), pp. 87–107. New York: Plenum Press.

Watson, P.L. (1983). *This Precious Foliage: A Study of the Aboriginal Psycho-active Drug Pituri*. Sydney: University of Sydney.

Weir, S. (1985). *Qat in Yemen: Consumption and Social Change*. New York: Dorset Press.

Wink, M. (1998a). Chemical ecology of alkaloids. In: *Alkaloids: Biochemistry, Ecology, and Medicinal Applications* (ed. M.F. Roberts & M. Wink), pp. 265–300. New York: Plenum Press.

Wink, M. (1998b). Modes of action of alkaloids. In: *Alkaloids: Biochemistry, Ecology, and Medicinal Applications* (ed. M.F. Roberts & M. Wink), pp. 301–326. New York: Plenum Press.

Wink, M. (1998c). A short history of alkaloids. In: *Alkaloids: Biochemistry, Ecology, and Medicinal Applications* (ed. M.F. Roberts & M. Wink), pp. 1–44. New York, Plenum Press.

Wink, M. (2000). Interference of alkaloids with neuroreceptors and ion channels. *Studies in Natural Products Chemistry*, **21**, 3–122.

Wink, M. (2003). Evolution of secondary metabolites from an ecological and molecular phylogenetic perspective. *Phytochemistry*, **64**, 3–19.

Wink, M. (2006). Importance of plant secondary metabolites for protection against insects and microbial infections. In: *Naturally Occurring Bioactive Compounds* (ed. M. Rai & M.C. Carpinella), pp. 251–268. Amsterdam: Elsevier.

Wink, M. & Schimmer, O. (1999). Molecular modes of action of defensive secondary metabolites. In: *Functions and Biotechnology of Plant Secondary Metabolites*, Annual Plant Reviews **Vol. 39** (ed. M. Wink), pp. 21–133. Oxford: Wiley-Blackwell.

Wise, R.A. (2000). Addiction becomes a brain disease. *Neuron*, **26**, 27–33.

World Health Organization (1981). Guidelines for surveillance, prevention and control of echinococcosis/hydatidosis. In: *Echinococcosis/Hydatidosis Surveillance, Prevention and Control* (ed. J. Eckert, M.A. Gemmell, & E.J.L. Souslby), p. 147. Geneva: FAO/UNEP/WHO.

Yen, D.E. (1977). Hoabinhian horticulture? The evidence and the questions from Northwest Thailand. In: *Sunda and Sahel* (ed. J. Allen, J. Golson, & R. Jones), pp. 567–600. New York: Academic Press.

Chapter 3

What are addictive substances and behaviours and how far do they extend?

Laura A. Schmidt

3.1 Introduction to addictive substances

Popular authors have used the concept of addiction to describe everything from working too hard, to businesses that function poorly, to whole societies dependent on foreign oil (Schaef, 1987; Schaef and Fassel, 1990). Within professional psychiatry, however, the boundaries around what constitutes an addictive disorder are carefully patrolled, if only to prevent this diagnostic class from becoming a 'catch-all of "disorders" ' (Petry, 2006). Indeed, as recently as the 1950s the World Health Organization still defined alcohol and tobacco, in contrast to illicit drugs, as 'habit forming' substances but not actually addictive (World Health Organization, 1957).

Today, however, discussions in professional circles reveal that the boundaries around addiction are expanding to embrace a wider range of habitual behaviours. On the one hand this means considering the addition of new substances to the list, such as sugar and 'hyper-palatable' foods loaded with salt, sugar, and fat. On the other hand, it means adding a whole new category of 'behavioural' or 'process' addictions represented by pathological gambling, along with Internet gaming and pornography. Growing preoccupation with these substances and behaviours has engendered widespread concern in many societies around the globe. Fifteen countries now tax sugar-sweetened beverages in an effort to address a dramatic growth in sugar consumption and related harms to health (Schmidt, 2014). And some countries in Asia have begun regulating Internet use following highly publicized cases of deaths from heart attacks in Internet cafés, gaming-related murder, and child neglect (Block, 2008; Ko et al., 2009).

This chapter tracks the 'net-widening' trend as professional psychiatrists consider new aspects of human cravings and habitual behaviours as candidates for addictive disorders. It is through this lens that we can see how the concept of addiction is itself changing and evolving. I argue that this net widening is a response to tangible changes unfolding in the information age, as globalized markets make a greater abundance of pleasurable substances and experiences available to more consumers on a 24/7 basis. Recent discussions around expanding addiction diagnoses reflect the response of psychiatry to the growing demand for ways to help individuals achieve hedonic balance in a social context that increasingly fails to support it.

3.2 **Defining addiction**

All potentially addictive experiences start with the consumption of something pleasurable. What distinguishes addiction is the failure to maintain equilibrium when it comes to seeking and experiencing a particular source of pleasure. What would normally be simply gratifying—a glass of wine, sexual arousal, a nice game of poker—becomes for the addict an object of unregulated excess, preoccupation, and compulsion. Ironically, it is the addict's very drive for satisfaction—satisfaction that cannot be stably achieved—that is at the root of his or her suffering. At its core, then, we can understand addiction as a disruption of 'hedonic balance'—an inability to achieve equilibrium in acts of seeking and experiencing of human pleasure (Steel et al., 2008). Maintaining hedonic balance is, in turn, at the core of what it means to experience a state of well-being.

The professional study of addiction cuts across many disciplines, and from this it follows that there are multiple approaches to defining addiction. Still, all definitions build upon the assumption that the problem starts with the habitual, heavy consumption of something pleasurable. Addiction also carries with it an attribution that the habitual use reflects an underlying compulsion—a 'disease of the will' or 'internal driving force' (Room, 1987; Valverde, 1998; Saunders, 2013). The technical criteria for addiction are usually codified in the psychiatric nomenclature under the diagnosis of 'dependence'. For example, in the fourth edition of American Psychiatric Association's *Diagnostic and Statistical Manual of Mental Disorders* (DSM-IV), published in 1994, clinical criteria for 'dependence' include: compulsive substance use despite harmful consequences; inability to stop using a drug; failure to meet work, social, or family obligations; and tolerance and withdrawal. The latter two criteria comprise 'physical dependence', in which the body adapts to the substance, requiring more of it to achieve a certain effect (tolerance) and eliciting substance-specific physical or mental symptoms if use is abruptly ceased (withdrawal).

Increasingly, addiction studies are concerned with both 'substance' and 'behavioural' or 'process' addictions (Potenza, 2006). Substance addictions are related to drugs, alcohol, tobacco, and arguably food, whereas process addictions relate to behaviours such as gambling, sexual activity, and Internet gaming. Debate over whether sugar and other hyper-palatable foods are addictive surrounded recent discussions over revising the diagnostic criteria for addictive disorders in the new edition of the *Diagnostic and Statistical Manual*, DSM-5 (Davis and Carter 2009; Smith and Robbins 2013). Those who support bringing sugar and other foods under the addiction rubric note that, like addicts, binge eaters experience a lack of control, continue overeating despite harm to their health, experience social, legal, and financial problems, and are often unsuccessful at attempts to cut back or reduce their consumption (Devlin, 2007; Gearhardt et al., 2011a,b). Detractors in the debate argue that binge-eating disorders are already covered elsewhere in the psychiatric nomenclature and question whether all of the criteria for dependence are observed in compulsive overeaters (Ziauddeen et al., 2012; Ziauddeen and Fletcher, 2013). While binge eating and other food compulsions remain outside the scope of the new addictive disorder class in DSM-5, the topic remains under active debate.

Candidates for 'behavioural' or 'process' addictions primarily include gambling, Internet gaming, and pornography (Holden 2001; Petry, 2007). Gambling and Internet gaming are fast-growing social problems, particularly in parts of Asia. Those affected are observed to spend large amounts of time online (upwards of 16 hours a day), and to suffer from a lack of sleep and shortage of social contacts as a result of their Internet preoccupation (Allison et al., 2006; Hussain and Griffiths, 2009). Mood modification, withdrawal symptoms, cravings, and relapse have been observed as well (Chappell et al., 2006; Charlton and Danforth, 2007; Wan and Chiou, 2007). In DSM-5 the new label for addiction, 'substance-related and addictive disorders', indicates that there is at least room for a gambling disorder under the addiction rubric (Hasin et al., 2013).

3.3 **Slouching towards a pan-addiction model**

Academic debates over the validity of formally defining new substances and behaviours as addictions consume many pages of today's medical journals, as well as lengthy discussions amongst expert panels revising the *International Classification of Diseases* (ICD) and DSM. Part-and-parcel of these discussions is the search for a broader explanatory model—a unifying 'pan-addiction model', if you will—that provides a single explanatory framework encompassing both substance and behavioural addictions. Efforts to move towards a more unified theory of addiction began in the mid-1980s, when the field shifted over to uniform or 'generic' criteria for all forms of substance dependence. As Hughes (2006) explains, 'the conceptualization that all drugs had several common features led to the use of the same criteria for dependence for all drugs'.

In their book *The Hidden Addiction*, Phelps and Nourse (1986) posited that all addictions stem from common genetic and biological roots. Interestingly, sugar was granted status as 'the basic addiction' because it 'precede[d] all others' and was the 'world's most widespread' substance of abuse (Phelps and Nourse, 1986, p. 73). Since then, a vast body of research using animal experiments and human neuroimaging studies has investigated common pathways for addiction in the brain. This growing body of research focuses on how substances of abuse and repetitive behaviours produce similar long-term changes in neurotransmitter levels and brain functioning (National Institute on Drug Abuse, 1999; Volkow and Li, 2005; Volkow et al., 2007).

If anything today comes close to a unifying pan-addiction model it is the 'reward deficiency hypothesis'. This model links substance and behavioural addictions by their similar impacts on the brain's limbic region—the brain's 'reward centre'—as well as some common effects on the higher-order brain functions of learning and memory and inhibitory controls over behaviour. Here it is argued that prolonged, heavy exposure to concentrated doses of a pleasurable substance or experience will produce changes in the neurotransmitter dopamine (Blumenthal and Gold, 2012). All natural rewards, like eating and sexual arousal, as well as most drugs of abuse, cause a release of dopamine, which is experienced as pleasure. Reward deficiency occurs when the brain changes to accommodate heavy, frequent dopamine spikes from the repetitive use of a psychoactive substance or arousing experience. Over repeated doses or experiences, dopamine levels naturally produced by the brain, and the number of dopamine receptors housed in the brain, decline significantly—a phenomenon referred to as 'dopamine down-regulation'. Ultimately, this produces a declining capacity to experience reward and pleasure, leading the addicted brain to compensate by craving, as well as driving the individual towards heavier and more frequent consumption of the addictive substance or experience (Blum et al., 2000; Volkow et al., 2007).

Neuroimaging studies (e.g. functional magnetic resonance imaging, fMRI), suggest that nearly all addictive drugs act either directly or indirectly upon the brain's reward system by heightening dopaminergic activity. In numerous fMRI studies, dopamine down-regulation has been observed with respect to a wide range of potential addictions: consumption of added sugar, gambling, as well as Internet gaming and pornography use (Olds and Milner, 1954; Brewer and Potenza, 2008; Volkow et al., 2011). Works document the loss of dopamine receptors in response to excessive sugar intake, and more generally in studies of people who compulsively overeat (Avena et al, 2008 a,b; Di Chiara and Imperato, 1988; Wang et al., 2001, 2004; Devlin, 2007). Studies with rats have also explored sugar craving, continued use despite harm (via non-lethal shocks), withdrawal, tolerance, and cross-sensitization (from sugar to stimulants and alcohol) (Ahmed, 2012). Similar patterns of results, consistent with the reward deficiency hypothesis, have also been observed in the brains of pathological gamblers (Petry, 2006) and habitual Internet gamers (Ko et al., 2009).

3.4 **Making sense of the widening scope of addiction**

What we observe today within psychiatry is far from the first movement to re-define new aspects of the human condition as psychiatric disorders. Indeed, the phenomenon of 'net widening' has been a long-standing preoccupation for the sociology of medicine. Sociologists have observed that, over the course of modern history, more and more forms of human difference and suffering have become redefined and treated as psychiatric and medical problems. Chronic inebriety itself, once viewed as a moral failing, was transformed into today's alcoholism, or rather 'dependence', in the early nineteenth century (Schneider, 1978). During the mid-twentieth century, disruptive schoolchildren became redefined as those afflicted by attention deficit and hyperactivity disorder (Conrad, 1975, 1977); other examples of net widening abound. Some sociologists go so far as to argue that, on the whole, medicine has 'nudged aside' or 'replaced' religion as the dominant moral ideology in modern societies (Roman, 1991). And there is now a long tradition of critics arguing for the adverse consequences of bringing so many aspects of the human condition under the label of psychiatric pathology (Szasz, 1963; Frances, 2013).

In sociological analyses, net widening is typically linked to the collective interests of professions—pressures to increase professional jurisdiction and therefore institutional control, the need to 'secure medical turf', and to increase consumer demand for professional services (Conrad and Schneider, 1980; Abbott, 1988; Conrad 2008). Robin Room argues that as medicine is increasingly subjected to privatization and marketization 'psychiatry has been more entre-preneurial and less inclined to decide collectively that cases lie outside its competence. This has encouraged inclusiveness in [diagnostic] criteria and thresholds, so it is unlikely that a clinician will have to turn away anyone appearing for treatment on the grounds that they do not qualify for the diagnosis' (Room, 2007, p. 52).

Taken at face value, today's discussions around expanding addictive disorders into new domains of behaviour could easily be interpreted as a standard case of professional net widening. After all, for years sociologists have criticized the addiction concept for its 'murkiness' (Roman and Blum, 1991), precisely because it allows for a certain 'malleability and expansiveness' in what constitutes an addiction (Conrad, 1992). Still, I would argue that what we are currently observing is far more a reaction by professional psychiatrists to changing social problems and rising demand than proactive entrepreneurism by a profession seeking to expand its jurisdiction and consumer market.

First, in many countries there is a chronic undersupply of beds for addiction treatment, as well as long waiting lists for care. In the United States, for example, it is estimated that only about 10% of those who qualify as having a substance use disorder actually obtain treatment for the problem (Schmidt et al., 2008). Secondly, nearly all of the proposed new candidates for addictions in question—from compulsive overeating, to gambling, to Internet gaming—are already listed in the psychiatric nomenclature under the grouping of 'impulse-control disorders' (Potenza, 2006; Sadock and Sadock, 2008). What might on the surface look like 'net widening' is in fact a debate about reshuffling already-existing diagnoses from one class of mental disorders to another (Block, 2008).

Finally, we cannot ignore the fact that the current net-widening discussion takes place amidst fast-moving, expanding epidemics of obesity, gambling, and Internet game use that have been targeted by governments around the world as major social problems. As societies face new, unfamiliar 'epidemics of the will' (Sedgwick, 1992), it is natural that they look to medicine, psychiatry, and other institutions of social control for solutions. I believe that recent discussions around expanding addiction diagnoses reflect psychiatry's response to growing demands for ways to help individuals achieve hedonic balance in a social context that increasingly fails to support it. To appreciate this one need look no farther than to the spate of new popular books on how to control one's sugar addiction: from Kessler's (2012) *Your Food is Fooling You* that describes 'how your brain is hijacked by sugar, fat and salt', to *Why Diets Fail: Because You're Addicted to Sugar* (Avena and Talbott, 2013), to *Obsessed: America's Food Addiction—and My Own* (Brzezinski, 2013), and to Robert Lustig's (2012) *New York Times* best seller, *Fat Chance: Beating the Odds Against Sugar, Processed Food, Obesity, and Disease*.

3.5 The social context of net widening today

It was not long ago that Coca Cola and other soft drinks were prescribed as 'replacement fluids' whose use should be encouraged by alcoholics in recovery. These so-called 'soft drinks' were promoted as 'sober pleasures' that might help alcoholics wean themselves off 'harder' drinks containing alcohol (Valverde, 1998, Chapter 7). Today, as we have seen, there is an active debate within psychiatry as to whether the sugar in Coca Cola constitutes an addictive substance in its own right. In this section, we look to how changing social conditions have given rise to new social problems, like overconsumption of sugar, which are currently candidates for professional disease designations as addictions. I argue that the key mechanisms underlying this include: (1) the commercial production and global marketing of *more concentrated* pleasure-inducing substances and experiences; (2) their *increased availability* and aggressive marketing to consumers; and (3) *declines in external social controls* that would otherwise limit their high concentration and widespread availability.

3.5.1 The dose makes the poison

In small doses, most potentially addictive substances and experiences are simple pleasures, and some (such as opium and cocaine) are even therapeutic. Substances only become 'hazardous' and 'addictive' when distilled down into concentrated form—into white powders—that significantly heighten the pleasure produced and generally induce a more powerful experience. When chewed or consumed in tea, coca leaves produce a mildly stimulating effect on a par with drinking a cup of coffee. But when the active ingredient in coca leaves is extracted and processed into the white-powder rock called 'crack', the very same substance assumes a 'high addiction potential' (Nutt et al., 2010).

'Drug hardening' occurs when producers move towards more industrial and commercialized modes of production and distribution (Bakalar and Grinspoon, 1984). Highly concentrated products prove easier to transport, thereby reaching wider markets, with more gratified consumers. Likewise, the traditional home brewing and craft production of alcohol has generally resulted in products containing lower concentrations of ethanol. It is largely in a context of industrial production and commercialization that highly concentrated products become possible and make sense, from the standpoint of ease of distribution and technological capacity to refine products in highly concentrated form (Schmidt and Room, 2012).

One factor that many of our new candidates for addiction share is that their production is heavily industrialized and commercialized, encouraging producers to package products in more concentrated forms. The sugar fructose is far from hazardous when produced, packaged, and consumed the way nature provides it, in fruit. It only becomes a health hazard when the essential sweetness of fructose is extracted from cane, beets, and corn and then added to packaged foods in very high concentrations (Lustig et al., 2012). A parallel to 'drug hardening' is arguably the case with Internet gambling, where on-line games are carefully engineered to trigger 'the chase' for greater returns at higher stakes (Petry, 2006). This may also apply to Internet games and pornography, which are increasingly engineered to entice players into faster-paced, more emotive, more compelling 'virtual lives' (Weinstone, 2002).

3.5.2 **Increased availability**

Babor et al. (2003) underscore the fact that addictive substances have many so-cial functions, among which is that they serve as commodities bought and sold in the marketplace. There are consequently many vested interests in the pro-duction and sale of alcohol, prescription drugs, and tobacco products, as well as hyper-palatable foods, gambling enterprises, Internet games, and pornography. These commodities generate profits for their producers, advertisers, and inves-tors, provide employment opportunities, and, increasingly, are traded on a glo-bal scale. Many of these commodities also bring generous tax revenues to the governments of nation states.

Today's globalizing economies introduce an unprecedented capacity for the large-scale production and marketing of highly concentrated pleasure-inducing substances and experiences. In the modern food-processing industry, sugar is added to a remarkable 73% of packaged foods, including foods that taste savoury and are marketed on the basis of being 'healthy' (Ng et al., 2012). Food scientists employed by the largest packaged food corporations use sophisticated labora-tory techniques to engineer foods for greater palatability and satiety inhibition (Moss, 2013). Ironically, the very brain imaging technologies developed in medi-cine to study addiction processes are today used in the laboratories of corporate food scientists to engineer hyper-palatable foods that make individuals crave, and therefore purchase, more. In a similar vein, growing worldwide access to the Internet makes pornography, gambling, and gaming available to individuals on a round-the-clock basis with virtually unfettered access (Chou et al., 2005).

3.5.3 **Social control structures in decay**

Social control structures are societal mechanisms that regulate individual be-haviour to gain conformity and compliance to the rules of a given society (Hor-witz, 1990). Traditional societies rely mostly on *informal* social controls embedded in customs and the conditions of daily life; these informal controls quite naturally place limits on the consumption of intoxicating substances and experiences. Take the case of traditional beer brewing in Africa, where indigen-ous beer is produced in small batches for bartering, work parties, and cere-monial uses. The technology for producing beer from grain is simple, intensive labour is required, and the beer does not remain potable for long, requiring that any excess must be immediately consumed. Due to limited means of storage and transport, in a traditional context, little alcohol travels far from the point of production (Schmidt and Room, 2012).

However, today, the production of alcohol, along with hyper-palatable foods, Internet games, and other intoxicants, is the business of multinational firms that ultimately view global populations as their markets (Jernigan, 1997; Room, 2013). What curbs and helps regulate individual consumption in this context are *formal, institutionalized structures of social control*, largely based in the legal and regulatory powers seated in nation states and agencies of global governance (e.g. the United Nations). With longstanding substances of abuse—alcohol, to-bacco, and psychoactive drugs—formal social controls, promulgated through national and global policies, have proven highly successful at regulating avail-ability, and therefore individual use. Public health protections such as taxation, advertising, and price controls are some of the most effective tools for curbing individual consumption of addictive substances and therefore mitigating re-lated harms to individuals and societies (Babor et al., 2003).

In today's world, the liberalization of markets, along with the increased glo-balization of trade and the growing affluence of societies, significantly con-strains the capacity of governments to impose formal controls that help individuals regulate their consumption behaviours. In an era of free markets and consumer sovereignty, the ability of governments to control the marketing of pleasurable substances and experiences has been compromised, at the na-tional level by courts or commissions enforcing internal free markets and at the international level by regional trade agreements and activities to liberalize trade between nations, for example under the auspices of the World Trade Organiza-tion (Room et al., 2008).

Governments are especially constrained in their ability to regulate many of the new candidates for addictions. In the case of sugar-laden and hyper-palatable foods, as much as 90% of global marketing occurs through direct foreign investment which is not regulated by international trade policies or transparent legal instruments that can be litigated in international courts (Taylor et al., 2014). Meanwhile, Internet gambling and pornography are de-livered to consumers via the only electronic medium not currently regulated (Robinson, 1999)—except by a handful of nation states (Zixiang, 1999).

3.6 **Conclusion**

Humans will always be driven to seek pleasure. But the means to get there on a regular basis—and through a wide range of concentrated, readily available prod-ucts and experiences—has at no time been greater than it is today. Amidst the powerful forces of a globalizing economy and the information age, along with market liberalization, consumers face relatively unfettered access to a wide range of pleasure-inducing substances and behaviours. I have argued that this social context places a greater burden on the individual to manage and self-regulate pleasure seeking. And that, in an environment in which an extraordinary range of concentrated pleasures are marketed on a 24/7 basis, with limited countervailing social controls, we can expect that more and more individuals will struggle to achieve some degree of hedonic balance and will look to medicine and psychiatry for help.

This wider social context can help us to understand changing conceptions of addiction within professional psychiatry. These broad social forces are leading the field to widen the scope of addictive disorders to include experiences, processes, and behaviours—to reconsider the longstanding tenet that a precondition for addiction must be the habitual consumption of some externally derived psychoactive agent. At the same time, these forces have spurred the search for a unifying pan-addiction model that might help the field organize around a shared definition of addiction—one that allows it to hold 'substance' and 'behavioural' addictions within a common framework of understanding.

It is unlikely that the demands on addiction psychiatry have been greater at any other time. But then again, neither have been the demands on individuals seeking balance in an age of intoxication.

References

Abbott, A. (1988). *The System of Professions: An Essay on the Division of Expert Labor*. Chicago, IL: University of Chicago Press.

Ahmed, S.H. (2012). Is sugar as addictive as cocaine? In: *Food and Addiction: A Comprehensive Handbook* (ed. K.D. Brownell & M.S. Gold), pp. 231–237. Oxford: Oxford University Press.

Allison, S.E., von Wahlde, L., Shockley, T., & Gabbard, G.O. (2006). The development of the self in the era of the internet and role-playing fantasy games. *American Journal of Psychiatry*, **163**, 381–385.

American Psychiatric Association (1994). *Diagnostic and Statistical Manual of Mental Disorders*, 4th edn. Washington, DC: American Psychiatric Press.

Avena, N.M. & Talbott, J.R. (2013). *Why Diets Fail (Because You're Addicted to Sugar): Science Explains How to End Cravings, Lose Weight, and Get Healthy*. New York: Random House LLC.

Avena, N.M., Bocarsly, M.E., Rada, P., Kim, A., & Hoebel, B.G. (2008a). After daily bingeing on a sucrose solution, food deprivation induces anxiety and accumbens dopamine/acetylcholine imbalance. *Physiology and Behavior*, **94**, 309–315.

Avena, N., Rada, P., & Hoebel, B. (2008b). Evidence for sugar addiction: behavioural and neurochemical effects of intermittent, excessive sugar intake. *Neuroscience Behavior Review*, **32**, 20–39.

Babor, T., Caetano, R., Casswell, S., et al. (2003). *Alcohol: No Ordinary Commodity—Research and Public Policy*. Oxford: Oxford University Press.

Bakalar, J.B. & Grinspoon, L. (1984). *Drug Control in a Free Society*. New York: Cambridge University Press.

Beckman, V. (1988). *Alcohol: Another Trap for Africa.* Örebro, Sweden: Libris Publishing.

Block, J. (2008). Issues for DSM-V: internet addiction. *American Journal of Psychiatry,* **165,** 306–307.

Blum, K., Braverman, E.R., Holder, J.M., et al. (2000). The reward deficiency syndrome: a biogenetic model for the diagnosis and treatment of impulsive, addictive and compulsive behaviors. *Journal of Psychoactive Drugs,* **32**(Suppl. 1): 1–112.

Blumenthal, D.M. & Gold, M.S. (2012). Relationships between drugs of abuse and eating. *Food and Addiction: A Comprehensive Handbook.* New York: Oxford University Press.

Brewer, J.A. & Potenza, M.N. (2008). The neurobiology and genetics of impulse control disorders: relationships to drug addictions. *Biochemical Pharmacology,* **75,** 63–75.

Brzezinski, M. (2013). *Obsessed: America's Food Addiction—and My Own.* New York: Weinstein Books.

Chappell, D., Eatough, V., Davies, M.N., & Griffiths, M. (2006). EverQuest—it's just a computer game right? An interpretative phenomenological analysis of online gaming addiction. *International Journal of Mental Health and Addiction,* **4**: 205–216.

Charlton, J.P. & Danforth, I.D.W. (2007). Distinguishing addiction and high engagement in the context of online game playing. *Computers in Human Behavior,* **23**: 1531–1548.

Chou, C., Condron, L., & Belland, J.C. (2005). A review of the research on internet addiction. *Educational Psychology Review,* **17**: 363–388.

Colson, E. & Scudder, T. (1988). *For Prayer and Profit: The Ritual, Economic, and Social Importance of Beer in Gwembe District, Zambia, 1950–1982.* Stanford, CA: Stanford University Press.

Conrad, P. (1975). Discovery of hyperkinesis: notes on the medicalization of deviant behavior. *Social Problems,* **23,** 12–21.

Conrad, P. (1977). Medicalization, etiology and hyperactivity: a reply to Whalen and Henker. *Social Problems,* **24,** 596–598.

Conrad, P. (1992). Medicalization and social control. *Annual Review of Sociology,* **18,** 209–232.

Conrad, P. (2008). *The Medicalization of Society: On the Transformation of Human Conditions into Treatable Disorders.* Baltimore, MD: Johns Hopkins University Press.

Conrad, P. & Schnedier, J. (1980). *Deviance and Medicalization: From Badness to Sickness.* St Louis, MO: Mosby.

Conrad, P. & Walsh, D.C. (1992). The new corporate health ethic: lifestyle and the social control of work. *International Journal of Health Services,* **22,** 89–111.

Davis, C. & Carter, J.C. (2009). Compulsive overeating as an addiction disorder. A review of theory and evidence. *Appetite,* **53,** 1–8.

Devlin, M.J. (2007). Is there a place for obesity in DSM-V? *International Journal of Eating Disorders,* **40,** S83–S88.

Eber, C. (1995). *Women and Alcohol in a Highland Maya Town: Water of Hope, Water of Sorrow.* Austin, TX: University of Texas Press.

Frances, A. (2013). *Saving Normal: An Insider's Revolt Against Out-of-Control Psychiatric Diagnosis, DSM-5, Big Pharma and the Medicalization of Ordinary Life.* New York: Morrow, William.

Di Chiara, G. & Imperato, A. (1988). Drugs abused by humans preferentially increase synaptic dopamine concentrations in the mesolimbic system of freely moving rats. *Proceedings of the National Academy of Sciences of the United States of America*, **85**, 5274–5278.

Gearhardt, A.N., Grilo, C.M., DiLeone, R.J., Brownell, K.D., & Potenza, M.N. (2011a). Can food be addictive? Public health and policy implications. *Addiction*, **106**, 1205–1377.

Gearhardt, A.N., Yokum, S., Orr, P.T., Stice, E., Corbin, W.R., & Brownell, K.D. (2011b). Neural correlates of food addiction. *Archives of General Psychiatry*, **68**, 808–816.

Hasin, D., O'Brien, C.P., Auriacombe, M., et al. (2013). DSM-5 criteria for substance use disorders: recommendations and rationale. *American Journal of Psychiatry*, **170**, 834–851.

Holden, C. (2001). 'Behavioral' addictions: do they exist? *Science*, **294**, 980–982.

Horwitz, A.V. (1990). *The Logic of Social Control*. New York: Plenum Press.

Hughes, J.R. (2006). "Should criteria for drug dependence differ across drugs?." *Addiction* 101.s1 : 134–141.

Hussain, Z. & Griffiths, M.D. (2009). The attitudes, feelings, and experiences of online gamers: a qualitative analysis. *CyberPsychology and Behavior*, **12**, 747–753.

Jernigan, D. (1997). *Thirsting for Markets: The Global Impact of Corporate Alcohol*. San Rafael, CA: Marin Institute for the Prevention of Alcohol and Other Drug Problems.

Kessler, D.A. (2012). *Your Food is Fooling You: How Your Brain is Hijacked by Sugar, Fat, and Salt*. New York: Macmillan.

Ko, C.-H., Liu, G.-C., Hsiao, S., et al. (2009). Brain activities associated with gaming urge of online gaming addiction. *Journal of Psychiatric Research*, **43**, 739–747.

Levine, H. (1978). The discovery of addiction: changing conceptions of habitual drunkenness in America. *Journal of Studies on Alcohol*, **39**, 143–174.

Lustig, R.H. (2012). *Fat Chance: Beating the Odds Against Sugar, Processed Food, Obesity, and Disease*. New York: Hudson Street Press.

Lustig, R.H., Schmidt, L.A., & Brindis, C.D. (2012). The toxic truth about sugar. *Nature*, **487**, 27–29.

Maula, J. (1997). *Small-Scale Production of Food and Traditional Alcoholic Beverages in Benin and Tanzania: Implications for the Promotion of Female Entrepreneurship*. Helsinki: Finnish Foundation for Alcohol Studies.

Moss, M. (2013). *Salt, Sugar, Fat: How the Food Giants Hooked Us*. New York: Random House.

National Institute on Drug Abuse (1999). *Principles of Drug Addiction Treatment: A Research-Based Guide*, 2nd edn. Bethesda, MD: National Institute on Drug Abuse, National Institutes of Health.

Ng, S.W., Slining, M.M., & Popkin, B.M. (2012). Use of caloric and noncaloric sweeteners in US consumer packaged foods, 2005–2009. *Journal of the Academy of Nutrition and Dietetics*, **112**, 1828–1834.

Nutt, D.J., King, L.A., & Phillips, L.D. (2010). Drug harms in the UK: a multicriteria decision analysis. *Lancet*, **376**, 1558–1565.

Olds, J. & Milner, P. (1954). Positive reinforcement produced by electrical stimulation of septal area and other regions of rat brain. *Journal of Comparative and Physiological Psychology* 47, 419–427.

Petry, N.M. (2006). "Should the scope of addictive behaviors be broadened to include pathological gambling?." *Addiction* 101.s1: 152–160.

Phelps, J.K. & Nourse, A.E. (1986). *The Hidden Addiction and How to Get Free*, 1st edn. Boston, MA: Little Brown.

Potenza, M.N. (2006). "Should addictive disorders include non-substance-related conditions?." *Addiction* 101.s1: 142–151.

Robinson, G.O. (1999). *Regulating the Internet*. Social Science Research Network: Legal Essays. URL: <http://papers.ssrn.com/sol3/papers.cfm?abstract_id=205038>.

Roman, P.M. (1991). Problem definitions and social movement strategies: the disease concept and the hidden alcoholic revisited. In: *Alcohol: the Development of Sociological Perspectives on Use and Abuse* (ed. P.M. Roman), pp. 235–253. New Brunswick, NJ: Rutgers Center of Alcohol Studies.

Roman, P.M. & Blum, T.C. (1991). *The Medicalized Conception of Alcohol-Related Problems: Some Social Sources and Some Social Consequences of Murkiness and Confusion*. New Brunswick, NJ: Rutgers University Press.

Room, R. (1987). Bring back inebriety?: a response to "no 'alcoholism' please, we're British". *British Journal of Addiction*, 82, 1064–1068.

Room, R. (2007). Cultural and societal influences on substance use diagnoses and criteria. In: *Diagnostic Issues in Substance Use Disorders: Refining the Research Agenda for DSM-V* (ed. J.B. Saunders, M.A. Schuckit, P.J. Sirovatka, & D.A. Regier), pp. 45–60. Arlington, VA: American Psychiatric Association.

Room, R. (2013). Sociocultural aspects of alcohol consumption. In: *Alcohol: Science, Policy and Public Health* (ed. P. Boyle, P. Boffetta, A.B. Lowenfels, et al.), pp. 38–45. Oxford: Oxford University Press.

Room, R., Schmidt, L.A., Rehm, J., & Makela, P. (2008). International regulation of alcohol. *British Medical Journal*, 337, a2364.

Room, R., Hellman, M., & Stenius, K. (2014) Addiction: the dance between concepts and terms. *International Journal of Alcohol and Drug Research* (in press).

Sadock, B.J. & Sadock, V.A. (2008). *Kaplan & Sadock's Concise Textbook of Clinical Psychiatry*, 3rd edn. Philadelphia, PA: Lippincott Williams & Wilkins.

Saunders, J.B. (2013). The concept of substance use disorders. A commentary on 'Defining substance use disorders: do we really need more than heavy use' by Rehm et al. *Alcohol and Alcoholism* 48, 644–645.

Schaef, A.W. (1987). *When Society Becomes an Addict*, 1st edn. San Francisco: Harper & Row.

Schaef, A.W. & Fassel, D. (1990). *The Addictive Organization*. San Francisco: Harper.

Schivelbusch, W. (1992). *Tastes of Paradise: A Social History of Spices, Stimulants, and Intoxicants*. New York: Vintage Books.

Schmidt, L.A. (2014). New unsweetened truths about sugar. *JAMA Internal Medicine*, 174, 525–526.

Schmidt, L.A. & Room, R. (2012). Alcohol and the process of economic development: contributions from ethnographic research. *International Journal of Alcohol and Drug Research*, 1, 41–55.

Schmidt, L., Greenfield, T., & Mulia, N. (2006). Unequal Treatment: Racial and Ethnic Disparities in Alcoholism Treatment Services. *Alcohol Research and Health*, **29**(1): 49–54.

Schneider, J.W. (1978). Deviant drinking as disease: alcoholism as a social accomplishment. *Social Problems*, **25**, 361–372.

Sedgwick, E.K. (1992). Epidemics of the will. In: *Incorporations* (ed. J. Crary & S. Kwinter), pp. 582–595. New York: Zone.

Smith, D.G. & Robbins, T.W. (2013). The neurobiological underpinnings of obesity and binge eating: a rationale for adopting the food addiction model. *Biological Psychiatry*, **73**, 804–810.

Sonnenstuhl, W.J. (1986). *Inside an Emotional Health Program: A Field Study of Workplace Assistance for Troubled Employees*. Ithaca, NY: Cornell University Press.

Steel, P., Schmidt, J., & Shultz, J. (2008). Refining the relationship between personality and subjective well-being. *Psychological Bulletin*, **134**, 138–161.

Szasz, T.S. (1963). *Law, Liberty and Psychiatry*. New York: Macmillan.

Taylor, A.L., Parento, E.W., & Schmidt, L.A. (2014). The increasing weight of regulation: countries combat the global obesity epidemic. *Georgetown Law Faculty Publications and Other Works*, **90**. Paper 1329. URL: <http://scholarship.law.georgetown.edu/facpub/1329>.

Valverde, M. (1998). *Diseases of the Will: Alcohol and the Dilemmas of Freedom*. Cambridge: Cambridge University Press.

Volkow, N.D. & Li, T.-K. (2005). Drugs and alcohol: treating and preventing abuse, addiction and their medical consequences. *Pharmacology and Therapeutics*, **108**, 3–17.

Volkow, N.D., Fowler, J.S., Wang, G.-J., Swanson, J.M., & Telang, F. (2007). Dopamine in drug abuse and addiction: results of imaging studies and treatment implications. *Archives of Neurology*, **64**, 1575–1579.

Volkow, N.D., Wang, G.-J., Fowler, J,S., Tomasi, D., & Telang, F. (2011). Addiction: beyond dopamine reward circuitry. *Proceedings of the National Academy of Sciences of the United States of America*, **108**, 15037–15042.

Wan, C.-S. & Chiou, W.-B. (2007). The motivations of adolescents who are addicted to online games: a cognitive perspective. *Adolescence*, **42**, 179–197.

Wang, G.-J., Volkow, N.D., Logan, J., et al. (2001). Brain dopamine and obesity. *Lancet*, **357**, 354–357.

Wang, G.-J., Volkow, N.D., Thanos, P.K., & Fowler, J.S. (2004). Similarity between obesity and drug addiction as assessed by neurofunctional imaging: a concept review. *Journal of Addictive Diseases*, **23**, 39–53.

Watters, E. (2010). *Crazy Like Us: The Globalization of the American Psyche*. New York: Simon and Schuster.

Weinstone, A. (2002). Welcome to the pharmacy: addiction, transcendence, and virtual reality. In: *High Anxieties: Cultural Studies in Addiction* (ed. J.F. Brodie & M. Redfield), pp. 161–174. Berkeley, CA: University of California Press.

World Health Organization (1957). *Expert Committee on Addiction-Producing Drugs, 7th Report*. World Health Organization Technical Report Series 116. Geneva: World Health Organization.

Ziauddeen, H. & Fletcher, P.C. (2013). Is food addiction a valid and useful concept? *Obesity Reviews*, **14**, 19–28.

Ziauddeen, H., Farooqi, I.S., & Fletcher, P.C. (2012). Obesity and the brain: how convincing is the addiction model? *Nature Reviews Neuroscience*, **13**, 279–286.

Zixiang, T. (1999). Regulating China's Internet: convergence toward a coherent regulatory regime. *Telecommunications Policy*, **23**, 261–276.

Chapter 4

Well-being as a framework for understanding addictive substances

Laura Stoll and Peter Anderson

4.1 Introduction to well-being

This chapter proposes the use of societal well-being and its domains as a framework for a better understanding of addictive substances and behaviours. We begin with an overview of the developments in measuring societal well-being, especially in the UK, we consider why this is necessary, and describe the key domains of well-being, using those proposed by the Organisation for Economic Co-operation and Development's (OECD) Better Life Index. We then describe the two-way links between these domains of societal well-being and addictions. Finally, we discuss the implications of using well-being as the basis for improved governance of addictions, outlining a shift from a criminal-based to a health and well-being-based approach to illegal drugs.

4.2 Societal well-being

Over the past few years there has been a growing interest in using measures of well-being in public policy as a complement to traditional measures of economic success. This is a culmination of several decades of academic research, alongside a growing political recognition that we need to adopt a better definition of progress and a more holistic way of measuring it than gross domestic product (GDP).

Today, the countries of the world rank themselves in terms of GDP, which has become the most common shorthand for national welfare. Reactions to increases or decreases in GDP growth reveal that politicians have gradually come to rely on this indicator as a signal of whether public policy is leading a country in the right (or wrong) direction. But GDP was not designed with this purpose in mind. The period 1930–1950 saw the first modern national accounting systems and the start of official and regular national accounting in a small number of countries. These developments were closely linked to the economic circumstances of the times: the economic crisis of the 1930s and the Second World War and its aftermath (Bos, 2011). These specific economic circumstances shaped the development of national accounting, establishing overall productivity as the key measure of a country's general success. Over time the measurement itself began to shape our conceptual understanding (Tooze, 2001) and GDP became widely interpreted as a proxy for societal progress.

GDP has been criticized as a measure of welfare on several counts: it fails to take account of the distribution of income within countries; it includes expenditure due to negative events, for example natural disasters, which tend to boost GDP; it ignores other aspects of welfare, such as health and education; it fails to acknowledge the value of unpaid work; and it does not account for the environmental costs of some activities that increase GDP. In addition to these criticisms, evidence has revealed that its relationship to improvements in reported (subjective) well-being is substantially weaker than has traditionally been assumed. In his now oft-cited paper, 'Does economic growth improve the human lot? Some empirical evidence', the American economist Richard Easterlin (1974) showed that although at any given time income and well-being are correlated, both at the level of the country (richer countries tend to have higher average levels of well-being) and of the individual (richer individuals tend to have higher levels of well-being), over time economic growth in a country does not necessarily lead to a rise in average levels of happiness. This finding was dubbed the 'Easterlin paradox'.

Although the Easterlin paradox has not gone unchallenged (e.g. by Stevenson and Wolfers, 2008), the finding, coupled with evidence from psychology suggesting that only a small proportion of the variation in subjective well-being is attributable to material circumstances (Lyubomirsky et al., 2005), significantly weakens the traditional link between GDP and well-being, strengthening the call for better measures of progress. As we enter a period of increasing economic, social, and environmental uncertainty, this need becomes ever greater and more urgent. A myopic obsession with economic growth has meant that we have tended to ignore its negative impacts on our well-being, for example longer working hours. Add to this some of its consequences for the environment, such as pollution, and the case for very different measures of progress and policy evaluation becomes compelling.

Easterlin's paper sparked a new academic interest in subjective well-being that grew most rapidly from the mid-1990s onwards, fuelled by the availability of large-scale social survey data. Psychologists, and later economists, used these data to explore the statistical relationships between measures of subjective well-being and a variety of personal, social, and economic factors. This study of well-being as a science built upon a long philosophical tradition dating back to the Ancient Greeks of considering what the 'good life' requires (McMahon, 2006), and has attracted interest from sociologists and political theorists as well as psychologists and economists.

It is only in the last 10 years that there has been a corresponding level of interest from policy-makers at a national level. This was partly in response to long-standing concerns about using GDP as a measure of national welfare but also in response to the criticism that macro-economic statistics did not reflect how ordinary people felt about their own lives, especially during the economic crisis (OECD, 2011).

In the UK, well-being has been on the policy agenda since 2000, when the Local Government Act gave local authorities in England and Wales the power to 'promote the economic, social and environmental well-being of their area', acknowledging that policy should be concerned with a broad range of positive outcomes. In 2005 the national sustainable development strategy stated that a key component of sustainable development included 'promoting personal well-being, social cohesion and inclusion and creating equal opportunity for all'. This led to the first official attempt to define well-being in UK policy, headed by the cross-governmental Whitehall Wellbeing Working Group (W3G) that commissioned research to help conceptualize and define well-being. From this work a 'shared understanding' of well-being was published in 2007 (Newton, 2007).

Alongside these UK developments, two large international conferences were held in 2007, hosted and attended by organizations such as OECD, the European Commission (EC), and the United Nations (UN), and both called for broader measures of societal progress.

Further significant research on well-being was commissioned by the UK Government Office for Science as a Foresight Project on Mental Capital and Wellbeing. The report, published in 2008, outlined the findings of an extensive 2-year study that examined the policy factors influencing well-being (BIS, 2008).

In 2008, French president Nicolas Sarkozy launched the Commission on the Measurement of Economic Performance and Social Progress (commonly called the 'Stiglitz Commission') led by Nobel prize-winners Joseph Stiglitz and Amartya Sen. It was driven by 'increasing concerns . . . about the adequacy of current measures of economic performance . . . [and] about the relevance of these figures as measures of societal wellbeing, as well as measures of economic, environmental, and social sustainability' (Stiglitz et al., 2009). The commission's report gained huge international attention and set the agenda for European statistical offices. The report recommended that subjective measures of quality of life should be collected by governments, and played an important part in creating a strong base of political and policy-making support for measuring subjective well-being.

In October 2010, the UK Prime Minister David Cameron announced that the Office for National Statistics (ONS) was going to start collecting data on the subjective well-being of the UK population, and, in a connected programme of work, would collaborate with the public and experts to construct an index of national well-being (Cameron, 2010). The inclusion of measures of subjective well-being in the ONS flagship national survey made the UK the first country to collect national-level data on subjective well-being; an equally important innovation was the 'public debate' that saw the ONS engage with a wide range of stakeholders to use these and other data to create a new measure of national progress (ONS, 2011).

Cross-national momentum has continued—in 2011 a UN General Assembly declaration invited member states 'to pursue the elaboration of additional measures that better capture the importance of the pursuit of happiness and well-being in development with a view to guiding their public policies'. Several countries, including Australia, Norway, Germany, Italy, Spain, Canada, and Slovenia, have responded to this and are working to develop and use measures of well-being in policy and politics (Kroll, 2011; OECD, 2011).

Several international initiatives have also been established. In 2011 the EC created the European Statistical System Committee (ESSC) to work towards developing a set of quality of life indicators for the European Union (EU). In 2012 the UN hosted a high-level meeting in New York on well-being and happiness, attended by representatives from many national governments. From this an 'International Expert Working Group for a New Development Paradigm' has been formed, to work towards the creation of a new global well-being and sustainability-based economic paradigm (Alkire, 2013). To coincide with the meeting, the *World Happiness Report* was published by a group of academics, the first in a set of annual analyses of global well-being (Helliwell et al., 2012, 2013).

4.2.1 Defining well-being

As with many emerging sciences, the science of well-being has struggled with definitional issues, and debate still continues, particularly regarding the distinction between factors that are fundamental parts of the concept itself and those that are necessary for, but external to, well-being, as well as the most appropriate way of measuring well-being for policy-making.

As part of the Foresight Project on Mental Capital and Wellbeing, the New Economics Foundation (NEF) produced a 'dynamic model of well-being', a model which attempted to align the various definitions of individual well-being. The model, which has since been slightly adapted (Fig. 4.1) can be used to understand the division between those who define well-being as subjective (i.e. the top two boxes in Fig. 4.1) and classify other social, economic, environmental, or quality of life factors as determinants or drivers of subjective well-being, and those who consider that subjective well-being represents one independent aspect of well-being alongside a range of other domains, such as health, material conditions, income, etc. (i.e. all of Fig. 4.1).

There has also been much discussion about the best way to measure well-being. It is clear that the term subjective well-being captures more than just the hedonic aspect of well-being (good feelings from day to day)and that it also requires the meeting of various human psychological needs, such as the ability to pursue one's goals and to maintain good social relationships (Ryan and Deci, 2001). This is often referred to as eudaimonic well-being. Therefore a set of measures of well-being including both hedonic and eudaimonic ones is necessary to understand the true breadth of people's lived experience. And, despite

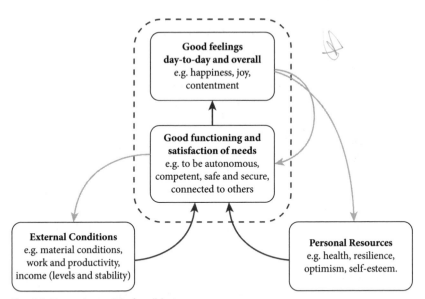

Fig. 4.1 Dynamic model of well-being.

Adapted from Foresight Mental Capital and Wellbeing Project, Final Project report, The Government Office for Science, London, UK, © Crown Copyright 2008, licence under the Open Government Licence v.2.0, available from https://www.gov.uk/government/uploads/system/uploads/attachment_data/file/292450/mental-capital-wellbeing-report.pdf. Originally adapted with permission from Measuring well-being in policy: issues and applications, Copyright © 2008 New Economics Foundation, available from http://b.3cdn.net/nefoundation/575659b4f333001669_ohm6iiogp.pdf

some conceptual disagreement, most people agree that when it comes to assessing well-being at a societal level, a comprehensive framework that includes a range of components *including* subjective well-being is necessary to provide an adequate picture of the well-being of a population.

4.2.2 Domains of well-being

To understand overall societal well-being, and to help to identify and analyse the factors that may influence personal (subjective) well-being, several academics and organizations have produced a series of domains (often also called dimensions or components) of well-being. There is a high degree of consistency around the domains included—they tend to be a mix of individual factors such as personal health and community/environmental factors such as governance.

The Stiglitz Commission identified eight dimensions of well-being: material living standards (income, consumption, and wealth); health; education; personal activities, including work; political voice and governance; social connections and relationships; environment (present and future conditions); and insecurity (economic as well as physical). The OECD used 11 domains to construct its Better Life Index: housing; income; jobs; community; education; environment; civic engagement; health; life satisfaction; safety; and work–life balance. Bhutan's measure of Gross National Happiness (heavily drawn on by the International Expert Working Group for a New Development Paradigm) uses nine domains: psychological well-being (domain satisfaction, positive and negative emotions, spirituality and mind-training); good health: education; living standards; environmental diversity and resilience; good governance; time use; community vitality; and cultural diversity and resilience. The UK ONS used its public consultation to construct a index using ten domains: personal well-being; our relationships; health; what we do (a mixture of employment and non-work activity); where we live (both housing and the local environment); personal finance; the economy; education and skills; governance; and the natural environment. And the EU quality of life indicators are grouped according to the following domains: material living conditions; productive or main activity; health; education; leisure and social interactions; economic and physical safety; governance and basic rights; natural and living environment; and overall experience of life.

For the purposes of this chapter we focus on the OECD's Better Life Index domains, which fit conceptually into their Framework for Measuring Wellbeing and Progress (based on the recommendations made by the Stiglitz Commission) which organizes the domains into three groups: material conditions; quality of life; and sustainability (Fig. 4.2). The Better Life Index covers the first two groups, leaving sustainability of well-being over time to be defined and measured using the OECD Green Growth Strategy Indicators.

Under material living conditions the Better Life Index includes income and wealth, jobs and earnings, and housing. Income and wealth capture people's current and future consumption possibilities and the relationship between income and well-being is well established in the well-being literature (Stoll et al., 2012). Most evidence from both individual-level and country-level analyses reveals diminishing marginal returns to income: once a certain level of national or individual income is obtained, increases in income do not translate into increases—or only into small increases—in well-being. The availability and quality of jobs are both relevant for well-being, not only by supplying the income that people require but also by providing the opportunity to fulfil their ambitions and build self-esteem. National and international research shows that unemployment is strongly negatively correlated with several measures of subjective well-being (Stoll et al., 2012). Finally, housing and housing quality are necessary in meeting basic needs but also to lead to a sense of privacy, personal security, and personal space.

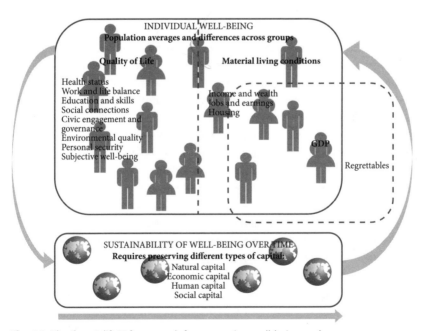

Fig. 4.2 The 'how's life?' framework for measuring well-being and progress.

Reproduced with permission from OECD (2011), How's Life?: Measuring Well-being, OECD Publishing, http://dx.doi.org/10.1787/9789264121164-en

The quality of life group includes health status, work–life balance, education and skills, civic engagement and governance, social connections, environmental quality, personal security, and subjective well-being. Good health, both objectively assessed and self-rated, is strongly correlated with subjective well-being and is also important for performing a range of activities relevant to well-being, including work. In addition, there is evidence of a strong effect of subjective well-being on health (Diener and Chan, 2011).

Education has been viewed as a resource for raising the living standards of individuals and society as a whole. At the individual level, many (but not all) studies have found that more education is often associated with higher subjective well-being, when controlling for other variables (particularly income and health) (Stoll et al., 2012). Being able to reconcile work and life is also important for the well-being of those who have both a job and a family and, more generally, being able to spend time on leisure activities boosts subjective well-being. Interestingly, there is some evidence to suggest an inverse U-shaped relationship between hours worked and subjective well-being (Meier and Stutzer, 2008, Van Praag and Ferrer-i-Carbonell, 2010).

Civic engagement and quality of governance matter for well-being, and countries with high levels of subjective well-being generally have higher levels of democracy and democratic participation (Helliwell and Huang, 2008). Social connectedness is a basic human need, and strong social networks and time spent socializing are positively associated with subjective well-being (Stoll et al., 2012). A strong social network may also help fulfil other important goals, such as finding work.

The quality of their local environment affects people's health and subjective well-being and influences their ability to do a number of essential activities. Likewise, an environment in which people can feel secure is important to people's subjective well-being. Unsurprisingly perhaps, evidence shows that crime is negatively associated with subjective well-being, both for victims and for residents in areas with a high crime rate (Lelkes, 2006).

Finally, a consideration of how people feel in terms of their day-to-day feelings, their overall evaluations of life, and eudaimonic aspects of well-being, such as feelings of autonomy and competence, should form a central part of a well-being framework, allowing policy-makers to monitor people's lived experience more directly. With advancements in measurement there is a good understanding of how a combination of different subjective well-being questions can be used to capture the range of underlying concepts necessary for a more complete understanding of experienced well-being. Viewing these measures alongside the entire range of domains can also help to understand how objective living circumstances interact to affect how people feel and function in their everyday lives.

4.3 **Two-way links between domains of societal well-being and addictions**

We continue by describing the two-way links between elements of the domains of societal well-being and addictions, using three examples. Our first example is how domains of quality of life and material living conditions can impact on the harm done by addictive substances and behaviours. Our second example is how prohibition can lead to a range of losses of well-being for individuals and societies, using the case of cannabis. And, our third example is how quality of life and material living conditions can interact with people undergoing opioid substitution treatment for heavy opioid use.

4.3.1 **Quality of life, material conditions and their impact on the harm done by addictive substances and behaviours**

Here we show that the level of quality of life and material living conditions may increase the harm done by addictive substances over and above the direct harm that the substance itself can do the health and well-being of an individual. More importantly, societal moral responses to substance use, and a lack of societal concern about the overall well-being and material living conditions of heavy drug users, are also important determinants of harm over and above the direct harm from the substance itself.

As Gell et al. (2014) have shown, the social and cultural context within which licit and illicit drug use take place is important in determining how societies understand what is considered harmful behaviour. Harms to the individual can be caused by how societies handle substance use; for example, the criminalization of illicit drugs can result in the production of unregulated substances that may contain harmful agents. On the other hand, harms to society can result from an individual's substance use; for example, the lost economic productivity that can result from alcohol-related ill-health and premature death.

The harms experienced as a result of addictive substances may be influenced by how societies perceive drug use. As such, within a given culture or society, the harm related to the use of a substance may change over time. A 'moral panic' occurs when a condition, episode, person, or group is suddenly regarded as a threat to societal values and interests (Cohen, 1972). This can cause harm through public hostility towards deviants, resulting in social exclusion, and the awarding of unusually harsh punishments for deviant behaviour, resulting in civic disengagement (Critcher, 2008). Under these circumstances behaviour that might previously have been considered risky becomes harmful because of society's changed reaction to it. As Gell et al. (2014) point out, a well-studied example of a 'moral panic' is the public reaction to crack cocaine use that occurred in the United States in the mid-1980s. The determinants of this negative societal reaction included an overall decline in the public's acceptance of illegal drug use, growing interest of the media and action groups in illegal drug use, and over-dramatization of the actual prevalence of illegal drug use, with a subsequent disproportionate concern among politicians and lawmakers. The negative social reaction was exacerbated by the novelty of crack cocaine and overdoses that occurred among some prominent athletes. The harms that resulted from the negative social reaction included a crackdown in law enforcement and a crisis reaction among the population, both of which increased the overall harm done by crack cocaine to the well-being of individuals and societies (Goode and Ben-Yehuda, 1994).

In addition to threats posed by negative societal reactions, societal norms may influence societal responses to addictive substances, and the harm experienced from them. Addictive substances can be highly moralized about and are often subject to prohibitory or strict regulatory frameworks which vary from place to place and from time to time. Engagement with addictive substances can convey strong social meaning and may lead to stigma, which can be particularly focused on the marginalized 'misusers' as opposed to the supposedly more responsible mainstream users (Room, 2011). This can lead to punitive societal responses which are potentially harmful to well-being in themselves and, conversely, a lack of intervention in mainstream behaviour which allows harms to occur unchecked. For example, if caught using drugs in a country with a zero tolerance approach to the use of illicit substances, individuals may be subject to criminal sanctions with potential negative implications for their quality of life and material living conditions. Countries may also change drug laws or the response of law enforcers to substance use over time, perhaps resulting in the reclassification of a drug or a law enforcement crackdown, with implications for the experience of harm for those individuals continuing to use particular substances.

Drug control policy also frames and influences drug users' health, for example through laws around the provision or lack of access to clean needles and syringes (Campbell and Shaw, 2008). Lack of access to clean needles is one example of how it may not be drug use in itself that causes health problems but a lack of services that societies offer to drug users that would enable people to take drugs in less harmful ways (Bourgois et al., 1997). The extent to which harm reduction is pursued as a policy objective in a given society thus influences the experience of consequences of negative well-being resulting from the use of an addictive substance.

Deprivation, poverty, and social exclusion are all forms of social and economic marginalization. Individuals and groups may be marginalized along divisions such as economic status, ethnicity, and education, with engagement in harmful substance use often, although not always, seen to occur along similar societal divisions. Indicators of social marginalization such as not being in the workforce and not being stably housed are strong predictors for harmful substance use. Premature death from substance use is associated with indicators of marginalization—lower education, lower income, and lower housing stability all contribute significantly to predicting death from an alcohol-specific condition (Makela, 1999). Reasons for the social class gradient in mortality and other negative consequences related to alcohol might be due to groups with a higher socioeconomic status having more resources to protect themselves. Additionally, people in higher socioeconomic groups are usually advantaged in terms of having a family, which may be a motivating factor in the decision to do something about a substance use problem before severe consequences occur. Different drug usage and the clustering of risk factors (such as malnutrition, poor access to health services, and low income) in some populations (Schmidt et al., 2010) may also explain why some groups suffer harm from addictive substances while others do not.

Treatment and control systems also influence the marginalization experienced by substance users. Individuals in substance treatment are often excluded from society and employment or are on the periphery of society for the duration of their treatment. Following treatment, people may not adequately reintegrate into society, having undergone treatment in an environment in which their everyday lives may have been constrained. Drug policy can also keep users in a marginalized position, for example by criminalizing the distribution and use of many addictive substances, thus criminalizing and facilitating punishment of the behaviour of those with drug dependences (Campbell and Shaw, 2008). Thus, individuals engaging in heavy substance use may experience a cycle of marginalization that is difficult to break.

Societal responses to 'deviant' heavy drug use may also result in the formation of subcultures of individuals who group together in response to social exclusion. Societal exclusion can result when agencies that deal with drug-related problems impose a label on particular forms of deviance or social problems. Individuals exposed to labelling may take on the associated identity and develop groupings (Goode, 2004), perhaps as a form of defence or adjustment. The subcultures that develop are often marginalized from wider society. For example, following a criminal conviction, an individual may find it impossible to secure work and may therefore be forced into a life of crime to survive. Thus, marginalization is a determinant of harmful substance use. Further, harmful substance use may result in further marginalization.

Finally, there is evidence for a negative impact of unemployment on harmful substance use. Unemployed people from the United States, Australia, the UK, and Finland have between two to four times the risk of harmful substance use as employed people (Henkel, 2011). Long-term unemployment also increases the risk of alcohol-related deaths for both men and women (Garcy and Vagero, 2012), while plant closures increase the risk of hospitalization due to alcohol-related disorders and alcohol-related death (Eliason and Storrie, 2009).

4.3.2 Well-being losses from prohibition—the example of cannabis

Here we show how prohibition of cannabis leads to losses in well-being for individuals and societies in the domains of quality of life, material living conditions, and sustainability of well-being over time over and above the direct harm that cannabis use itself can do to the health and well-being of individuals and societies. We also describe how prohibition can result in discrimination against segments of the population leading to further harm to well-being over and above the direct harm that can result from cannabis.

Cannabis is a generic term for preparations (e.g. marijuana, hashish, and hash oil) derived from the plant *Cannabis sativa*. Cannabis use can be associated with some acute and chronic harms to health, but is a much less hazardous product than alcohol or smoked tobacco products. Twenty-three million Europeans (6.8% of all 15–64-year-olds) have used cannabis in the past year and about 12 million (3.6% of all 15–64-year-olds) in the last month (Trautmann et al., 2013).

In terms of the sustainability of economic well-being over time, prohibition has placed control of a multi-billion Euro market in cannabis in the hands of organized criminal networks and unregulated markets. In the EU and Norway, for example, the cannabis used corresponds to a retail value of between €18 and €30 billion per year (Trautmann et al., 2013). Many commercial cannabis-growing operations in the EU are run by criminal organizations which rarely restrict their activities to one criminal area, and their involvement in the cannabis trade increases the likelihood of an association developing between cannabis production and other criminal activities. Many European countries have reported increases in criminal activities, including violence and intimidation, linked to cannabis production (EMCDDA, 2012b).

Prohibition also drains public funds into criminal justice systems, has high opportunity costs, and forfeits potential tax revenues. The total annual government expenditure on drug policy in the UK, for example, is around £1.1 billion annually (Davies et al., 2011). The majority of this expenditure is on treatment, with only around £300 million spent on enforcement. By contrast, it is estimated that the total government expenditure on drug-related offending across the criminal justice system is more than ten times this figure, at £3.4 billion. Drug law enforcement budgets translate into reduced options for other areas of expenditure—whether other enforcement priorities, other drug-related public health interventions (such as education, prevention, harm reduction, and treatment), or wider social policy spending. Further opportunity costs accrue from the productivity and economic activity that is forfeited as a result of the mass imprisonment of drug offenders. Lost tax revenue is another opportunity cost. The Dutch coffee shops, for example, with a turnover of €2 billion pay over €400 million in tax annually (EMCDDA, 2012b).

At an individual and community level, adverse social effects include stigma and discrimination against drug users and negative effects that drug users' behaviours have on community well-being and public safety. Many who receive a criminal record due to cannabis possession or sale experience negative consequences in terms of their civil rights, employment, accommodation, interpersonal relationships, driving licences, and other stigmas associated with criminality.

There are sizeable gaps in many European countries between formal cannabis policy and cannabis policy as implemented (Reuter, 2009). One key factor relates to whom responsibility for policy enforcement is entrusted. Different policies, for example, 'officially' assign discretionary power to regional police authorities, enforcement officials, prosecutorial officials, and/or judicial officials. These officials may opt for a more punitive or more permissive approach, depending on their own or their organization's agenda.

Such discretionary power has resulted in discriminatory enforcement leading to civic disengagement and social exclusion of parts of society. Cannabis laws have been selectively enforced by police officers, for example, who identify certain groups for cannabis control and 'stop and search' checks.

In England and Wales, the 2011/2012 Crime Survey found that the proportions of 16–59-year-olds using any illicit drug during the previous year were 9.4% for those classified as being of white ethnicity, 5.1% for those classified as black, and 3.1% for those classified as Asian. The respective proportions for cannabis use were 7.3, 4.3, and 2.2% (Home Office, 2012). UK law allows police to stop and search an individual if they have 'reasonable grounds' to believe that they will find controlled drugs, an offensive weapon or firearm, a sharp article, prohibited fireworks, stolen goods, articles which could be used to commit a crime, articles which could be used to commit a terrorist attack, or articles that could cause criminal damage. In 2009/10, the stop and search rate for drugs across people living in the Greater London area was 34 stop searches for drugs per 1000 residents. For white people there were 24 stop searches for drugs per

1000 residents. For black people there were 66 stop searches for drugs per 1000 residents. Thus black people in London were stopped and searched for drugs at nearly three times the rate of white people. Asian people were subject to stop and search for drugs at 1.5 times the rate of white people (Eastwood et al., 2013).

For the very small percentage of people who are found with drugs after being stopped and searched by police, there are a number of criminal justice responses that can be deployed. These responses are: cannabis warning which does not form part of a person's criminal record; a Penalty Notice for Disorder which is an on-the-spot £80 fine and does not form part of a criminal record; a caution instead of charging and referring a person to court for prosecution, which forms part of a criminal record; and a charge, in which the matter will be referred to the courts to be dealt with. In the Greater London area black people are charged at five times the rate of white people and receive cannabis warnings at three times the rate. This jump in disproportionality at the charge stage demonstrates that a black person is more likely to receive a harsher police response for possession of cannabis.

4.3.3 Living conditions among patients in opioid substitution treatment

Here we show that heavy opioid users have a poorer quality of life and material living conditions before entering opioid substitution treatment (OST), how a poorer quality of life and material living conditions are predictors of poorer treatment outcomes, and how treatment, although generally improving quality of life and material living conditions, can affect them negatively by withdrawing people from the labour market.

The most common type of treatment in Europe for people who are heavy users of opioids is OST, typically integrated with psychosocial care and provided at specialist outpatient centres, by general practitioners, or by a shared-care arrangement with specialist treatment centres (EMCDDA, 2012a). As the most used OST, methadone maintenance treatment (MMT) has been found to reduce illicit opiate use, opioid-related death, behaviour putting people at risk of HIV, and drug and property-related criminal behaviours (Marsch, 1998; Brugal et al., 2005; Soyka et al., 2012). In this subsection we describe how social and environmental factors, such as employment, have a strong impact on OST.

4.3.3.1 Living conditions among patients entering treatment

Heavy opioid users entering treatment tend to have poor mental and physical health (Luty and Arokiadass, 2008). Their heavy drug use also leads to social and relationship problems that prevent people achieving their desired goals. For example, criminality restricts their employment, and heavy drug use damages relationships with their family and significant others. The impairment of quality of life among people entering MMT tends to be higher than that for people with other clinical conditions such as chronic obstructive pulmonary disease or coronary artery disease (Ryan and White, 1996; De Maeyer et al., 2010). Clients admitted to OST are frequently unemployed, although they often have stable accommodation (Smyth et al., 2005; Millson et al., 2006); however, OST seems to exacerbate the problem because entering OST often leads to loss of a job or the inability to work (Richardson et al., 2012).

4.3.3.2 Living conditions as predictors of treatment

Having a supportive relationship, particularly with a drug-free individual, a satisfying job, good housing status, a higher level of education, and personal coping skills are important determinants of success in OST (Abrahams, 1979; Nosyk et al., 2011; Baharom et al., 2012). Lower depression scores, higher level of education, and being married make stable employment more likely among clients in OST (Zanis et al., 1994). A good level of education is also associated with improved health-related quality of life of patients in OST (Baharom et al., 2012).

A good relationship with family, living with a partner, strong social support from family or friends, income, employment, and absence of a criminal history are all associated with better retention in treatment (Torrens et al., 1996; del Rio et al., 1997; Brown and Zuelsdorff, 2009; Butler et al., 2010; Lin et al., 2011; Yang et al., 2013). However, the type of therapy is one of the strongest predictors of retention in treatment, with abstinence-oriented therapy showing the lowest retention compared with MMT (Salamina et al., 2010).

Social and environmental support (alongside pharmacological treatment) are important factors affecting improvement in the patient's quality of life when in OST treatment (De Maeyer et al., 2011). However, although OST can help individuals stabilize their situations and participate in society, several negative consequences, for example dependence, can be associated with its use and may affect quality of life.

4.3.3.3 Impact of treatment on living conditions

OST has been shown to improve clients' quality of life, with improved mental and physical health and social functioning and reduced criminality (Maremmani et al., 2007; Ponizovsky and Grinshpoon, 2007; Reimer et al., 2011; Chen et al., 2012; Torrens et al., 2013). OST also leads to improvements in material living conditions, including accommodation and employment (Sand and Romelsjö, 2005).

Clients report that the positive factors of being in OST include improvements in their clinical condition, the ability to change their standard of living, not being involved in crime, improvements in their economic and material capital, and rebuilding of family and social bonds. On the other hand, clients report that treatments are 'very addictive' and erect many hurdles in their lives. Treatment are often reported as long and, in most cases, clients are obliged to attend a centre and be monitored more often than they would like (Sanders et al., 2013).

4.4 **Governance**

We continue by illustrating how a well-being framework can describe the different approaches to governance of addictive substances across Europe, highlighting the many existing deficiencies. Governance can be described as 'the processes and structures of public policy decision making and management that engage people constructively across the boundaries of public agencies, levels of government, and/or the public, private and civic spheres in order to carry out a public purpose that could not otherwise be accomplished' (Emerson et al., 2012, p. 2).

Ysa et al. (2014) have documented the current approaches to governing addictive substances in European countries in order to learn from them, to find out if there are different typologies, and ultimately to help reframe the governance of addictive substances in Europe by identifying existing weaknesses and shortcomings and helping to define innovative and more integrative approaches. They categorized countries on the basis of strategy and structure (Fig. 4.3), with strategy being the content of the policy and the focus and priorities of each country when governing addictive substances, and structure focusing on the organization and the involvement of public, non-profit, and private stakeholders in the different stages of the governance of addictions.

At one extreme of the 'strategy' concept they placed the 'safety and disease approach'; this reflects an individualistic approach criminalizing the drug user who is regarded as a diseased person and/or an offender. Furthermore, countries with this vision normally gave more weight to supply reduction policies especially focused on the traffic of illicit substances and controlled by security-oriented ministries. Such countries had strict penalties and did not make sophisticated distinctions between penalties depending on the substance. At the other extreme, they placed countries with a 'well-being and relational management approach', characterized by having high levels of social acceptance for tackling drugs and addictions. This meant that their citizens in general had a greater understanding of drug use and drug addicts. In such countries, individual actions were respected as long as they did not risk the freedom of another individual. Furthermore, the 'well-being and relational management approach'

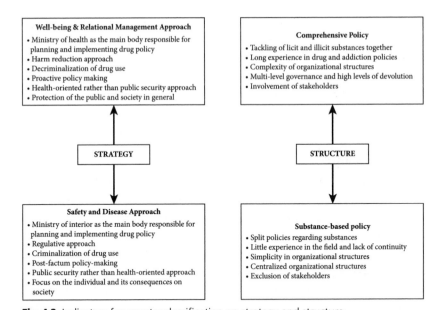

Fig. 4.3 Indicators for country classification on strategy and structure.

Adapted from Ysa, T. et al., Governance of Addictions: European Public Policies, Oxford University Press, Oxford, UK, Copyright © 2014, by permission of Oxford University Press.

embraced the three trends of decriminalization, harm-reduction, and regulation. Hence, these countries decriminalized drug use and in some instances even drug possession in small quantities. They also embraced a social vision by taking into account the social consequences of substance consumption and substance addictions and dealing with them by means of harm reduction policies. Finally, most of these countries' policies were based on the evidence of empirical research and had the aim of protecting the public and society in general through regulation.

In the case of 'structure', the authors differentiated countries based on their policy-making and their organizational structures when dealing with substances and addictions. At one extreme were countries with 'substance-based policy', including those with different policies for different substances, those with little experience in the field, and those with some inconsistencies due to their lack of continuity regarding policies on addictive substances. In this sense they were considered to be followers of EU guidelines, establishing their structures and policies in alignment with those promoted by the EU. Another characteristic of countries with 'substance-based policy' was that they were organized on the basis of problems related to addiction and drugs. Furthermore, it seemed that policies and structures were only developed when a problem appeared—hence they did not anticipate problems but lagged behind trends in addictive substances (i.e. policy-making was reactive). At the other extreme were countries described as having a 'comprehensive policy'. This meant that they embraced holistic political strategies including both substances (either licit or illicit) and behaviours. Moreover, these countries had long experience of policies on drugs and addiction—this normally leads to more complex and transverse structures, i.e. more ministries and departments involved and higher levels of interdependence when dealing with drug-related problems. Based on this classification, cluster analyses found four models or groupings of countries (Table 4.1):

◆ Model 1: these countries embraced to a certain extent the three trends of decriminalization, harm reduction, and regulation. None of them included a well-being perspective in their aims; none of them had supply reduction as one of the top priorities in their aims; and all of them decriminalized possession of drugs. Nevertheless, there was little implementation of evidence-based policies for licit substances. All countries had established an ad hoc coordinating body for addictions policies. The ministry of health tended to be the responsible institution. Countries were characterized by the devolution of the implementation process, and a long history of legislating on illicit drugs.

◆ Model 2: these countries tended to control licit substances through regulations limiting the sale and use of tobacco and alcohol. Their policies regarding illicit substances were still closer to a safety and disease strategy than to a well-being and relational management one. All of the countries had organized an ad hoc body to deal with addictions, had devolved implementation

Table 4.1 Governance models for drug policy: characteristics and countries

Model	Characteristics	Countries
1	A 'well-being and relational management' strategy with a comprehensive structure. Focus on illicit substances	Belgium, Czech Republic, Germany, Italy, Luxemburg, Netherlands, Portugal, and Spain
2	Strict regulation on licit substances (tobacco and alcohol)	Finland, France, Ireland, Norway, Sweden, and the UK
3	Most divergent countries of the sample. They do not follow a clear trend	Austria, Bulgaria, Cyprus, Denmark, Poland, and Slovenia
4	Have not embraced the three trends. They have a 'safety and disease' strategy combined with a 'substance-based structure'	Estonia, Greece, Hungary, Latvia, Lithuania, Malta, Romania, and Slovakia

to decentralized structures, and did not have 'addiction' as such as an object-ive in their national strategies. Most of the countries in this group tackled licit and illicit substances together, involved not-for-profit organizations in the decision-making process, and had a long history of legislating on drug-related issues.

- Model 3: these countries had different approaches, with no clear trend. None of the countries decriminalized possession nor did they have injection rooms as a harm reduction policy; their tobacco policies tended to be weak. They tended to have the ministry of health as the institution responsible for tackling drug and addiction issues and prioritized treatment and prevention issues before supply reduction ones. Thus, they tended to have a safety and disease strategy rather than a well-being and relational management one. These countries were more scattered in structure than in strategy. They did not tackle licit and illicit substances together; hence they focused on the sub-stances rather than on addictions. None of the countries involved not-for-profit and private organizations in the decision-making process. Most countries devolved policy-making and implementation to decentralized structures.

- Model 4 is closer to a 'safety and disease approach' than to a 'well-being and relational management' one. Countries in this cluster shared traditional drug and addiction policies and had not yet embraced a public-health per-spective. They still regarded drugs and addictions as an issue to be tackled through a security-oriented perspective. Thus, their focus was on supply re-duction; regarding demand, they looked at prevention and treatment, with harm reduction measures as residuals. In all but one country, the ministry of the interior or the prime minister had responsibility for addictions policies. Alcohol policies have been stricter in recent years, but tobacco was loosely regulated. Countries were mainly reactive and tended to follow European trends by producing very similar strategies and action plans to those ap-proved by the EU. Countries tended to have an ad hoc coordinating body, but not-for-profit and private organizations were not involved in decision making, there was no devolution of policy-making and implementation to decentralized structures, and the concept of addiction was excluded from the aims.

What is striking from the analysis is that there are enormous opportunities for improved governance from the perspective of societal well-being in all countries. Although Model 1 countries had passed laws that decriminalized the use and possession of illicit substances and, at the same time, gave much importance to harm reduction policies, to fully embrace a 'well-being and relational management' strategy these countries need to improve their evidence-based regulations for the licit substances of alcohol and tobacco. Although Model 2 countries had implemented strict but evidence-based regulations aimed at reducing the harm done by alcohol and tobacco, and enhancing societal well-being, their policies regarding illicit substances were still closer to a safety and disease strategy than to a well-being and relational management one. Model 3 and 4 countries have a long way to go to embrace decriminalization, regulation, and harm reduction policies.

References

Abrahams, J.L. (1979). Methadone maintenance patients' self-perceived factors responsible for successful rehabilitation. *International Journal of the Addictions*, **14**, 1075–1081.

Alkire, S. (2013). *Well-being, Happiness and Public Policy*. Oxford Poverty and Human Development Initiative (OPHI) Research in Progress 37a. URL: <http://www.ophi.org.uk/ophi-research-in-progress-37a/>.

Baharom, N., Hassan, M.R., Ali, N., & Shah, S.A. (2012). Improvement of quality of life following 6 months of methadone maintenance therapy in Malaysia. *Substance Abuse Treatment, Prevention and, Policy*, **7**, 32.

BIS (Department for Business, Innovation and Skills) (2008). *Mental Capital and Wellbeing: Making the Most of Ourselves in the 21st Century*. Final report of the Foresight project. London: The Government Office for Science. URL:<https://www.gov.uk/government/uploads/system/uploads/attachment_data/file/292453/mental-capital-wellbeing-summary.pdf>.

Bos, F. (2011). *Three Centuries of Macro-economic Statistics*. MPRA Paper 35391. Munich: University Library of Munich. URL: <http://mpra.ub.uni-muenchen.de/35391/>.

Bourgois, P., Lettiere, M., & Quesada, J. (1997). Social misery and the sanctions of substance abuse: confronting HIV risk among homeless heroin addicts in San Francisco. *Social Problems*, **44**, 155–173.

Brown, R.T. & Zuelsdorff, M. (2009). Treatment retention among African-Americans in the Dane County Drug Treatment Court. *Journal of Offender Rehabilitation*, **48**, 336–349.

Brugal, M.T., Domingo-Salvany, A., Puig, R., Barrio, G., García de Olalla, P., & de la Fuente, L. (2005). Evaluating the impact of methadone maintenance programmes on mortality due to overdose and aids in a cohort of heroin users in Spain. *Addiction*, **100**, 981–989.

Butler, S.F., Black, R.A., Serrano, J.M., Wood, M.E., & Budman, S.H. (2010). Characteristics of prescription opioid abusers in treatment: prescription opioid use history, age, use patterns, and functional severity. *Journal of Opioid Management*, **6**, 239–241.

Cameron, D. (2010). PM speech on wellbeing. URL: <https://www.gov.uk/government/speeches/pm-speech-on-wellbeing>.

Campbell, N. & Shaw, S. (2008). Incitements to discourse: illicit drugs, harm reduction and the production of ethnographic subjects. *Cultural Anthropology*, **23**, 21–39.

Chen, C.Y., Ting, S.Y., Tan, H.K., & Yang, M.C. (2012). A multilevel analysis of regional and individual effects on methadone maintenance treatment in Taiwan. *Value Health*, **15**(1 Suppl.), S60–S64.

Cohen, S. (1972). *Folk Devils and Moral Panics: The Creation of the Mods and the Rockers* Oxford: Basil Blackwell.

Critcher, C. (2008). Moral panic analysis: past, present and future. *Sociology Compass*, **2**, 1127–1144.

Davies, C., English, L., Stewart, C., Lodwick, A., McVeigh, J., & Bellis, M. (eds.) (2011). *United Kingdom Drug Situation: Annual Report to the EMCDDA 2011.* URL: <http://www.emcdda.europa.eu/attachements.cfm/att_191569_EN_UnitedKingdom_2011.pdf> (accessed 21 February 2014).

De Maeyer, J., Vanderplasschen, W., & Broekaert, E. (2010). Quality of life among opiate-dependent individuals: a review of the literature. *International Journal of Drug Policy*, **21**, 364–380.

De Maeyer, J., Vanderplasschen, W., Lammertyn, J., van Nieuwenhuizen, C., Sabbe, B., & Broekaert, E. (2011). Current quality of life and its determinants among opiate-dependent individuals five years after starting methadone treatment. *Quality of Life Research*, **20**, 139–150.

Diener, E. & Chan, M.Y. (2011). Happy people live longer: subjective well-being contributes to health and longevity. *Applied Psychology: Health and Well-Being*, **3**, 1–43.

Easterlin, R. (1974). Does economic growth improve the human lot? Some empirical evidence. In: *Nations and Households in Economic Growth: Essays in Honor of Moses Abramowitz* (ed. P.A. David & M.W. Reder), pp. 89–125. New York: Academic Press.

Eastwood, N., Shiner, M., & Bear, D. (2013). *The Numbers in Black and White: Ethnic Disparities in the Policing and Prosecution of Drug Offences in England and Wales.* Release Report no. 2. London: LSE Consulting. URL: <http://www.lse.ac.uk/businessAndConsultancy/LSEConsulting/pdf/ReleaseReport.pdf> (accessed 21 February 2014).

Eliason, M. & Storrie, D. (2009). Does job loss shorten life? *Journal of Human Resources*, **44**, 277–302.

EMCDDA (2012a). *2012 Annual Report on the State of the Drugs Problem in Europe.* Lisbon: European Monitoring Centre for Drugs and Drug Addiction. URL: <http://www.emcdda.europa.eu/publications/annual-report/2012>.

EMCDDA (2012b). *EMCDDA Insights: Cannabis Production and Markets in Europe.* Lisbon: European Monitoring Centre for Drugs and Drug Addiction. URL: <http://www.emcdda.europa.eu/publications/insights/cannabis-market> (accessed 21 February 2014).

Emerson, K., Nabatchi, T., & Balogh, S. (2012). An integrative framework for collaborative governance. *Journal of Public Administration Research Theory*, **22**, 1–31.

Garcy, A. & Vagero, D. (2012). The length of unemployment predicts mortality, differently in men and women, and by cause of death: a six year mortality follow-up of the Swedish 1992–1996 recession. *Social Science and Medicine*, **74**, 1911–1920.

Gell, L., Holmes, J., Bühringer, G., et al. (2014). *Determinants of Harmful Substance Use and Harmful Gambling: An Interdisciplinary Review.* URL: <http://www.alicerap.eu/>

Goode, E. & Ben-Yehuda, N. (1994). *Moral Panics: The Social Construction of Deviance* Malden, MA: Blackwell.

Goode, E. (2004). *Deviant Behaviour.* Upper Saddle River, NJ: Pearson.

Helliwell, J. & Huang, H.F. (2008). How's your government? International evidence linking good government and well-being. *British Journal of Political Science*, **38**, 595–619.

Helliwell, J., Layard, R., & Sachs, J. (eds.) (2012). *World Happiness Report*. New York: Earth Institute, Columbia University.

Helliwell, J., Layard, R., & Sachs, J. (eds.) (2013). *World Happiness Report*. New York: Earth Institute, Columbia University.

Henkel, D. (2011). Unemployment and substance use: a review of the literature (1990–2010). *Current Drug Abuse Reviews*, 4, 4–27.

Home Office (2012). *Drug Misuse Declared: Findings From the 2011/12 Crime Survey for England and Wales*. URL: <https://www.gov.uk/government/statistics/drug-misuse-declared-findings-from-the-2011-to-2012-crime-survey-for-england-and-wales-csew-second-edition> (accessed 4 April 2014).

Kroll, C. (2011). *Measuring Progress and Well-Being: Achievements and Challenges of a New Global Movement*. Berlin: Friedrich Ebert Stiftung.

Lelkes, O. (2006). Knowing what is good for you. Empirical analysis of personal preferences and the 'objective good'. *Journal of Socio-Economics*, 35, 285–307.

Lin, C., Wu, Z., & Detels, R. (2011). Family support, quality of life and concurrent substance use among methadone maintenance therapy clients in China. *Public Health*, 125, 269–274.

Luty, J. & Arokiadass, S.M. (2008). Satisfaction with life and opioid dependence. *Substance Abuse Treatment, Prevention and Policy*, 3, 2.

Lyubomirsky, S., Sheldon, K.M., & Schkade, D. (2005). Pursuing happiness: the architecture of sustainable change. *Review of General Psychology*, 9, 111–131.

McMahon, D.M. (2006). *The Pursuit of Happiness: A History From the Greeks to the Present*. London: Penguin Books.

Makela, P. (1999). Alcohol-related mortality as a function of socio-economic status. *Addiction*, 94, 867–886.

Maremmani, I., Pani, P.P., Pacini, M., & Perugi, G. (2007). Substance use and quality of life over 12 months among buprenorphine maintenance-treated and methadone maintenance-treated heroin-addicted patients. *Journal of Substance Abuse and Treatment*, 33, 91–98.

Marsch, L.A. (1998). The efficacy of methadone maintenance interventions in reducing illicit opiate use, HIV risk behavior and criminality: a meta-analysis. *Addiction*, 93, 515–532.

Meier, S. & Stutzer, A. (2008). Is volunteering rewarding in itself? *Economica*, 75, 39–59.

Millson, P., Challacombe, L., Villeneuve, P.J., et al. (2006). Determinants of health-related quality of life of opiate users at entry to low-threshold methadone programs. *European Addiction Research*, 12, 74–82.

Newton, J. (2007). *Wellbeing Research: Synthesis Report*. London: Defra. URL: <http://archive.defra.gov.uk/sustainable/government/documents/Wellbeingresearchsynthesisreport.pdf>.

Nosyk, B., Guh, D.P., Sun, H., et al. (2011). Health related quality of life trajectories of patients in opioid substitution treatment. *Drug and Alcohol Dependence*, 118, 259–264.

OECD (2011). *How's Life?: Measuring Well-being*. Paris: OECD Publishing. URL: <http://dx.doi.org/10.1787/9789264121164-en>.

ONS (2011). *Measuring National Well-being: A Discussion Paper on Domains and Measures*. Cardiff: ONS. URL: <http://www.ons.gov.uk/ons/rel/wellbeing/measuring-national-

well-being/discussion-paper-on-domains-and-measures/measuring-national-well-being---discussion-paper-on-domains-and-measures.html>.

Perlman, M. & Marietta, M. (2005). The politics of social accounting: public goals and the evolution of the national accounts in Germany, the United Kingdom and the United States. *Review of Political Economy*, 17, 211–230.

Ponizovsky, A.M. & Grinshpoon, A. (2007). Quality of life among heroin users on buprenorphine versus methadone maintenance. *American Journal of Drug and Alcohol Abuse*, 33, 631–642.

Reimer, J., Verthein, U., Karow, A., Schäfer, I., Naber, D., & Haasen, C. (2011). Physical and mental health in severe opioid-dependent patients within a randomized controlled maintenance treatment trial. *Addiction*, 106, 1647–1655.

Reuter, P. (2009). The unintended consequences of drug policies. In: *A Report on Global Illicit Drugs Markets 1998–2007* (ed. P. Reuter & F. Trautmann), pp. 233–252. Brussels: European Commission.

Richardson, L., Wood, E., Montaner, J., & Kerr, T. (2012). Addiction treatment-related employment barriers: the impact of methadone maintenance. *Journal of Substance Abuse and Treatment*, 43, 276–284.

del Rio, M., Mino, A., & Perneger, T.V. (1997). Predictors of patient retention in a newly established methadone maintenance treatment programme. *Addiction*, 92, 1353–1360.

Room, R. (2011). Addiction and personal responsibility as solutions to the contradictions of neoliberal consumerism. *Critical Public Health*, 21, 141–151.

Ryan, C.F. & White, J.M. (1996). Health status at entry to methadone maintenance treatment using the SF-36 health survey questionnaire. *Addiction*, 91, 39–45.

Ryan, R.M. & Deci, E.L. (2001). On happiness and human potentials: a review of research on hedonic and eudaimonic well-being. *Annual Review of Psychology*, 52, 141–166.

Salamina, G., Diecidue, R., Vigna-Taglianti, F., et al. (the VEdeTTE Study Group) (2010). Effectiveness of therapies for heroin addiction in retaining patients in treatment: results from the VEdeTTE study. *Substance Use and Misuse*, 45, 2076–2092.

Sand, M. & Romelsjö, A. (2005). *Opiatmissbrukare Med och utan Behandling i Stockholms Län*. SoRAD Report no. 30. Stockholm: SoRAD, Stockholm University.

Sanders, J.J., Roose, R.J., Lubrano, M.C., & Lucan, S.C. (2013). Meaning and methadone: patient perceptions of methadone dose and a model to promote adherence to maintenance treatment. *Journal of Addiction Medicine*, 7, 307–313.

Schmidt, L., Makela, P., Rehm, J., & Room, R. (2010). Alcohol: equity and social determinants. In: *Equity, Social Determinants and Public Health Programmes* (ed. E. Blas & A. Kurup), pp. 11–39. Geneva: World Health Organization.

Smyth, B.P., Barry, J., Lane, A., et al. (2005). In-patient treatment of opiate dependence: medium-term follow-up outcomes. *British Journal of Psychiatry*, 187, 360–365.

Soyka, M., Träder, A., Klotsche, J., et al. (2012). Criminal behavior in opioid-dependent patients before and during maintenance therapy: 6-year follow-up of a nationally representative cohort sample. *Journal of Forensic Science*, 57, 1524–1530.

Stevenson, B. & Wolfers, J. (2008). Economic growth and subjective well-being: reassessing the Easterlin paradox. *Brookings Papers on Economic Activity, Economic Studies Program, the Brookings Institution*, 39(1), 1–102.

Stiglitz, J.E., Sen, A., & Fitoussi, J.-P. (2009). *Report by the Commission on the Measurement of Economic Performance and Social Progress.* URL: <http://www.stiglitz-sen-fitoussi.fr/en/index.htm>.

Stoll, L., Michaelson, J., & Seaford, C. (2012). *Well-being Evidence for Policy: A Review.* London: nef.

Tooze, J.A. (2001). *Statistics and the German State, 1900–1945: The Making of Modern Economic Knowledge.* Cambridge: Cambridge University Press.

Torrens, M., Castillo, C., & Pérez-Solá, V. (1996). Retention in a low-threshold methadone maintenance program. *Drug and Alcohol Dependence,* **41**, 55–59.

Torrens, M., Fonseca, F., Castillo, C., & Domingo-Salvany, A. (2013). Methadone maintenance treatment in Spain: the success of a harm reduction approach. *Bulletin of the World Health Organization,* **91**, 136–141.

Trautmann, F., Kilmer, B., & Turnbull, P. (eds.) (2013). *Further Insights into Aspects of the EU Illicit Drugs Market.* Luxembourg: Publications Office of the European Union.

Van Praag, B.M.S. & Ferrer-i-Carbonell, A. (2010). Happiness economics: a new road to measuring and comparing happiness. *Foundations and Trends in Microeconomics* **6**, 1–97.

Yang, F., Lin, P., Li, Y., et al. (2013). Predictors of retention in community-based methadone maintenance treatment program in Pearl River Delta, China. *Harm Reduction Journal,* **10**, 3.

Ysa, T., Colom, J., Albareda, A., Ramon, A., Carrión, M., & Segura, L. (2014). *Governance of Addictions: European Public Policies.* Oxford: Oxford University Press.

Zanis, D.A., Metzger, D.S., & McLellan, A.T. (1994). Factors associated with employment among methadone patients. *Journal of Substance Abuse and Treatment,* **11**, 443–447.

Chapter 5

The effects of addictive substances and addictive behaviours on physical and mental health

Kevin D. Shield and Jürgen Rehm

5.1 Overview of how addictive substances and behaviours affect physical and mental health

The use of addictive substances and engagement in addictive behaviours go back to the beginning of recorded history, are postulated to have contributed to human evolution (Hill and Newlin, 2002), and occur worldwide. Furthermore, compulsive and addictive behaviours that are characterized by an impulse, drive, or temptation to perform the behaviour are also hypothesized to be the result of evolutionary pressures (Anselme and Robinson, 2013). It is theorized that people engage in the use of addictive substances and in addictive behaviours to feel good, to feel better, to do things in better ways, out of curiosity, and 'because others are doing it' (Oetting and Beauvais, 1986). After beginning substance use or engaging in an addictive behaviour an individual's vulnerability to becoming addicted to the substance or behaviour is dependent on numerous complex and interacting genetic and environmental factors (Swadi, 1999). Furthermore, the extent of use of addictive substances varies greatly on a spectrum from just use to dependence, while engagement in addictive behaviours ranges on a scale from sporadic behaviour to a behavioural disorder (American Psychiatric Association, 2013).

The use of addictive substances and engagement in addictive behaviours result in numerous consequences for the physical and mental health of the person using the substance and/or engaging in the behaviour and for people in their immediate and extended social network. The impact, or burden, of these causally related physical and mental health consequences can be measured by examining data on mortality, potential years of life lost, years lived with disability (a measure of the duration of a disabling condition and the magnitude of the disability), and disability-adjusted life years (DALYs; a measure of overall disease burden—one DALY can be thought of as one lost year of 'healthy' life).

A clear understanding of the role and relative magnitude of the risk factors leading to diseases, conditions, and injuries and the effective and affordable interventions that can prevent them should guide the development of health policies and programmes (Babor, 2010). The magnitude of the burden of addictive substances and behaviours, especially the use of tobacco, alcohol, illicit drugs, and non-medical drug use, is large, and these represent some of the major risk factors for the global burden of disease (Murray and Lopez, 1997). This has been recognized by numerous organizations (WHO, 2008), and addressing these risk factors has been designated as a global health priority. Specifically, the World Health Organization (WHO) has designated both tobacco use and alcohol use as two of the four key modifiable risk factors that contribute to the global burden of non-communicable diseases, and has proposed actions to reduce the burdens they cause (Babor, 2010; WHO, 2011).

This chapter outlines the diseases, conditions, and injuries that are causally related to addictive substances and behaviours (namely, tobacco, alcohol, illicit drug use, non-medical drug use, and gambling disorder) and the resulting health burdens attributable to them.

5.2 Diseases, conditions, and injuries causally related to addictive substances

The relationship between the use of addictive substances and the risk of negative and positive physical and psychological conditions has long been recognized (CDC, 2010b). Although the effects of tobacco, alcohol, illicit drugs, and non-medical drug use, as well as engagement in addictive behaviours, have similar psychological effects in terms of dependence they also have very different physiological and psychological effects *other than* dependence. The diseases, conditions, and injuries that are causally related to the use of addictive substances and behaviours can be classified as: (1) those entirely attributable to addictive substances and behaviours (i.e. diseases, conditions, and injuries that would not be present if the exposure did not exist); and (2) those for which addictive substances and behaviours are a component cause (i.e. the addictive substances and behaviours are neither sufficient nor necessary for a disease, condition, or injury). In both cases exposure to addictive substances and behaviours increases the risk of the incidence of or mortality from a disease, condition, or injury (Rothman et al., 2008).

5.2.1 **Tobacco**

Tobacco smoking, including cigarettes, other forms of tobacco use, and exposure to second-hand smoke, is a worldwide global health problem. It is the third leading cause of the global burden of disease (Lim et al., 2012) and significantly increases the risk of infectious and parasitic diseases, pulmonary diseases, conditions arising during the perinatal period, malignant neoplasms, diabetes mellitus, neuropsychiatric conditions, and cardiovascular diseases. The increased risk of these diseases and conditions accumulates with use and depends on the age of the person when they started smoking, the average number of cigarettes smoked per day, the characteristics of the cigarette (such as tar and nicotine content), and smoking behaviours such as inhalation characteristics (Ezzati et al., 2004).

5.2.1.1 Infectious and parasitic diseases

The chronic inhalation of smoke alters a wide range of functions of the innate and adaptive immune system (Sopori, 2002). There are over 5300 compounds in tobacco smoke and many constituents have been shown to modulate the function of immune cells.

◆ Impact on innate immunity. The lungs are an important route of exposure to environmental pathogens and antigens. Although smoking increases the number of alveolar macrophages by several fold, changes in the activity of these cells lead to multiple health consequences. Alveolar macrophages in smokers produce higher levels of oxygen radicals and have a higher myeloperoxidase content, thereby increasing their ability to kill intracellular pathogens (Reynolds, 1987; Sopori et al., 1994). However, despite these changes the alveolar macrophages have decreased levels of inflammatory cytokines, and thus a reduced ability to phagocytise and kill bacteria (Martin and Warr, 1977; King et al., 1988). In animal models, cigarette smoke has been shown to impair the function of natural killer cells (a type of lymphoid cell that regulates tumour growth) (Ferson et al., 1979); mice show a reduced resistance to implanted tumours when exposed to cigarette smoke (Holt, 1987).

◆ Impact on adaptive immunity. Concentrations of leukocytes are increased in smokers; however, the function of these leukocytes is greatly impaired, such that when exposed to influenza, smokers have lower titrates and a decreased half-life of influenza-specific antibodies. Specifically, animal studies have shown that when exposed to antigens, increased concentrations of cigarette smoke are associated with a reduced antibody response (Holt, 1987; Sopori et al., 1994).

5.2.1.2 Pulmonary diseases

Tobacco smoking is causally related to chronic obstructive pulmonary disease, pneumoconiosis, asthma, chronic bronchitis, and emphysema, with smokers experiencing an increased risk of these diseases in a dose–response manner with the risk of emphysema plateauing at a smoking history of between fifty and a hundred pack-years (one pack-year being equivalent to smoking twenty cigarettes a day for a year) (Hogg, 2004). The risk of pulmonary disease decreases for people who stop smoking, reducing the pathogenetic processes leading to chronic obstructive pulmonary disease (Hogg, 2004). Tobacco smoke overwhelms the natural defence mechanisms that protect against inhaled agents. It increases the risk of pulmonary diseases by increasing oxidative stress (injury), leading to chronic pulmonary disease and by creating a protease–antiprotease imbalance leading to emphysema (Schulz et al., 2000).

5.2.1.3 Conditions arising during the perinatal period

Exposure of the father, mother, and developing foetus to tobacco has an impact on the risk of conditions arising during the perinatal period. Periconceptional smoking can lead to cleft lip (with or without cleft palate) (Little et al., 2004), and maternal exposure to tobacco smoke (specifically carbon monoxide) during pregnancy can lead to foetal loss, pre-term delivery, and low birth weight, and may cause neurological deficits (Longo, 1976, 1977). Maternal exposure to tobacco smoke interferes in the transformation of spiral arteries in the uterus and the formation of the placenta (Brosens et al., 1972), as well as having immunosuppressive effects in the mother and a negative impact on the maternal body's inflammatory response (van der Vaart et al., 2005), which can lead to miscarriage and pre-term delivery. Exposure to tobacco smoke can also lead to genetic polymorphisms in genes such as transforming growth factor-alpha, increasing the risk of oral clefting (van Rooij et al., 2001). Maternal exposure to tobacco smoke can cause histopathological changes in the foetus, particularly in the lung and brain, leading to impaired lung and brain functioning (Makin et al., 1991; Nelson et al., 1999). There is evidence that in men exposure to tobacco smoke can effect chromosomal changes and damage the DNA in sperm cells, affecting fertility and pregnancy viability and possibly leading to developmental conditions in offspring (Shen et al., 1997; Potts et al., 1999).

5.2.1.4 Malignant neoplasms

Since the 1950s there has been sufficient evidence to classify tobacco as a carcinogen (Doll, 1998). In 1986 the International Agency for Research on Cancer (IARC) working group determined that there was enough evidence to classify tobacco smoke as a multipotent carcinogenic mixture that can cause cancer in many different organs. In the particulate and vapour phases, tobacco smoke contains more than 5300 compounds, of which more than 70 are known carcinogens that initiate and/or promote cancer (Rodgman and Perfetti, 2009; IARC, 2012). The IARC monograph on tobacco smoking concluded that oesophageal cancer, nasopharyngeal cancer, pancreatic cancer, kidney and other urinary organ cancers, bladder cancer, stomach cancer, leukaemia, liver cancer, tracheal, bronchial, and lung cancers, cervical cancer, colon and rectal cancer, and mouth cancer are causally related to tobacco smoking. However, evidence suggests a lack of carcinogenicity for cancers of the breast and endometrium (IARC, 2004). The carcinogens in cigarette smoke act through two main pathways: (1) formation of DNA adducts (a piece of DNA covalently bonded to a carcinogen) and (2) binding to cell surface receptors. The binding of these carcinogens to cell surface receptors leads to a decrease in apoptosis but also to an increase in angiogenesis and transformation, thus promoting the proliferation of cancerous cells. In addition to directly increasing the risk of cancer, tobacco products also contain tumour promoters and co-carcinogens, which enhance carcinogenesis (Hecht, 2003).

5.2.1.5 Diabetes mellitus

A meta-analysis of the effect of tobacco use on the risk of developing non-insulin-dependent diabetes mellitus has shown that smoking increases the risk of diabetes mellitus in a dose–response manner (Willi et al., 2007). Exposure to tobacco is hypothesized to act through the effects of nicotine or other components of cigarette smoke on beta cells of the pancreas, causing a decrease in insulin secretion by acting on nicotinic acetylcholine receptors on beta cells and increasing the apoptosis of beta cells (Talamini et al., 1999; Xie et al., 2009).

5.2.1.6 Neuropsychiatric conditions

Prolonged tobacco use can lead to tobacco dependence, caused and sustained by nicotine. The main negative effects of tobacco dependence are due to the health effects of tobacco smoking, because the long-term use of nicotine medications does not appear to cause harm (American Psychiatric Association, 2013). However, nicotine withdrawal symptoms include affective disturbance (including irritability and anger), anxiety, a depressed mood, restlessness, sleep disturbance, and an increased appetite (Hasin et al., 2000; American Psychiatric Association, 2013).

5.2.1.7 Cardiovascular diseases

Tobacco use is major a cause of ischaemic heart disease, cerebrovascular disease, atrial fibrillation and flutter, aortic aneurysm, and peripheral vascular disease (CDC, 2010b). The risk relationship between cardiovascular diseases and tobacco smoke is generally non-linear, with the dose–response relationship between tobacco smoke and cardiovascular diseases having a sharp increase at low levels of exposure (including to second-hand smoke), the rate of this increase in risk diminishing as the average number of cigarettes smoked per day increases (Law and Wald, 2003). Smokers who stop smoking and do not have ischaemic heart disease experience a reduction in their risk of cardiovascular disease; however, there currently is no evidence that among smokers a reduction in the number of cigarettes smoked per day or stopping smoking using a nicotine alternative reduces the risk of cardiovascular disease (Murray et al., 1996).

Tobacco use increases the risk of cardiovascular diseases through multiple biological pathways. Specifically, tobacco exposure causes acute myocardial ischaemia (Benowitz and Gourlay, 1997) leading to injury and dysfunction of endothelial cells in both the coronary and peripheral arteries (Celermajer et al., 1996; Campisi et al., 1998), increases the risk of thrombosis (Dullaart et al., 1994), and changes the atherogenic lipid profile (increasing triglycerides and decreasing high-density lipoprotein cholesterol) (Eliasson et al., 1994). Exposure to tobacco smoke also produces a chronic inflammatory state of the cardiovascular system, thereby contributing to the atherogenic disease processes, and produces insulin resistance and chronic inflammation, leading to the acceleration of macrovascular and microvascular complications (Burke and FitzGerald, 2003).

5.2.2 **Alcohol**

Alcohol has been part of human culture for all of recorded history, and almost all societies where alcohol is consumed have experienced a net detrimental effect on health as a result (McGovern, 2009). Alcohol's relationship to health has been recognized for many centuries, both as a risk factor and as a remedy (Cochrane et al., 2003). The industrialization of production and the globalization of marketing and promotion of alcohol have led to a global increase in alcohol consumption and in its related health harms.

The relationship between alcohol consumption and the resulting physical and mental health conditions is complex because alcohol has a beneficial effect on some diseases and a negative effect on others; however, at the population level, alcohol consumption has always been observed to have an overall negative impact on health. Alcohol consumption is causally linked to over 200 three-digit disease codes in the tenth revision of the ICD (see Rehm et al. (2010) for a complete list of diseases, conditions, and injuries). These conditions include: infectious and parasitic diseases; respiratory infections; conditions arising during the perinatal period; malignant neoplasms; diabetes mellitus; neuropsychiatric conditions; cardiovascular diseases; digestive diseases; unintentional injuries; and intentional injuries.

The three main characteristics of drinking that impact on alcohol-attributable mortality and morbidity are: (1) the overall volume of alcohol consumed; (2) consumption patterns; and (3) the quality of the alcoholic beverage. These factors impact health primarily by: (1) toxic and beneficial biochemical effects; (2) intoxication; and (3) dependence. For an overview of these intermediate mechanisms see Rehm et al. (2003).

5.2.2.1 Overall mortality

Alcohol consumption is hypothesized to have a J-shaped dose–response relationship with all-cause mortality; the hypothesized protective effect stems from a decrease in the risk of ischaemic heart disease, stroke, and diabetes—in each case for non-binge-drinkers who consume relatively little alcohol (Skog, 1996). However, the existence of this J-shaped curve is controversial due to multiple measurement errors, including the suitability and measurement of the reference lifetime abstainers and the heterogeneity of binge-drinking for people with approximately the same average daily alcohol consumption (Skog, 1996).

5.2.2.2 Infectious and parasitic diseases

Alcohol consumption causally impacts the risk of contracting tuberculosis (TB), pneumonia, and HIV/AIDS, as well as the risk of mortality from these infectious diseases, through multiple pathways.

The dose-dependent association between the consumption of alcohol and the risk of TB has long been acknowledged (Lönnroth et al., 2009; Rehm et al., 2009). Recent estimates of this association indicate a strong and consistent association, with an approximately three-fold increased risk of TB for heavy drinkers compared with the general population (Lönnroth et al., 2009). There are two possible biological pathways for how alcohol consumption increases the risk of TB. First, alcohol-related immunosuppression increases susceptibility to infection as well as conversion to active TB (Szabo and Mandrekar, 2009). Secondly, drinkers tend to consume alcohol in social environments that facilitate the spread of TB infection (Rehm et al., 2009). Alcohol consumption also affects the course of disease for individuals with TB by lowering adherence to medication treatment regimens and decreasing the likelihood of seeking medical assistance (Hendershot et al., 2009; Parry et al., 2009).

The consumption of alcohol is considered to be a major contributor to the risk of developing pneumonia, by inhibiting the immune system (Szabo et al., 1995; Heermans, 1998; Neuman, 2003; Gamble et al., 2006; Zhang et al., 2008; Szabo and Mandrekar, 2009). A meta-analysis observed a dose–response effect of alcohol on the risk of community-acquired pneumonia, and found that people with alcohol use disorders had eight times the risk of contracting community-acquired pneumonia compared with people who abstained from alcohol (Samokhvalov et al., 2010b). As with TB, in addition to weakening the immune system there is evidence that alcohol consumption lowers adherence to medication treatment regimens and decreases the likelihood of seeking medical assistance (Hendershot et al., 2009; Parry et al., 2009).

Alcohol consumption is causally related to the risk of acquiring HIV/AIDS as well as the disease course and mortality caused by HIV/AIDS. One reason for this is because alcohol consumption has a causal relationship to an increased chance of engaging in unprotected sexual intercourse. The role of alcohol consumption in increasing the risk of acquiring HIV from the use of injected drugs is less clear because alcohol affects executive function; however, the role of alcohol in the sharing of injection equipment has not been determined (Stall and Leigh, 1994; Dingle and Oei, 1997; Fisher et al., 2007; Baliunas et al., 2010; Shuper et al., 2010; Rehm et al., 2012). Alcohol consumption has also been shown to affect susceptibility to HIV infection by weakening the immune system (Braithwaite et al., 2005; Neuman et al., 2006; Shuper et al., 2009; Baliunas et al., 2010; Hahn and Samet, 2010; Shuper et al., 2010), and there is sufficient evidence that alcohol worsens the disease course of HIV/AIDS and can subsequently increase the likelihood of death by affecting adherence to antiretroviral treatment (Braithwaite et al., 2005, 2007; Hendershot et al., 2009; Azar et al., 2010; Gmel et al., 2011).

5.2.2.3 Conditions arising during the perinatal period

Alcohol affects the foetus by increasing prostaglandin levels, inhibiting progesterone synthesis (a regulator of prostaglandin), decreasing blood levels of progesterone (Ahluwalia et al., 1992; Wimalasena, 1994), and increasing the risk of premature birth (Challis and Olson, 1988; Cook and Randal, 1998). Additionally, exposure of the foetus to the alcohol metabolite acetaldehyde affects the placenta, causing foetal hypoxia, impaired cell proliferation, and delayed foetal development (Abel, 1982). Thus, heavy episodic and heavy (in volume) consumption of alcohol by a woman during pregnancy is causally related to low birth weight, preterm birth, and to the foetus being small for its gestational age (Patra et al., 2011). However, the impact of the pattern of alcohol consumption during different phases of pregnancy is not clear—studies have found conflicting results on the effects of moderate alcohol consumption during early pregnancy (Little et al., 2008).

5.2.2.4 Malignant neoplasms

The action of ethanol (the most active and abundant carcinogen in alcoholic beverages) as a carcinogen is not fully understood for all cancers, because the biological pathway by which alcohol affects the risk of developing cancer depends on the target organ. Additional factors that determine and/or mediate the relationship between consumption of ethanol and the risk of developing cancer include variants of alcohol dehydrogenase, aldehyde dehydrogenase, cytochrome P450 2E1, concentrations of oestrogen, and changes in foliate metabolism and DNA repair (Boffetta and Hashibe, 2006). For example, the risk of developing oesophageal cancer and other gastrointestinal cancers with alcohol consumption is greater for individuals who have at least one *alcohol dehydrogenase 2 (ALDH2)* Lys487 allele (this allele is more prevalent in Asian populations) (Eng et al., 2007; Brooks et al., 2009).

A relationship between the consumption of ethanol and the incidence of cancer was first suggested in 1910, when it was observed that patients with cancer of the oesophagus or the gastric cardia were more likely to be alcoholics (Lamy, 1910). The accumulation of evidence for a relationship between ethanol consumption and the incidence and disease course of cancer, and for a causal relationship between ethanol as a carcinogen—specifically for the development of cancers of the oral cavity, pharynx, larynx, oesophagus, liver, colorectal, and female breast—led the IARC to recognize ethanol as a carcinogen (IARC, 2008).

Alcohol may also play a role in the development of prostate cancer, with a meta-analysis observing that ingestion of ethanol increases the risk of prostate cancer (Dennis, 2000; Middleton et al., 2009; Rota et al., 2012). However, further research is required to determine the exact biological pathway(s) via which ethanol contributes to the development of prostate cancer.

Observational evidence has also suggested that ethanol may be a carcinogen for the development of stomach cancer (Bagnardi et al., 2001; Tramacere et al., 2012a): two meta-analyses have found that ethanol is not related to an increased risk of developing gastric cardia adenocarcinoma (Tramacere et al., 2012a,d) but one found that ethanol was related to gastric non-cardia adenocarcinoma (Tramacere et al., 2012a). The protective mucosal lining of the stomach may prevent the metabolism of ethanol and thus protect against the carcinogenic effects of ethanol.

Furthermore, observational studies have found a non-significant positive association between ethanol consumption and endometrial (Bagnardi et al., 2001; Rota et al., 2012), ovarian (Bagnardi et al., 2001), and pancreatic cancers (Bagnardi et al., 2001); however, with the exception of ovarian cancer, the risk relationship between ethanol consumption and the risk for developing these cancers is modest at most. Thus, since previous studies examining the relationship between ethanol consumption and these cancers were underpowered, additional studies with large numbers of participants are needed to accurately assess the relationship (Bagnardi et al., 2001).

The relationship between ethanol consumption and bladder and lung cancers is the least clear, with a meta-analysis finding that ethanol is involved in the development of bladder and lung cancers (Bagnardi et al., 2001). However, a recent meta-analysis of studies which included people who had never smoked found no association between ethanol consumption and the risk of either bladder cancer (Pelucchi et al., 2012) or lung cancer (Bagnardi et al., 2001). Thus, the finding of a positive relationship between ethanol consumption and these cancers may be due, in part, to the exposure of study participants to tobacco smoke (Bagnardi et al., 2001; Pelucchi et al., 2012).

As insulin resistance may play a key role in the development of renal cancer (because an increased risk of renal cancer has been observed in individuals with diabetes) (Lindblad et al., 1999; Joh et al., 2011), light to moderate consumption of alcohol is thought to exert a protective effect for renal cancer by increasing insulin sensitivity (Facchini et al., 1994; Davies et al., 2002; Joosten et al., 2008). Furthermore, results from observational studies also suggest that alcohol may be a protective factor against the development of renal cell carcinoma (Bellocco et al., 2012; Song et al., 2012), Hodgkin's lymphoma (Tramacere et al., 2012c), and non-Hodgkin's lymphoma (Tramacere et al., 2012b). However, the biological mechanisms by which alcohol consumption exerts a protective effect against the risk of developing Hodgkin's and non-Hodgkin's lymphoma are currently unknown (Tramacere et al., 2012b,c). These previously observed protective effects of alcohol against the risk of developing cancer should be interpreted with caution—they are not considered causal since the biological mechanisms are not fully understood and confounding and/or misclassification of abstainers within observational studies may partly explain the observed protective effects.

5.2.2.5 Diabetes mellitus

Moderate alcohol consumption decreases the risk of type II diabetes (Baliunas et al., 2009), because alcohol consumption increases insulin sensitivity and counteracts the development of insulin resistance (a key part in the pathogenesis of type II diabetes) (Mayer et al., 1993; Kiechl et al., 1996; Lazarus et al., 1997; Davies et al., 2002; Wannamethee and Shaper, 2003; Sierksma et al., 2004; Wannamethee et al., 2004; Hendriks, 2007). Moderate alcohol consumption also increases metabolites such as acetaldehyde and acetate (Sarkola et al., 2002), increases high-density lipoprotein (Rimm et al., 1999), and exerts an anti-inflammatory effect (Imhof et al., 2001). These observations should be interpreted with caution, as the protective effect of moderate alcohol consumption on the development of diabetes may be due, in part, to moderate alcohol consumption being a marker for healthy lifestyle choices.

5.2.2.6 Neuropsychiatric conditions

Alcohol consumption is causally related to epilepsy and unipolar depressive disorders, and is hypothesized to be related to Alzheimer's disease and vascular dementia. Heavy consumers of alcohol have an increased risk of cerebral atrophy (Dam et al., 1985), cerebrovascular infarctions, lesions, head traumas, and changes in neurotransmitter systems and ionic balance (Dam et al., 1985; Freedland and McMicken, 1993; Rathlev et al., 2006; Barclay et al., 2008; Samokhvalov et al., 2010a), and repeated withdrawals from alcohol consumption lead to a lowering of the epileptogenic threshold (Ballenger and Post, 1978). Alcohol consumption is also causally linked to unipolar depressive disorders (Rehm et al., 2003); however, alcohol-attributable morbidity and mortality from unipolar depressive disorders cannot be calculated as they may be confounded by genetic predispositions and environmental factors or the use of alcohol for self-medication purposes (Grant and Pickering, 1997; Rehm et al., 2004).

People who consume low to moderate amounts of alcohol are hypothesized to have a lower risk of Alzheimer's disease and vascular dementia because they have a lower risk of ischaemic circulatory events (Tyas, 2001; Peters et al., 2008). However, the design, statistical analyses, and results of studies investigating the association between alcohol consumption and Alzheimer's disease and vascular dementia make it unclear if this relationship is causal (Panza et al., 2008; Peters et al., 2008).

5.2.2.7 Cardiovascular diseases

Alcohol consumption affects the cardiovascular system by means of multiple pathways. It has been observed to lead to the development of hypertension (except for women at lower levels of consumption), conduction disorders and other dysrhythmias, and cardiovascular disease (ischaemic stroke, at a higher volume of consumption, and haemorrhagic stroke). Alcohol consumption has a protective effect at lower volumes of consumption in the development of hypertension in women and for ischaemic heart disease and ischaemic stroke in both men and women. Differences in drinking patterns between men and women may explain these differences in the observed role of alcohol in the development of hypertension (Rehm et al., 2003). The biological pathways by which alcohol exerts its effects on the cardiovascular system are not always clear. Alcohol is known to act upon the cardiovascular system in four main ways: by increasing cellular signalling, blood concentrations of high-density lipoproteins, and dissolution of blood clots through enzyme action, and by decreasing the formation of blood clots by platelets (Zakhari, 1997).

Alcohol is involved in the development of hypertension by increasing the activity of the sympathetic nervous system, the constriction of blood vessels, and the contractile force of the heart (Zakhari, 1997). Another possible pathway for the effect of alcohol on hypertension is that alcohol decreases the sensitivity of baroreceptors, diminishing the ability of the body to regulate blood pressure (Zakhari, 1997). Because alcohol leads to the development of hypertension, a risk factor for haemorrhagic stroke, alcohol therefore also has a role in the risk of haemorrhagic stroke (Taylor et al., 2009). There are also differences in the alcohol-related risk of mortality and morbidity from hypertension and haemorrhagic stroke that may stem from a number of factors: (1) heavy drinkers tend to have other co-morbidities that increase the probability of a fatal event; (2) alcohol consumption may worsen the disease course by decreasing compliance with medication regimens; (3) the effects of alcohol on morbidity may be underestimated due to stigmatization of heavy alcohol consumption, which may decrease the probability that heavy drinkers will be treated for stroke; and (4) there may be a younger age at the time of stroke in morbidity studies.

Alcohol consumption has been found to play a role in the development of conduction disorders and dysrhythmias (Samokhvalov et al., 2010c) by causing a change in the electrical activity of the heart and by direct cardiotoxicity of alcohol, hyperadrenergic activity during drinking and withdrawal, impairment of vagal tone, and increasing in the intra-atrial conduction time (Balbão et al., 2009).

Alcohol plays a protective role in the development of ischaemic diseases and conditions at low levels of consumption, but is hypothesized to play a detrimental role in the development of ischaemic conditions at higher levels of consumption and for people who engage in binge-drinking. As previously mentioned, alcohol interacts with the ischaemic system by increasing levels of high-density lipoprotein, preventing blood clots, and increasing the rate at which blood clots are broken down. However, binge-drinking, even by people who normally consume low to moderate amounts of alcohol, increases the probability of clotting and ventricular fibrillation, leading to an increased risk of an ischaemic event. As with haemorrhagic stroke, meta-analyses have found that the effects of alcohol on ischaemic events differ for mortality and morbidity; alcohol has a larger protective effect for morbidity than for mortality (Roerecke and Rehm, 2012; Taylor et al., 2009). Despite the increased risk for ischaemic heart disease at higher levels of alcohol consumption that is seen in observational studies (Roerecke and Rehm, 2012), there is insufficient evidence of a detrimental effect of alcohol consumption on ischaemic heart disease for this effect to be considered causal.

5.2.2.8 Digestive diseases

Alcohol consumption is involved in the development of digestive diseases; in particular, alcohol consumption leads to liver diseases such as fatty liver, alcoholic hepatitis, and cirrhosis. Specifically, the breakdown of ethanol by means of oxidative and non-oxidative metabolic pathways in the liver produces free radicals, acetaldehyde, and fatty acid ethyl esters that negatively affect liver cells (Tuma and Casey, 2003). Alcohol consumption carries a higher risk of mortality than morbidity for cirrhosis of the liver as it is linked with worsening of the course of liver disease and a detrimental effect on the immune system (Rehm et al., 2010b).

Alcohol consumption can also lead to acute and chronic pancreatitis by acting via the same pathways that cause liver damage, namely the formation of free radicals, acetaldehyde, and fatty acid ethyl esters which damage pancreatic acinar cells (Vonlaufen et al., 2007). Heavy drinkers (more than, on average, four internationally standardized drinks per day, or 48 g of pure alcohol) have an elevated risk of pancreatitis, while people who consume low to moderate amounts of alcohol have a smaller elevated risk.

5.2.2.9 Unintentional injuries

The psychological effects of alcohol consumption play a causal role in both unintentional and intentional injuries.

The consumption of alcohol increases the risk of unintentional injuries due to its effect on cognitive and psychomotor processes, such as reaction time, impaired cognitive processing, and reduced coordination and vigilance (Moskowitz and Robinson, 1988; Krüger, 1993; Eckardt et al., 1998; USDHHS, 2000). In controlled experimental studies, the blood alcohol content (BAC) at which these symptoms appear has been shown to be between 0.04 and 0.05%, with this minimum being dependent on tolerance (Eckardt et al., 1998).

Acute consumption of alcohol is related to the risk of unintentional injuries, with an increased risk of injury due to alcohol starting at relatively low volumes of intake (i.e. below the maximum legal BAC limits for driving) (Taylor et al., 2010). The risks due to alcohol consumption are dependent on a person's tolerance to alcohol: people who have the highest risk of unintentional injuries are those who consume relatively large amounts on few binge-drinking occasions, and when the binge consumption amounts are markedly greater than the amounts of alcohol consumed on average occasions (Gruenewald and Nephew, 1994; Gruenewald et al., 1996; Treno et al., 1997; Treno and Holder, 1997).

5.2.2.10 Intentional injuries

The consumption of alcohol alters receptors in the brain and thus neurotransmission, affecting neurological pathways that increase the likelihood of aggressive behaviour and self-inflicted injuries. Alcohol affects serotonin and gamma-aminobutyric acid receptors in the brain (see Pihl et al., 1993) leading to a reduction in fear and anxiety responses to the social, physical, or legal consequences of one's actions (Pihl and Hoaken, 2001). This reduction in fear and anxiety responses results in increased risk-taking, as observed through animal research (Miczek et al., 1993) and experimental and observational research (Pihl et al., 1993; Graham et al., 2000). Second, alcohol also affects cognitive functions (Peterson et al., 1990), leading to impaired problem-solving capabilities and increased conflict situations (Sayette et al., 1993), and resulting in overly emotional responses or emotional instability (Pliner and Cappell, 1974). Other biological mechanisms by which alcohol consumption increases the risk of intentional injury include the drinker developing a narrow and tenacious focus on the present (Washburne, 1956; Graham et al., 2000) and an increasing concern with demonstrating personal power (especially in men) (McClelland et al., 1972; Tomsen, 1997; Graham et al., 2000).

Observational studies have found that the consumption of alcohol is consistently associated with an increase in violence (Graham and West, 2001) and self-inflicted harm (Taylor et al., 2010). Experimental research shows that alcohol consumption increases aggression (Bushman, 1997), with drinking to intoxication or drinking five or more drinks per occasion being the best predictor of getting into a fight (Room et al., 1995; Rossow, 1996; Dawson, 1997; Wells et al., 2000; Wells and Graham, 2003). Additionally, there is an association between drinking and being the victim of aggression, as intoxication may make the drinker an easy target for predators (Leppa, 1974; Marek et al., 1974; Miczek and Barry, 1977; Wells and Graham, 1999).

5.2.3 **Illicit and non-medical drug use**

Forms of use of illicit drugs and the non-medical use of drugs can be broadly categorized as use of opioids, cocaine, hallucinogen, inhalants, other stimulant, sedative, hypnotic, or anxiolytic drugs, and other psychoactive substances (see Table 5.1). As this category of drug use encompasses numerous psychoactive substances, it is related to numerous conditions depending on the drug category and substance. Additionally the effects of illicit and non-medical drug use can be due to the toxic effects of the substance or the intoxicating effects of the substance and either direct (due to acute and chronic use) or indirect.

The main direct effects of *acute* illicit and non-medical drug use include accidental injury, motor vehicle accidents, drug-induced psychotic symptoms and myocardial infarction. The main effects of *chronic* illicit and non-medical drug use are cardiovascular diseases, liver disease, pulmonary diseases, cancers, neurotoxic effects, psychotic disorders, common mental disorders, and suicide (see Table 5.2) (Degenhardt and Hall, 2012).

Table 5.1 Substance-related and addictive disorders.

Condition category	ICD 10 code	Condition
Substance-related disorders	F10	Alcohol-related disorders
	F11	Opioid-related disorders
	F12	Cannabis-related disorders
	F13	Sedative-, hypnotic-, or anxiolytic-related disorders
	F14	Cocaine-related disorders
	F15	Other stimulant-related disorders
	F15.929, F15.93	Caffeine-related disorders
	F16	Hallucinogen-related disorders
	F17	Nicotine dependence
	F18	Inhalant-related disorders
	F19	Other psychoactive substance-related disorder
Non-substance-related disorders	F63.0	Gambling disorder

Source: data from ICD-10 Version 2010, World Health Organization, Geneva, Switzerland, Copyright © 2014, available from http://apps.who.int/classifications/icd10/browse/2010/en

Government policies on use of illicit and non-medical drugs can also create harm for drug users, people within the social network of the drug user, and people who live in the environments where drugs are sold and used. Prohibitionist policies create social environments of risk that stigmatize drug users, decrease the effectiveness of harm reduction strategies, and increase health harms (Sellman, 2010; Stanbrook, 2012). Stigma and law enforcement efforts create social networks of drug users that have both beneficial and detrimental effects (Rhodes et al., 2005; Kirst, 2009). However, prohibitionist policies also deter people from seeking help for cannabis use; for example, in Portugal the percentage of people seeking help from social workers, lawyers, and medical professionals increased after decriminalization (Tavares et al., 2005) while the lifetime prevalence of cannabis use among students increased after decriminalization from 9.4% in 1999 to 15.1% in 2003 (Tavares et al., 2005). Prohibitionist policies also encourage marketers to sell and users to use more potent forms of illicit drugs that are either incorrectly advertised in terms what they are or are laced with harmful substances (Shesser et al., 1991). Prohibitionist policies that criminalize the possession of equipment used to take drugs, such as crack pipes and hypodermic needles, lead to harms by increasing the risk of infectious diseases such as HIV

Table 5.2 Major potential acute and chronic consequences of illicit drug use.

	Cannabis				Opioids				Amphetamines				Cocaine			
	Effect	Level of evidence	Size of effect	Reference	Effect	Level of evidence	Size of effect	Reference	Effect	Level of evidence	Size of effect	Reference	Effect	Level of evidence	Size of effect	Reference
Acute toxic effects (fatal overdose)	×	–	0	19,38	√	C	CMR 0.7	11	√	C	?	13, 39, 109	√	C	?	12, 39
Acute intoxication effects																
Accidental injury	?	–	–	19, 38	√	C	CMR 0.16	11	?	–	–	13, 39	?	–	–	12, 39
Motor vehicle accidents	√	D	?	19, 38, 41	?	–	–	41	?	–	–	13, 41	?	–	–	12, 41
Drug-induced psychotic symptoms	√	A	OR 2–3	19, 38, 21	×	–	0	39	√	A	?	37, 39	√	E	?	39, 84
Myocardial infarction	?	E	–	19, 38	×	–	0	39	√	E	?	37, 39	√	E	?	39
Dependence (lifetime risk %)	√	A	9%	61	√	A	23%	101	√	A	11%	101	√	A	16%	101
Adverse health effects of chronic use																
Cardiovascular pathology	?	–	–	19, 38	√	E	?	39	√	C	?	39	√	E	?	39
Liver disease	×	–	0	19,38	√	C	?	39	?	C	?	37, 39	?	–	–	39
Pulmonary disease	?	–	–	19, 38	√	E	?	39	?	C	?	39	?	–	–	39
Cancers	?	–	–	10, 19, 38	?	C	?	11,85	?	–	–	39	?	–	–	39

Table 5.2 (continued) Major potential acute and chronic consequences of illicit drug use.

	Cannabis				Opioids				Amphetamines				Cocaine			
Neurotoxic effects	?	C	–	19, 38	×	–	–	39	√	–	?	37	√	–	?	39
Psychotic disorders	√	B	OR 2–3	19, 20,23	×	–	0	39	√	D	?	86	√	D	?	84
Common mental disorders	?	B	–	19, 23	√	D	?	87	√	D	?	86	√	D	?	87
Suicide	×	B	0	10	√	C	CMR 0.12	11	?	–	?	37, 86, 87	–	–	?	37
Increased mortality (standardised mortality ratios)	×	B	1	10	√	C	14·7 (95% CI 12·8–16·5)*	11	√	C	6.2†	13	√	C	4.7–7.6‡	12

Levels of evidence: A, experimental or controlled evidence supports this finding; B, findings across cohorts, representative population-based; C, findings across cohorts of drug users; D, findings across cross-sectional studies, representative population-based, or case–control studies; E, cross-sectional associations in non-representative samples of drug users, case series suggesting outcome.

Abbreviations and symbols: CMR, crude mortality rate per 100 person-years; n/a, not applicable; OR, odds ratio; SMR, standardized mortality ratio; ×, this drug does not seem to have an effect on the outcome; √, the outcome might be increased by the use of this drug; ?, insufficient data exist for this drug and this outcome to allow conclusions about the association between the two.

*Pooled SMR estimated from random effects meta-analysis (very high heterogeneity existed across studies; stratifi ed analyses investigated this heterogeneity in further analyses and demographic and regional diff erences were clearly evident).

†Only one study from the Czech Republic reported SMRs (this should be interpreted with caution).

‡Range from several studies only—interpret with caution.

The references cited in the table are as follows:

10. Calabria, B., Degenhardt, L., Hall, W., & Lynskey, M. (2010). Does cannabis use increase the risk of death? Systematic review of epidemiological evidence on adverse effects of cannabis use. *Drug and Alcohol Review*, 29, 318–330.

11. Degenhardt, L., Bucello, C., Mathers, B., Ali, H., Hickman, M., & McLaren, J. (2011). Mortality among dependent users of heroin and other opioids: a systematic review and meta-analysis of cohort studies. *Addiction*, 106, 32–51.

12. Degenhardt, L., Singleton, J., Calabria, B., et al. (2011). Mortality among cocaine users: a systematic review of cohort studies. *Drug and Alcohol Dependence*, 113, 88–95.

13. Singleton, J., Degenhardt, L., Hall, W., & Zabransky, T. (2009). Mortality among people who use amphetamines: a systematic review of cohort studies. Drug and Alcohol Dependence, 105, 1–8.

Table 5.2 (continued) Major potential acute and chronic consequences of illicit drug use.

19. Hall, W. & Degenhardt, L. (2009). The adverse health and psychological effects of non-medical cannabis use. *Lancet*, 374, 1383–1391.

20. Arseneault, L., Cannon, M., Witton, J., & Murray, RM. (2004). Causal association between cannabis and psychosis: examination of the evidence. *British Journal of Psychiatry*, 184, 110–117.

21. Degenhardt, L., Hall, W.D., Lynskey, M., et al. (2009). Should we make burden of disease estimates for cannabis use as a risk factor for psychosis? *PLoS Medicine*, 6, e1000133.

23. Moore, T.H., Zammit, S., Lingford-Hughes, A., et al. (2007). Cannabis use and risk of psychotic or affective mental health outcomes: a systematic review. *Lancet*, 370, 319–328.

37. Darke, S., Kaye, S., McKetin, R., & Duflou, J. (2008). Major physical and psychological harms of methamphetamine use. *Drug and Alcohol Review*, 27, 253–262.

38. Hall, W., Degenhardt, L., & Lynskey, M. (2001). *The Health and Psychological Consequences of Cannabis Use*. Canberra: Australian Publishing Service.

39. Karch, S.B. (2002). *Karch's Pathology of Drug Abuse*, 3rd edn. Boca Raton, FL: CRC Press.

41. Kelly, E., Darke, S., & Ross, J. (2004). A review of drug use and driving: epidemiology, impairment, risk factors and risk perceptions. *Drug and Alcohol Review*, 23, 319–344.

61. Kandel, D., Yamaguchi, K., & Klein, L. (2006). Testing the gateway hypothesis. *Addiction*, 101, 470–472.

84. Satel, S., Southwick, S., & Gawin, F. (1991). Clinical features of cocaine-induced paranoia. *American Journal of Psychiatry*, 148: 495–498.

85. Randall, D., Degenhardt, L., Vajdic, C.M., et al. (2011). Increasing cancer mortality among opioid dependent persons in Australia—a new public health challenge for a disadvantaged population. *Australia and New Zealand Journal of Public Health*, 35, 220–225.

86. Marshall, B.D.L. & Werb, D. (2010). Health outcomes associated with methamphetamine use among young people: a systematic review. *Addiction*, 105, 991–1002.

87. Hall, W., Degenhardt, L., & Teesson, M. (2009). Understanding comorbidity between substance use, anxiety and affective disorders: broadening the research base. *Addictive Behaviors*, 34, 526–530.

101. Anthony, J.C., Warner, L., & Kessler, R. (1994). Comparative epidemiology of dependence on tobacco, alcohol, controlled substances, and inhalants: basic findings from the national co-morbidity survey. *Experimental and Clinical Psychopharmacology*, 2, 244–268.

109. Rossow, I. & Lauritzen, G. (1999). Balancing on the edge of death: suicide attempts and life-threatening overdoses among drug addicts. *Addiction*, 94, 209–219.

from the sharing of equipment (De et al., 2007). Prohibitionist policies also create black markets for illicit drugs. These markets are associated with criminal organizations that create public health problems for the communities in which they operate (Wilkins and Casswell, 2002; Asmussen, 2008; Room et al., 2010).

Conviction of illicit drug users creates social and public health harms, as people with criminal records are stigmatized (Schnittker and John, 2007) and find it difficult to enter legitimate labour markets (Bourgois, 2003). Imprisonment also has a negative impact on people within the social network of the prisoner, especially children (Gabel and Johnston, 1995). The proportion of arrests for cannabis possession and subsequent sentences differ according to race (Ramchand et al., 2006). Therefore the policy environment in which drugs are used can also lead to an increased amount of harm for the drug user, people within the drug user's social network, and people in the environment where drugs are being purchased or used.

5.2.4 Addictive behaviours

5.2.4.1 Gambling disorder

The fifth edition of the *Diagnostic and Statistical Manual of Mental Disorders* (DSM-5) lists gambling disorder as the only behavioural disorder for which there is evidence of it being an addictive behaviour. Repetitive engagement in gambling interferes with a person's functioning in other domains. In this respect, the harms from gambling resemble the harms from substance use disorders.

Gambling disorder is associated with poor physical and mental health, and people with gambling disorder utilize medical services at high rates (Erickson et al., 2005; Petry and Weinstock, 2007). Specific functional consequences of gambling disorder arise mainly from the person's involvement with gambling, which may lead to them jeopardizing or losing important relationships with family members or friends. Such problems result from someone lying repeatedly to cover the severity of their gambling problems or from requesting money to gamble or to pay off gambling debts. The employment or educational activities of the person with a gambling disorder also may be negatively affected, with gambling disorder resulting in absenteeism and poor work or school performance.

Gambling disorder is also associated with numerous co-morbidities, including substance use disorders, depressive disorders, anxiety disorders, and personality disorders, even after controlling for substance use disorders and tobacco use disorders (Shaffer and Korn 2002; Petry et al., 2005). The relationships between gambling disorders and psychological co-morbidities are complex, with some co-morbidities preceding a gambling use disorder and/or the gambling use disorder preceding some of these co-morbidities (especially anxiety disorders and substance use disorders) (Shaffer and Korn, 2002).

5.2.4.2 Other potentially addictive behaviours

Behaviours where there is not enough evidence to definitively classify them as addictive are listed under Section III of DSM-5. These conditions include: attenuated psychosis syndrome; depressive episodes with short-duration hypomania; persistent complex bereavement disorder; caffeine use disorder; Internet gaming disorder; neurobehavioural disorder associated with pre-natal alcohol exposure; suicidal behaviour disorder; and non-suicidal self-injury (American Psychiatric Association, 2013). Although research on these conditions is insufficient to deem them as addictive behavioural disorders, they can result in impairment or distress (American Psychiatric Association, 2013).

5.3 The health burden of addictive substances

The global burden of disease due to addictive substances is large and varies across time and geographical region, with tobacco causing the largest burden, alcohol the second largest, and illicit and non-medical drug use the third. Table 5.3 outlines the global burden of disease attributable to tobacco, alcohol, and drug use in 2010. From 1990 to 2010 the leading risk factors that have contributed to the global burden of disease as a whole have shifted from those mainly causing communicable diseases in children to those mainly causing non-communicable diseases in adults (World Health Organization, 2011); for example, cancer incidence is expected to increase by 57% between 2012 and 2032 (Stewart and Wild 2014). Furthermore this shift from infectious diseases to non-communicable diseases is expected to continue as low- and middle-income countries develop. As the use of addictive substances is more associated with non-communicable diseases than infectious diseases, the implementation of policies that decrease tobacco and alcohol exposure is a global health priority (World Health Organization, 2011). However, the burden of disease attributable to addictive factors is also dependent on exposure to particular addictive substances. Shifts in the burden of diseases caused by tobacco, alcohol, and drugs are attributable to a large shift in the prevalence of tobacco, alcohol, and drug use, the associated patterns of use, and the underlying causes of death and disability that are causally related to tobacco, alcohol and drug use.

5.3.1 Burden of tobacco use

In 2010 tobacco use was the third leading risk factor for health loss and mortality, responsible for the loss of 157 million DALYs and 6.3 million deaths. Of this burden 137 million DALYs were lost as a result of first-hand tobacco use, with

Table 5.3 Deaths and DALYs attributable to addictive substances in 2010

Cause	Deaths per 100,000 people			DALYs per 100,000 people		
	Total	Women	Men	Total	Women	Men
(1) Tobacco						
Total (all causes)	95.9	48.8	151.2	2,385.2	1,194.8	3,682.5
HIV/AIDS and tuberculosis	0.9	0.2	1.6	31.5	5.0	58.5
Diarrhoea, lower respiratory infections, meningitis, and other common infectious diseases	1.7	1.6	1.9	150.1	138.4	161.1
Neoplasms	22.5	9.9	37.4	486.5	207.2	794.8
Cardiovascular and circulatory diseases	51.0	25.2	80.8	1,177.9	520.4	1,888.5
Chronic respiratory diseases	18.5	11.8	26.8	486.7	317.5	676.8
Diabetes, urogenital, blood, and endocrine diseases	1.4	0.2	2.7	52.6	6.4	102.8
(2) Alcohol						
Total (all causes)	41.1	24.8	57.6	1,444.0	653.1	2,234.2
HIV/AIDS and tuberculosis	2.0	0.7	3.4	79.8	29.2	131.5
Diarrhoea, lower respiratory infections, meningitis, and other common infectious diseases	2.0	1.4	2.7	42.1	28.1	57.4
Neoplasms	5.1	2.6	8.0	132.0	66.3	201.9
Cardiovascular and circulatory diseases	12.7	13.3	11.4	220.3	206.4	229.1
Cirrhosis of the liver	7.5	4.5	10.6	219.3	121.4	319.1
Digestive diseases (except cirrhosis)	0.3	0.1	0.5	9.4	3.1	15.8

Table 5.3 (continued) Deaths and DALYs attributable to addictive substances in 2010.

Cause	Deaths per 100,000 people			DALYs per 100,000 people		
Neurological disorders	0.3	0.2	0.5	26.2	14.7	37.6
Mental and behavioural disorders	1.7	0.6	2.8	258.6	105.9	409.6
Diabetes, urogenital, blood, and endocrine diseases*	(0.4)	(0.6)	(0.1)	(16.4)	(28.6)	(3.0)
Transport injuries	2.9	1.0	4.8	155.5	57.6	251.7
Unintentional injuries other than transport injuries	3.0	0.5	5.6	137.8	24.4	252.1
Self-harm and interpersonal violence	4.0	0.5	7.5	179.3	24.7	331.2
(3) Illicit and non-medical drug use						
Total (all causes)	2.3	1.4	3.2	343.2	221.3	461.6
HIV/AIDS and tuberculosis	0.6	0.4	0.9	31.1	19.5	42.4
Other communicable, maternal, neonatal, and nutritional disorders	0.0	0.0	0.0	0.4	0.3	0.5
Neoplasms	0.1	0.0	0.1	2.4	1.4	3.4
Cirrhosis of the liver	0.2	0.1	0.2	5.7	4.2	7.2
Mental and behavioural disorders	1.1	0.6	1.6	287.5	184.8	387.0
Self-harm and interpersonal violence	0.3	0.2	0.4	16.1	11.2	21.0

*Alcohol has a protective effect for this disease category.

Source: data from Wang H., et al., Age-specific and sex-specific mortality in 187 countries, 1970–2010: a systematic analysis for the Global Burden of Disease Study 2010, The Lancet, Volume 380, Issue 9859, pp. 2071–94, Copyright © 2012 Elsevier; Lozano R. et al, Global and regional mortality from 235 causes of death for 20 age groups in 1990 and 2010: a systematic analysis for the Global Burden of Disease Study 2010, The Lancet, Volume 380, Issue, pp. 2095–128. Copyright © 2012 Elsevier; Murray C.J., et al., Disability-adjusted life years (DALYs) for 291 diseases and injuries in 21 regions, 1990–2010: a systematic analysis for the Global Burden of Disease Study 2010, The Lancet, Volume 380, Issue 9859, pp. 2197–223, Copyright © 2012 Elsevier; and Lim S.S., et al., Pharmacotherapy of dependence: improving translation from the bench to the clinic, Animal and Translational Models for CNS Drug Discovery, pp. 91–106, Academic Press, Burlington MA, USA, Copyright © 2008.

second-hand smoke causing a loss of 20 million DALYs. Men where more affected by first-hand tobacco use, with men losing 106 million DALYs and women losing 31 million DALYs to this cause. Conversely women were more affected by second-hand smoke, with women losing 10.0 million DALYs and men losing 9.9 million DALYs to second-hand smoking. The burden of tobacco varied greatly by age. In terms of DALYs lost per 100,000 people attributable to tobacco use, babies aged 0 to 27 days were affected the most, followed by people aged 70 to 79 years. In terms of the percentage of all DALYs lost as a result of tobacco use, those aged 60 to 69 years were affected the most.

The burden of tobacco use varied greatly by country and was largest in eastern Europe and Central Asia because the population prevalence of smoking among men and women is comparatively the highest in these regions (World Health Organization 2013). Western, eastern and central sub-Saharan Africa experienced the least harm from tobacco smoking, with this region having a comparatively lower prevalence of smoking and people in this region experiencing less harm from non-communicable diseases related to tobacco use compared with other regions (World Health Organization, 2011). Figures 5.1 and 5.2 outline the burden of deaths and DALYS lost attributable to global tobacco use in 2010.

The burden of disease attributable to tobacco use decreased from a loss of 3379 DALYs per 100,000 people in 1990 to 2385 DALYs per 100,000 people in

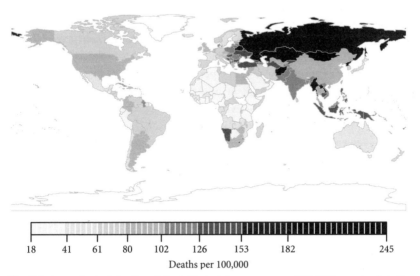

Fig. 5.1 Age-adjusted deaths attributable to tobacco use per 100,000 people globally in 2010.

Reproduced with permission from Institute for Health Metrics and Evaluation (IHME). GBD Compare. Seattle, WA: IHME, University of Washington, 2013. Available from http://vizhub. healthdata.org/gbd-compare (Accessed 1 February 2014).

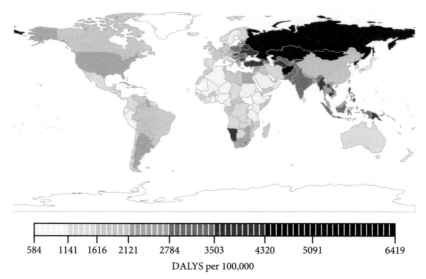

| 584 | 1141 | 1616 | 2121 | 2784 | 3503 | 4320 | 5091 | 6419 |

DALYS per 100,000

Fig. 5.2 Age-adjusted disability-adjusted life years (DALYs) lost attributable to tobacco use per 100,000 people globally in 2010.

Reproduced with permission from Institute for Health Metrics and Evaluation (IHME). GBD Compare. Seattle, WA: IHME, University of Washington, 2013. Available from http://vizhub. healthdata.org/gbd-compare (Accessed 1 February 2014).

2010 (figures adjusted for population data). This decrease in the DALYs lost as a result of tobacco use is observed for both men and women, but is only found when correcting for population structure—the burden of tobacco use is actually increasing in absolute terms. The percentage of DALYs lost attributable to tobacco use increased from 6.1% in 1990 to 6.3% in 2010, representing an increase of 4.0%; this increase, however, was only observed for men.

Tobacco use mostly exerts its health effects through cardiac and circulatory diseases (49.1% of all tobacco-attributable DALYs lost), with chronic respiratory diseases being responsible for the second highest number (20.3%), neoplasms third (20.2%), lower respiratory infections and other common infectious diseases fourth (6.9%), diabetes fifth (2.2%), and TB sixth (1.3%).

5.3.2 Burden of alcohol consumption

In 2010 alcohol consumption was the fifth leading risk factor for loss of health and the ninth leading risk factor for mortality, and was responsible for the loss of 97 million DALYs and 2.7 million deaths. Figures 5.3 and 5.4 outline the global burden of deaths and lost DALYS, respectively, attributable to alcohol consumption in 2010. Men experienced a much greater alcohol-attributable burden of disease, with 2234.2 DALYs lost to alcohol consumption per 100,000

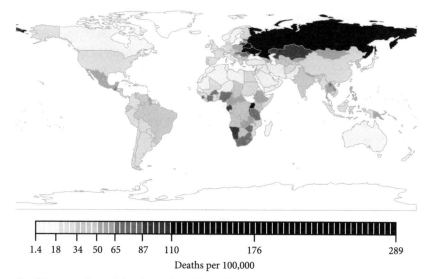

1.4 18 34 50 65 87 110 176 289

Deaths per 100,000

Fig. 5.3 Age-adjusted deaths attributable to alcohol consumption per 100,000 people globally in 2010.

Reproduced with permission from Institute for Health Metrics and Evaluation (IHME). GBD Compare. Seattle, WA: IHME, University of Washington, 2013. Available from http://vizhub. healthdata.org/gbd-compare (Accessed 1 February 2014).

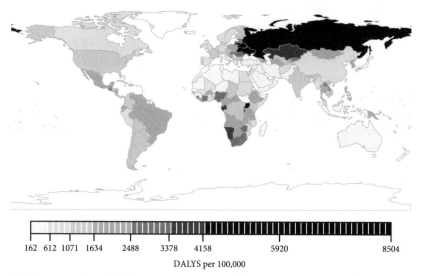

162 612 1071 1634 2488 3378 4158 5920 8504

DALYS per 100,000

Fig. 5.4 Age-adjusted disability-adjusted life years (DALYs) lost attributable to alcohol consumption per 100,000 people globally in 2010.

Reproduced with permission from Institute for Health Metrics and Evaluation (IHME). GBD Compare. Seattle, WA: IHME, University of Washington, 2013. Available from http://vizhub. healthdata.org/gbd-compare (Accessed 1 February 2014).

men. The corresponding figure for women was a loss of 653.1 DALYs per 100,000 women. The burden of alcohol consumption per 100,000 people was greatest in those aged 50 and above; however, as a percentage of all DALYs lost alcohol had the largest impact on those aged 35 to 64 years.

As with smoking, the greatest burden of alcohol consumption globally was in eastern Europe and Central Asia, with this burden mainly due to the volume of alcohol consumed and the harmful ways in which people consume alcohol. For instance in Russia alcohol is the second largest cause of burden of disease, being responsible for 23.6% of all DALYs lost (19.2% of all DALYs for women and 26.9% for men) (diet is the first cause). Although Russian men and women consume more alcohol then in other countries the way in which they consume it increases the risk of diseases such as cirrhosis of the liver and ischaemic heart disease (Leon et al., 2007; Zaridze et al., 2014).

As with tobacco, when correcting for population structure the burden of alcohol consumption has decreased from 1637 DALYs lost per 100,000 people in 1990 to 1444 DALYs per 100,000 people in 2010, with this decrease being observed among both men and women. Although the burden of disease per 100,000 people (population adjusted) has decreased, the percentage of DALYs lost as a result of alcohol consumption increased from 2.9% in 1990 to 3.9% in 2010, an increase of 32.5%. This increase can be explained by an increase in alcohol consumption in developing countries (previous research has shown that alcohol consumption is strongly correlated with the gross domestic product of a country, adjusted for purchase power parity; Shield et al., 2011) and a shift in deaths and burden of disability from infectious diseases to non-communicable diseases.

Alcohol consumption exerted most of its health effects through mental and behavioural disorders (18.1% of all alcohol-attributable DALYs), with cirrhosis of the liver being responsible for 15.0% of all alcohol-attributable DALYs, and cardiovascular and circulatory diseases for 14.9%. The impact of alcohol varied greatly by condition group, with infectious diseases being responsible for 8.4% of all alcohol-attributable DALYs, non-communicable diseases for 58.3% of all alcohol-attributable DALYs, and injuries for 33.3% of all alcohol-attributable DALYs.

These estimates should be interpreted with caution as they are limited by several factors. First, alcohol abuse and foetal alcohol syndrome were not included as a condition, and drinking during pregnancy as a risk factor for low birth weight was not included. Thus the burden of disease attributable to alcohol consumption is likely to be underestimated.

5.3.3 Burden of illicit and non-medical drug use

In 2010 illicit and non-medical drug use was the fifteenth leading risk factor for health loss and the eighteenth leading risk factor for mortality, responsible for the loss of 24 million DALYs and 0.16 million deaths. Men experienced much more harm attributable to illicit and non-medical drug use (461.6 DALYs lost per 100,000 men) compared with women (221.3 DALYs lost per 100,000 women). Figures 5.5 and 5.6 outline the global burden of deaths and DALYS, respectively, attributable to illicit drug in 2010. The main burden (DALYs lost per 100,000 people) of illicit and non-medical drug use occurred in children aged 0 to 6 years followed by adults aged 20 to 34 years. This age distribution is due to the high prevalence of substance use among adults aged 20 to 34 years and to substance use among pregnant women. In terms of the percentage of all DALYs attributable to illicit and non-medical drug use, people aged 20 to 34 years were most affected.

The burden of illicit and non-medical drug use was the greatest in North America, Australasia, eastern Europe, and western Europe; however, the country most affected was the United Arab Emirates, where 4.6% of all DALYs lost were attributable to illicit and non-medical drug use. The burden of each drug category was not consistent across regions, with cocaine dependence being most prevalent in high-income North America followed by tropical Latin America, the Caribbean, southern Latin America and Andean Latin America, whereas the prevalence of cannabis, amphetamine, and opioid dependence was highest in Australasia.

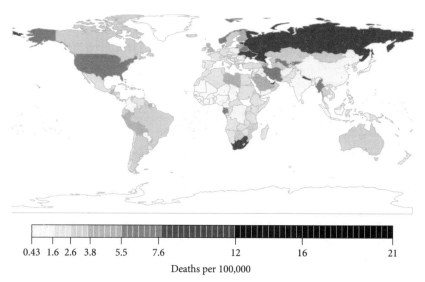

Fig. 5.5 Age-adjusted deaths attributable to illicit and non-medical drug use per 100,000 people globally in 2010.

Reproduced with permission from Institute for Health Metrics and Evaluation (IHME). GBD Compare. Seattle, WA: IHME, University of Washington, 2013. Available from http://vizhub. healthdata.org/gbd-compare (Accessed 1 February 2014).

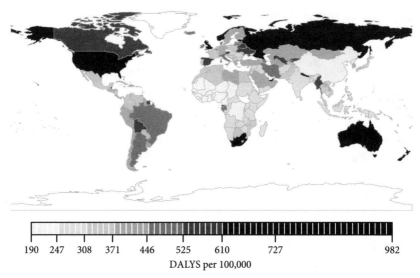

Fig. 5.6 Age-adjusted disability-adjusted life years (DALYs) lost attributable to illicit and non-medical drug use per 100,000 people globally in 2010.

Reproduced with permission from Institute for Health Metrics and Evaluation (IHME). GBD Compare. Seattle, WA: IHME, University of Washington, 2013. Available from http://vizhub. healthdata.org/gbd-compare (Accessed 1 February 2014).

The majority of the health effects due to the use of illicit and non-medical drugs were from mental and behavioural disorders (84.0% of all DALYs attributable to illicit and non-medical drug use), HIV (8.9%), self-harm (4.7%), and other non-communicable diseases (2.4%).

5.3.4 Who experiences the most harms from substance abuse and addictive behaviours

Attaining greater equity in health is one of the WHO's top priorities, and the achievement of various global health and development targets without an equitable distribution across populations and sub-populations is of limited value (World Health Organization, 2010). However, there is a surprising dearth of literature on the social determinants of loss of health and the resulting health inequities caused by substance abuse and addictive behaviours.

The magnitude of the harms caused by substance abuse and addictive behaviours is dependent on the prevalence, patterns of substance use and addictive behaviours, and the underlying vulnerability to and mortality from diseases, conditions, and injuries that are causally related to substance use and addictive behaviours.

In the United States it has been estimated that black and Native American populations experience much more alcohol-attributable harm than whites and

Pacific islanders, showing that an alcohol-related health disparity exists across racial groups in the United States (Shield et al., 2013). Racial disparities have also been observed in the United States for tobacco use and tobacco-attributable deaths, with black and Native American populations having the greatest exposure to tobacco smoke and experiencing the greatest tobacco-attributable harms (CDC, 1998, 2010a).

People with certain genotypes can experience a greater risk of developing a disease or condition than individuals with other genotypes for the same level of exposure to addictive substances. For example, certain variants of the *CYP1A1* and *GSTM1* genes have been found to be associated with a modest increase in the risk of cancer when carriers are exposed to tobacco smoke (Spivack et al., 1997; Bartsch et al., 2000; Houlston, 2000; Benhamou et al., 2002; Caporaso et al., 2002). There is also evidence that variants in genes for metabolizing enzymes such as *GSTT1*, *CYP1A1*, and *GSTM1* increase the risk of lowered birth weight and shorter gestation with tobacco exposure (Nukui et al., 2004; Kurahashi et al., 2005). Additionally, variants in the dehydrogenase gene *ALDH2* (commonly known as the 'flushing gene') and the alcohol dehydrogenase genes *ADH1B* and *ADH1C* (which are all more prevalent in East Asian populations) alter the metabolism of alcohol, leading to increased levels of the carcinogen acetaldehyde after the consumption of alcohol and thus to an increased risk of gastrointestinal cancers (Higuchi et al., 1994; Eng et al., 2007). For example, heavy drinkers who have these genetic polymorphisms have an estimated eighty times greater risk of developing oesophageal cancer compared with abstainers (Lewis and Smith, 2005; Druesne-Pecollo et al., 2009; Oze et al., 2011; Cadoni et al, 2012). Although not calculated in the Global Burden of Disease Study 2010, population differences in the frequencies of genotypes that modify the risk of addictive substances can create health loss inequities among sub-populations and between countries. This is especially important for countries like South Korea and Japan, where 30.0% and 33.7%, respectively, of all deaths are due to cancer and 29% and 46%, respectively, of all people have at least one copy of the genetic variant for *ALDH2* (Eng et al., 2007).

The global risk factor rankings provide a good picture of health loss around the world, but given that these figures differ by age, sex, race, and ethnicity they should not be considered exclusively. Additional analyses, such as sub-group population analyses investigating the distribution of health loss due to health inequities, should also be performed. As the information provided by Global Burden of Disease Study is limited there is a need for sub-national burden of disease studies to determine the underlying causes of health loss (i.e. risk factors) by additional dimensions other than age, for example by income, education, and race/ethnicity (Almeida et al., 2001).

5.4 **Conclusion**

Addictive substances and behaviours are causally related to numerous diseases, conditions, and injuries, which in turn create a large health burden. Results from the Global Burden of Disease Study 2010 suggest that the leading risk factors contributing to the global burden of disease attributable to addictive substances and behaviours changed substantially between 1990 and 2010. In particular, although the actual number of DALYs lost per 100,000 people attributable to addictive substances has decreased since 1990, the percentage of all DALYs lost that is attributable to addictive substances has increased. This observation is consistent with a decrease in the absolute number of DALYs lost per 100,000 people (adjusting for population structure) and a decrease in the absolute number of DALYs lost per 100,000 people attributable to addictive substances. However, the relative decrease in the total number of DALYs lost per 100,000 people has been greater than the relative decrease in the total number of DALYs lost per 100,000 people attributable to addictive substances. Given the increase in the relative importance of addictive substances since 1990 there is a need to develop and implement population health interventions that address this burden and the health inequalities it creates. The health effects of pathological gambling disorder are currently unknown. This is because it has only been designated as a behavioural disorder since publication of DSM-5 and more research on the physical and mental health effects of this disorder is needed to quantify its impact at the population level. Additional research will also be required if addictive behaviours other than pathological gambling disorder are recognized as addictive behavioural disorders in the future.

Acknowledgements

The estimates presented in this chapter are from the Global Burden of Disease Study 2010. See Lim et al. (2012) for an overview of the methodology used to calculate the burden attributable to addictive substances and Wang et al. (2012), Lozano et al. (2012), and Murray et al. (2012) for the underlying estimates of mortality and morbidity.

References

Abel, E.L. (1982). Consumption of alcohol during pregnancy: a review of effects on growth and development of offspring. *Human Biology*, **54**, 421–453.

Ahluwalia, B., Smith, D., Adeyiga, O., et al. (1992). Ethanol decreases progesterone synthesis in human placental cells: mechanism of ethanol effect. *Alcohol*, **9**, 395–401.

Almeida, C., Braveman, P., Gold, M.R., et al. (2001). Methodological concerns and recommendations on policy consequences of the World Health Report 2000. *Lancet*, **357**, 1692–1697.

American Psychiatric Association (2013). *Diagnostic and Statistical Manual of Mental Disorders*, 5th edn (text revision). Arlington, VA: American Psychiatric Association.

Anselme, P. & Robinson, M.J. (2013). What motivates gambling behavior? Insight into dopamine's role. *Frontiers in Behavioral Neuroscience*, 7, 182.

Asmussen, V. (2008). Cannabis policy: tightening the ties in Denmark. In: *A Cannabis Reader: Global Issues* and *Local Experiences*, Monograph Series 8, Vol. 1, pp. 157–168. Lisbon: European Monitoring Centre for Drugs and Drug Addiction.

Azar, M.M., Springer, S.A., Meyer, J.P., & Altice, F.L. (2010). A systematic review of the impact of alcohol use disorders on HIV treatment outcomes, adherence to antiretroviral therapy and health care utilization. *Drug and Alcohol Dependence*, **112**, 178–193.

Babor, T. (2010). *Drug Policy and the Public Good*. Oxford: Oxford University Press.

Bagnardi, V., Blangiardo, M., La Vecchia, C., & Corrao, G. (2001). Alcohol consumption and the risk of cancer: a meta-analysis. *Alcohol Research and Health*, **25**, 263–270.

Balbão, C.E.B., de Paola, A.A.V., & Fenelon, G. (2009). Effects of alcohol on atrial fibrillation: myths and truths. *Therapeutic Advances in Cardiovascular Disease*, **3**, 53–63.

Baliunas, D., Taylor, B., Irving, H., et al. (2009). Alcohol as a risk factor for type 2 diabetes—a systematic review and meta-analysis. *Diabetes Care*, **32**, 2123–2132.

Baliunas, D., Rehm, J., Irving, H., & Shuper, P. (2010). Alcohol consumption and risk of incident human immunodeficiency virus infection: a meta-analysis. *International Journal of Public Health*, **55**, 159–166.

Ballenger, J.C. & Post, R.M. (1978). Kindling as a model for alcohol withdrawal syndromes. *British Journal of Psychiatry*, **133**, 1–14.

Barclay, G.A., Barvour, J., Stewart, S., et al. (2008). Adverse physical effects of alcohol misuse. *Advances in Psychiatric Treatment*, **14**, 139–151.

Bartsch, H., Nair, U., Risch, A., Rojas, M., Wikman, H., & Alexandrov, K. (2000). Genetic polymorphism of CYP genes, alone or in combination, as a risk modifier of tobacco-related cancers. *Cancer Epidemiology, Biomarkers and Prevention*, **9**, 3–28.

Bellocco, R., Pasquali, E., Rota, M., et al. (2012). Alcohol drinking and risk of renal cell carcinoma: results of a meta-analysis. *Annals of Oncology*, **23**, 2235–2244.

Benhamou, S., Lee, W.J., Alexandrie, A.K., et al. (2002). Meta- and pooled analyses of the effects of glutathione-S-transferase M1 polymorphisms and smoking on lung cancer risk. *Carcinogenesis*, **23**, 1343–1350.

Benowitz, N.L. & Gourlay, S.G. (1997). Cardiovascular toxicity of nicotine: implications for nicotine replacement therapy. *Journal of the American College of Cardiology*, **29**, 1422–1431.

Boffetta, P. & Hashibe, M. (2006). Alcohol and cancer. *Lancet Oncology*, 7, 149–156.

Bourgois, P. (2003). *In Search of Respect: Selling Crack in El Barrio*. London: Cambridge University Press.

Braithwaite, R.S., McGinnis, K.A., Conigliaro, J., et al. (2005). A temporal and dose-response association between alcohol consumption and medication adherence among veterans in care. *Alcoholism: Clinical and Experimental Research*, **29**, 1190–1197.

Braithwaite, R.S., Conigliaro, J., Roberts, M.S., et al. (2007). Estimating the impact of alcohol consumption on survival for HIV+ individuals. *AIDS Care*, **19**, 459–466.

Brooks, P.J., Enoch, M.A., Goldman, D., et al. (2009). The alcohol flushing response: an unrecognized risk factor for esophageal cancer from alcohol consumption. *PLoS Medicine*, **6**, 258–263.

Brosens, I.A., Robertson, W.B., & Dixon, H.G. (1972). The role of the spiral arteries in the pathogenesis of preeclampsia. *Obstetrics and Gynecology Annual*, **1**, 177–191.

Burke, A. & FitzGerald, G.A. (2003). Oxidative stress and smoking-induced vascular tissue injury. *Progress in Cardiovascular Diseases*, **46**, 79–90.

Bushman, B. (1997). Effects of alcohol on human aggression: validity of proposed mechanisms. In: *Recent Developments in Alcoholism, Vol. 13, Alcohol and Violence* (ed. M. Galanter), pp. 227–244. New York: Plenum Press.

CDC (1998). *1998 Surgeon General's Report: Tobacco Use Among U.S. Racial/Ethnic Minority Groups*. Atlanta, GA: US Department of Health and Human Services. URL: <http://www.cdc.gov/tobacco/data_statistics/sgr/sgr_1998>.

CDC (2010a). Racial disparities in smoking-attributable mortality and years of potential life lost—Missouri, 2003–2007. *Morbidity and Mortality Weekly Report*, **59**, 1518–1522.

CDC (2010b). *How Tobacco Smoke Causes Disease: The Biology and Behavioral Basis for Smoking-Attributable Disease. A Report of the Surgeon General*. Atlanta, GA: Centers for Disease Control and Prevention.

Cadoni, G., Boccia, S., Petrelli, L., Di Giannantonio, P., Arzani, D., & Giorgio, A. (2012). A review of genetic epidemiology of head and neck cancer related to polymorphisms in metabolic genes, cell cycle control and alcohol metabolism. *Acta Otorhinolaryngologica Italia*, **32**, 1–11.

Campisi, R., Czernin, J., Schöder, H., et al. (1998). Effects of long-term smoking on myocardial blood flow, coronary vasomotion, and vasodilator capacity. *Circulation*, **98**, 119–125.

Caporaso, N.E. (2002). Why have we failed to find the low penetrance genetic constituents of common cancers? *Cancer Epidemiology, Biomarkers and Prevention*, **11**, 1544–1549.

Celermajer, D.S., Adams, M.R., Clarkson, P., et al. (1996). Passive smoking and impaired endothelium-dependent arterial dilatation in healthy young adults. *New England Journal of Medicine*, **334**, 150–154.

Challis, J. & Olson, D. (1988). Parturition. In: *The Physiology of Reproduction* (ed. E. Knobil & J. Neill), pp. 2177–2216. New York: Raven Press.

Cochrane, J., Chen, H., Conigrave, K.M., & Hao, W. (2003). Alcohol use in China. *Alcohol and Alcoholism*, **38**, 537–542.

Cook, J.L. & Randal, C.L. (1998). Ethanol and parturition: a role for prostaglandins. *Prostaglandins, Leukotrienes, and Essential Fatty Acids*, **58**, 135–142.

Dam, A.M., Fuglsang-Frederikse, A., Svarre-Olsen, U., & Dam, M. (1985). Late-onset epilepsy: etiologies, types of seizure, and value of clinical investigation, EEG, and computerized tomography scan. *Epilepsia*, **26**, 227–231.

Davies, M.J., Baer, D.J., Judd, J.T., et al. (2002). Effects of moderate alcohol intake on fasting insulin and glucose concentrations and insulin sensitivity in postmenopausal women: a randomized controlled trial. *Journal of the American Medical Association*, **287**, 2559–2562.

Dawson, D. (1997). Alcohol, drugs, fighting and suicide attempt/ideation. *Addiction Research*, **5**, 451–472.

De, P., Cox, J., Boivin, J.F., Platt, R.W., & Jolly, A.M. (2007). The importance of social networks in their association to drug equipment sharing among injection drug users: a review. *Addiction*, **102**, 1730–1739.

Degenhardt, L. & Hall, W. (2012). Extent of illicit drug use and dependence, and their contribution to the global burden of disease. *Lancet*, **379**, 55–70.

Dennis, L. (2000). Meta-analysis for combining relative risks of alcohol consumption and prostate cancer. *Prostate*, **42**, 56–66.

Dingle, G.A. & Oei, T.P. (1997). Is alcohol a cofactor of HIV and AIDS? Evidence from immunological and behavioral studies. *Psychological Bulletin*, **122**, 56–71.

Doll, R. (1998). Uncovering the effects of smoking: historical perspective. *Statistical Methods in Medical Research*, **7**, 87–117.

Druesne-Pecollo, N., Tehard, B., Mallet, Y., Gerber, M., Norat, T., & Hercberg, S. (2009). Alcohol and genetic polymorphisms: effect on risk of alcohol-related cancer. *Lancet Oncology*, **10**, 173–180.

Dullaart, R.P., Hoogenberg, K., Dikkeschei, B.D., & van Tol, A. (1994). Higher plasma lipid transfer protein activities and unfavorable lipoprotein changes in cigarette-smoking men. *Arteriosclerosis and Thrombosis*, **14**, 1581–1585.

Eckardt, M., File, S., Gessa, G., et al. (1998). Effects of moderate alcohol consumption on the central nervous system. *Alcoholism: Clinical and Experimental Research*, **22**, 998–1040.

Eliasson, B., Attvall, S., Taskinen, M.R., & Smith, U. (1994). The insulin resistance syndrome in smokers is related to smoking habits. *Arteriosclerosis and Thrombosis*, **14**, 1946–1950.

Eng, M.Y., Luczak, S.E., & Wall, T.L. (2007). ALDH2, ADH1B, and ADH1C genotypes in Asians: a literature review. *Alcohol Research and Health*, **30**, 22–27.

Erickson, L., Molina, C.A., Ladd, G.T., Pietrzak, R.H., & Petry, N.M. (2005). Problem and pathological gambling are associated with poorer mental and physical health in older adults. *International Journal of Geriatric Psychiatry*, **20**, 754–759.

Ezzati, M., Lopez, A.D., Rodgers, A., & Murray, C.J. (2004). *Comparative Quantification of Health Risks. Global and Regional Burden of Disease Attributable to Selected Major Risk Factors*. Geneva: World Health Organization.

Facchini, F., Chen, Y.D., & Reaven, G.M. (1994). Light-to-moderate alcohol intake is associated with enhanced insulin sensitivity. *Diabetes Care*, **17**, 115–119.

Ferson, M., Edwards, A., Lind, A., Milton, G.W., & Hersey, P. (1979). Low natural-killer-cell activity and immunoglobulin levels associated with smoking in human subjects. *International Journal of Cancer*, **23**, 603–609.

Fisher, J.C., Bang, H., & Kapiga, S.H. (2007). The association between HIV infection and alcohol use: a systematic review and meta-analysis of African studies. *Sexually Transmitted Diseases*, **34**, 856–863.

Freedland, E.S. & McMicken, D.B. (1993). Alcohol-related seizures, part I: pathophysiology, differential diagnosis and evaluation. *Journal of Emergency Medicine*, **11**, 463–473.

Gabel, K. & Johnston, D. (1995). *Children of Incarcerated Parents*. New York: Lexington Books.

Gamble, L., Mason, C.M., & Nelson, S. (2006). The effects of alcohol on immunity and bacterial infection in the lung. *Medicine et Maladies Infectieuses*, **36**, 72–77.

Gmel, G., Shield, K.D., & Rehm, J. (2011). Developing a method to derive alcohol-attributable fractions for HIV/AIDS mortality based on alcohol's impact on adherence to antiretroviral medication. *Population Health Metrics*, **9**, 5.

Graham, K. & West, P. (2001). Alcohol and crime. In: *International Handbook of Alcohol Dependence and Problems* (ed. N. Heather, T.J. Peters, & T. Stockwell), pp. 439–470. London: John Wiley and Sons.

Graham, K., West, P., & Wells, S. (2000). Evaluating theories of alcohol-related aggression using observations of young adults in bars. *Addiction*, **95**, 847–863.

Grant, B.F. & Pickering, R.P. (1997). Familial aggregation of DSM-IV alcohol disorders: examination of the primary-secondary distinction in a general population sample. *Journal of Nervous and Mental Disease*, **185**, 335–343.

Gruenewald, P., Mitchell, P., & Treno, A. (1996). Drinking and driving: drinking patterns and drinking problems. *Addiction*, **91**, 1637–1649.

Gruenewald, P. & Nephew, T. (1994). Drinking in California: theoretical and empirical analyses of alcohol consumption patterns. *Addiction*, **89**, 707–723.

Hahn, J.A. & Samet, J.H. (2010). Alcohol and HIV disease progression: weighing the evidence. *Current HIV/AIDS Reports*, **7**, 226–233.

Hasin, D., Paykin, A., Meydan, J., & Grant, B. (2000). Withdrawal and tolerance: prognostic significance in DSM-IV alcohol dependence. *Journal of Studies on Alcohol*, **61**, 431–438.

Hecht, S.S. (2003). Tobacco carcinogens, their biomarkers and tobacco-induced cancer. *Nature Reviews Cancer*, **3**, 733–744.

Heermans, E.H. (1998). Booze and blood: the effects of acute and chronic alcohol abuse on the hematopoietic system. *Clinical Laboratory Science*, **11**, 229–232.

Hendershot, C.S., Stoner, S.A., Pantalone, D.W., & Simoni, J.M. (2009). Alcohol use and antiretroviral adherence: review and meta-analysis. *Journal of Acquired Immune Deficiency Syndromes*, **52**, 180–202.

Hendriks, H.F.J. (2007). Moderate alcohol consumption and insulin sensitivity: observations and possible mechanisms. *Annals of Epidemiology*, **17**, S40–S42.

Higuchi, S., Matsushita, S., Imazeki, H., Kinoshita, T., Takagi, S., & Kono, H. (1994). Aldehyde dehydrogenase genotypes in Japanese alcoholics. *Lancet*, **343**, 741–742.

Hill, E.M. & Newlin, D.B. (2002). Evolutionary approaches to addiction: introduction. *Addiction*, **97**, 375–379.

Hogg, J.C. (2004). Pathophysiology of airflow limitation in chronic obstructive pulmonary disease. *Lancet*, **364**, 709–721.

Holt, P.G. (1987). Immune and inflammatory function in cigarette smokers. *Thorax*, **42**, 241–249.

Houlston, R.S. (2000). CYP1A1 polymorphisms and lung cancer risk: a meta-analysis. *Pharmacogenetics*, **10**, 105–114.

Imhof, A., Froehlich, M., Brenner, H., et al. (2001). Effect of alcohol consumption on systemic markers of inflammation. *Lancet*, **357**, 763–767.

Institute of Health Metrics and Evaluation (2013). *Data Visualizations*. Seattle, WA: Institute of Health Metrics and Evaluation. URL: <http://www.healthmetricsandevaluation.org/tools/data-visualizations>.

IARC (2004). Tobacco smoke and involuntary smoking. *IARC Monographs on the Evaluation of Carcinogenic Risks to Humans*, Vol. **83**. Lyon: IARC.

IARC (2008). *World Cancer Report 2008*. Lyon: IARC.

IARC (2012). Tobacco smoking. *IARC Monographs on the Evaluation of Carcinogenic Risks to Humans*, Vol. 100E. Lyon: IARC.

Joh, H.K., Willet, W.C., & Cho, E. (2011). Type 2 diabetes and the risk of renal cell cancer in women. *Diabetes Care*, **34**, 1552–1556.

Joosten, M.M., Beulens, J.W., Kersten, S., & Hendriks, H.F. (2008). Moderate alcohol consumption increases insulin sensitivity and ADIPOQ expression in postmenopausal women: a randomised, crossover trial. *Diabetologia*, **51**, 1375–1381.

Kiechl, S., Willeit, J., Poewe, W., et al. (1996). Insulin sensitivity and regular alcohol consumption: large, prospective, cross sectional population study (Bruneck study). *British Medical Journal*, **313**, 1040–1044.

King, T.E. Jr, Savici, D., & Campbell, P.A. (1988). Phagocytosis and killing of *Listeria monocytogenes* by alveolar macrophages: smokers versus nonsmokers. *Journal of Infectious Diseases*, **158**, 1309–1316.

Kirst, M. (2009). Social capital and beyond: a qualitative analysis of social contextual and structural influences on drug-use related health behaviors. *Journal of Drug Issues*, **39**, 653–676.

Krüger, H.P. (1993). Effects of low alcohol dosages: a review of the literature. In: *Alcohol, Drugs and Traffic Safety, T92: Proceedings of the 12th International Conference on Alcohol, Drugs, and Traffic Safety, Cologne, 28 September–2 October 1992* (ed. H.D. Utzelmann, G. Berghaus, & G. Kroj), pp. 763–778. Cologne: Verlag TUV Rheinland.

Kurahashi, N., Sata, F., Kasai, S., et al. (2005). Maternal genetic polymorphisms in CYP1A1, GSTM1 and GSTT1 and the risk of hypospadias. *Molecular Human Reproduction*, **11**, 93–98.

Lamy, L. (1910). Étude clinique et statistique de 134 cas de cancer de l'oesophage et du cardia. *Archives des Maladies de L'Appareil Digestif*, **4**, 451–475.

Law, M.R. & Wald, N.J. (2003). Environmental tobacco smoke and ischemic heart disease. *Progress in Cardiovascular Diseases*, **46**, 31–38.

Lazarus, R., Sparrow, D., & Weiss, S.T. (1997). Alcohol intake and insulin levels. The Normative Aging Study. *American Journal of Epidemiology*, **145**, 909–916.

Leon, D.A., Saburova, L., Tomkins, S., et al. (2007). Hazardous alcohol drinking and premature mortality in Russia: a population based case-control study. *Lancet*, **369**, 2001–2009.

Leppa, S. (1974). *A Review of Robberies in Helsinki in 1963–1973*. Helsinki: Research Institute of Legal Policy.

Lewis, S.J. & Smith, G.D. (2005). Alcohol, ALDH2, and esophageal cancer: a meta-analysis which illustrates the potentials and limitations of a Mendelian randomization approach. *Cancer Epidemiology, Biomarkers, and Prevention*, **14**, 1967–1971.

Lim, S.S., Vos, T., Flaxman, A.D., et al. (2012). A comparative risk assessment of burden of disease and injury attributable to 67 risk factors and risk factor clusters in 21 regions, 1990–2010: a systematic analysis for the Global Burden of Disease Study 2010. *Lancet*, **380**, 2224–2260.

Lindblad, P., Chow, W.H., Chan, J. et al. (1999). The role of diabetes mellitus in the aetiology of renal cell cancer. *Diabetologia*, **42**, 107–112.

Little, J., Cardy, A., & Munger, R.G. (2004). Tobacco smoking and oral clefts: a meta-analysis. *Bulletin of the World Health Organization*, **82**, 213–218.

Little, J., McKinzie, D., Setnik, B., Shram, M., & Em, S. (2008). Pharmacotherapy of dependence: improving translation from the bench to the clinic. In: *Animal and Translational Models for CNS Drug Discovery* (ed. R.A. McArthur & F. Borsini), pp. 91–106. Burlington, MA: Academic Press.

Longo, L.D. (1976). Carbon monoxide: effects on oxygenation of the fetus in utero. *Science,* **194**, 523–525.

Longo, L.D. (1977). The biological effects of carbon monoxide on the pregnant woman, fetus, and newborn infant. *American Journal of Obstetrics and Gynecology,* **129**, 69–103.

Lönnroth, K., Jaramillo, E., Williams, B.G., et al. (2009). Drivers of tuberculosis epidemics: the role of risk factors and social determinants. *Social Science and Medicine,* **68**, 2240–2246.

Lozano, R., Naghavi, M., Foreman, K., et al. (2012). Global and regional mortality from 235 causes of death for 20 age groups in 1990 and 2010: a systematic analysis for the Global Burden of Disease Study 2010. *Lancet,* **380**, 2095–2128.

McClelland, D., Davis, W., Kalin, R., & Wanner, E. (1972). *The Drinking Man: Alcohol and Human Motivation.* Toronto: Collier-Macmillan.

McGovern, P. (2009). *Uncorking the Past: The Quest for Wine, Beer, and Other Alcoholic Beverages.* Berkeley, CA: University of California Press.

Makin, J., Fried, P.A., & Watkinson, B. (1991). A comparison of active and passive smoking during pregnancy: long-term effects. *Neurotoxicology and Teratology,* **13**, 5–12.

Marek, Z., Widacki, J., & Hanausek, T. (1974). Alcohol as a victimogenic factor in robberies. *Forensic Science,* **4**, 119–123.

Martin, R.R. & Warr, G.A. (1977). Cigarette smoking and pulmonary macrophages. *Hospital Practice,* **12**, 97–104.

Mayer, E.J., Newman, B., Quesenberry, C.P. Jr, et al. (1993). Alcohol consumption and insulin concentrations. Role of insulin in associations of alcohol intake with high-density lipoprotein cholesterol and triglycerides. *Circulation,* **88**, 2190–2197.

Miczek, K. & Barry, H. (1977). Effects of alcohol on attack and defensive–submissive reactions in rats. *Psychopharmacology,* **52**, 231–237.

Miczek, K., Weerts, E., & DeBold, J. (1993). Alcohol, benzodiazepine-GABA receptor complex and aggression: ethological analysis of individual differences in rodents and primates. *Journal of Studies on Alcohol. Supplement,* **11**, 170S–179S.

Middleton, F.K., Chikritzhs, T., Stockwell, T., et al. (2009). Alcohol use and prostate cancer: a meta-analysis. *Molecular Nutrition and Food Research,* **53**, 240–255.

Moskowitz, H. & Robinson, C. (1988). *Effects of Low Doses of Alcohol on Driving-Related Skills: A Review of the Evidence.* Washington, DC: National Highway Traffic Safety Administration.

Murray, C.J. & Lopez, A.D. (1997). Global mortality, disability, and the contribution of risk factors: Global Burden of Disease Study. *Lancet,* **349**, 1436–1442.

Murray, R.P., Bailey, W.C., Daniels, K., et al. (1996). Safety of nicotine polacrilex gum used by 3,094 participants in the Lung Health Study Research Group. *Chest,* **109**, 438–445.

Murray, C.J., Vos, T., Lozano, R., et al. (2012). Disability-adjusted life years (DALYs) for 291 diseases and injuries in 21 regions, 1990–2010: a systematic analysis for the Global Burden of Disease Study 2010. *Lancet,* **380**, 2197–2223.

Nelson, E., Jodscheit, K., & Guo, Y. (1999). Maternal passive smoking during pregnancy and fetal developmental toxicity. Part 1: gross morphological effects. *Human and Experimental Toxicology*, **18**, 252–256.

Neuman, M. (2003). Cytokines—central factors in alcoholic liver disease. *Alcohol Research and Health*, **27**, 307–316.

Neuman, M.G., Monteiro, M., & Rehm, J. (2006). Drug interactions between psychoactive substances and antiretroviral therapy in individuals infected with human immunodeficiency and hepatitis viruses. *Substance Use and Misuse*, 41, 1395–1463.

Nukui, T., Day, R.D., Sims, C.S., Ness, R.B., & Romkes, M. (2004). Maternal/newborn *GSTT1* null genotype contributes to risk of pre-term, low birthweight infants. *Pharmacogenetics*, **14**, 569–576.

Oetting, E.R. & Beauvais, F. (1986). Peer cluster theory: drugs and the adolescent. *Journal of Counseling and Development*, **65**, 17–22.

Oze, I., Matsuo, K., Wakai, K., Nagata, C., Mizoue, T., & Tanaka, K. (2011). Alcohol drinking and esophageal cancer risk: an evaluation based on a systematic review of epidemiologic evidence among the Japanese population. *Japanese Journal of Clinical Oncology*, **41**, 677–692.

Panza, F., Capurso, C., D'Introno, A., et al. (2008). Vascular risk factors, alcohol intake, and cognitive decline. *Journal of Nutrition, Health, and Aging*, **12**, 376–381.

Parry, C.D.H., Rehm, J.R., Poznyak, V., & Room, R. (2009). Alcohol and infectious diseases: are there causal linkages? *Addiction*, **104**, 331–332.

Patra, J., Bakker, R., Irving, H., et al. (2011). Dose–response relationship between alcohol consumption before and during pregnancy and the risks of low birthweight, preterm birth and small for gestational age (SGA)-a systematic review and meta-analyses. *BJOG: International Journal of Obstetrics and Gynaecology*, **118**, 1411–1421.

Pelucchi, C., Galeone, C., Tramacere, I., et al. (2012). Alcohol drinking and bladder cancer risk: a meta-analysis. *Annals of Oncology*, **23**, 1586–1593.

Peters, R., Peters, J., Warner, J., et al. (2008). Alcohol, dementia and cognitive decline in the elderly: a systematic review. *Age and Ageing*, **37**, 505–512.

Peterson, J., Rothfleisch, J., Zelazo, P., & Pihl, R. (1990). Acute alcohol intoxication and neuropsychological functioning. *Journal of Studies on Alcohol*, **51**, 114–122.

Petry, N.M., Stinson, F.S., & Grant, B.F. (2005). Comorbidity of DSM-IV pathological gambling and other psychiatric disorders: results from the National Epidemiologic Survey on Alcohol and Related Conditions. *Journal of Clinical Psychiatry*, **66**, 564–574.

Petry, N.M. & Weinstock, J. (2007). Internet gambling is common in college students and associated with poor mental health. *American Journal on Addictions*, **16**, 325–330.

Pihl, R. & Hoaken, P. (2001). Biological bases of addiction and aggression in close relationships. In: *The Violence and Addiction Equation. Theoretical and Clinical Issues in Substance Abuse and Relationship Violence* (ed. C. Wekerle & M. Wall), pp. 25–43. New York: Brunner-Routledge.

Pihl, R., Peterson, J., & Lau, M. (1993). A biosocial model of the alcohol–aggression relationship. *Journal of Studies on Alcohol. Supplement*, **11**, 128S–139S.

Pliner, P. & Cappell, H. (1974). Modification of affective consequences of alcohol: a comparison of social and solitary drinking. *Journal of Abnormal Psychology*, **83**, 418–425.

Potts, R.J., Newbury, C.J., Smith, G., Notarianni, L.J., & Jefferies, T.M. (1999). Sperm chromatin damage associated with male smoking. *Mutation Research*, **423**, 103–111.

Ramchand, R., Pacula, R.L., & Iguchi, M.Y. (2006). Racial differences in marijuana-users' risk of arrest in the United States. *Drug and Alcohol Dependence*, **84**, 264–272.

Rathlev, N.K., Ulrich, A.S., Delanty, N., et al. (2006). Alcohol-related seizures. *Journal of Emergency Medicine*, **31**, 157–163.

Rehm, J., Room, R., Graham, K., et al. (2003). The relationship of average volume of alcohol consumption and patterns of drinking to burden of disease—an overview. *Addiction*, **98**, 1209–1228.

Rehm, J., Room, R., Monteiro, M., et al. (2004). Alcohol use. In: *Comparative Quantification of Health Risks: Global and Regional Burden of Disease Attributable to Selected Major Risk Factors* (ed. M. Ezzati, A.D. Lopez, A. Rodgers, & C.J.L. Murray), pp. 959–1109. Geneva: World Health Organization.

Rehm, J., Samokhvalov, A.V., Neuman, M.G., et al. (2009). The association between alcohol use, alcohol use disorders and tuberculosis (TB). A systematic review. *BMC Public Health*, **9**, 450.

Rehm, J., Taylor, B., Mohapatra, S., et al. (2010). Alcohol as a risk factor for liver cirrhosis—a systematic review and meta-analysis. *Drug and Alcohol Review*, **29**, 437–445.

Rehm, J., Shield, K.D., Joharchi, N., & Shuper, P.A. (2012). Alcohol consumption and the intention to engage in unprotected sex: systematic review and meta-analysis of experimental studies. *Addiction*, **107**, 51–59.

Reynolds, H.Y. (1987). Bronchoalveolar lavage. *American Review of Respiratory Disease*, **135**, 250–263.

Rhodes, T., Singer, M., Bourgois, P., Friedman, S., & Strathdee, S. (2005). The social structural production of HIV risk among injecting drug users. *Social Science and Medicine*, **61**, 1026–1044.

Rimm, E., Williams, P., Fosher, K., et al. (1999). Moderate alcohol intake and lower risk of coronary heart disease: meta-analysis of effects on lipids and haemostatic factors. *British Medical Journal*, **19**, 1523–1528.

Rodgman, A. & Perfetti, T.A. (2009). Alphabetical component index. In: *The Chemical Components of Tobacco and Tobacco Smoke* (ed. A. Rodgman & T.A. Perfetti), pp. 1483–1784. Boca Raton, FL: CRC Press.

Roerecke, M. & Rehm, J. (2012). The cardioprotective association of average alcohol consumption and ischaemic heart disease: a systematic review and meta-analysis. *Addiction*, **107**, 1246–1260.

van Rooij, I.A.L.M., Wegerif, M.J.M., Roelofs, H.M.J., et al. (2001). Smoking, genetic polymorphisms in biotransformation enzymes, and nonsyndromic oral clefting: a gene-environment interaction. *Epidemiology*, **12**, 502–507.

Room, R., Bondy, S., & Ferris, J. (1995). Risk of harm to oneself from drinking, Canada 1989. *Addiction*, **90**, 499–513.

Room, R., Fischer, B., Hall, W., Lenton, S., & Reuter, P. (2010). *Cannabis Policy: Moving Beyond Stalemate*. Oxford: Oxford University Press.

Rossow, I. (1996). Alcohol related violence: the impact of drinking pattern and drinking context. *Addiction*, **91**, 1651–1661.

Rota, M., Pasquali, E., Scotti, L., et al. (2012). Alcohol drinking and epithelial ovarian cancer risk. A systematic review and meta-analysis. *Gynecologic Oncology*, **125**, 758–763.

Rothman, K.J., Greenland, S., & Lash, T.L. (2008). *Modern Epidemiology*, 3rd edn. Philadelphia, PA: Lippincott Williams & Wilkins.

Samokhvalov, A.V., Irving, H., Mohapatra, S., & Rehm, J. (2010a). Alcohol consumption, unprovoked seizures and epilepsy: a systematic review and meta-analysis. *Epilepsia*, **51**, 1177–1184.

Samokhvalov, A.V., Irving, H.M., & Rehm, J. (2010b). Alcohol consumption as a risk factor for pneumonia: systematic review and meta-analysis. *Epidemiology and Infection*, **138**, 1789–1795.

Samokhvalov, A V., Irving, H.M., & Rehm, J. (2010c). Alcohol as a risk factor for atrial fibrillation: a systematic review and meta-analysis. *European Journal of Cardiovascular Prevention and Rehabilitation*, **17**, 706–712.

Sarkola, T., Iles, M.R., Kohlenberg-Mueller, K., & Eriksson, C.J. (2002). Ethanol, acetaldehyde, acetate, and lactate levels after alcohol intake in white men and women: effect of 4-methylpyrazole. *Alcoholism: Clinical and Experimental Research*, **26**, 239–245.

Sayette, M., Wilson, T., & Elias, M. (1993). Alcohol and aggression: a social information processing analysis. *Journal of Studies on Alcohol*, **54**, 399–407.

Schnittker, J. & John, A. (2007). Enduring stigma: the long-term effects of incarceration on health. *Journal of Health and Social Behavior*, **48**, 115–130.

Schulz, H., Brand, P., & Heyder, J. (2000). Particle deposition in the respiratory tract. In: *Particle–Lung Interactions. Lung Biology in Health and Disease Vol. 143* (ed. P. Gehr & J. Heyder), pp. 229–290. New York: Marcel Dekker.

Sellman, D. (2010). The 10 most important things known about addiction. *Addiction*, **105**, 6–13.

Shaffer, H.J. & Korn, D.A. (2002). Gambling and related mental disorders: a public health analysis. *Annual Review of Public Health*, **23**, 171–212.

Shen, H.-M., Chia, S.-E., Ni, Z.-Y., New, A.-L., Lee, B.-L., & Ong, C.-N. (1997). Detection of oxidative DNA damage in human sperm and the association with cigarette smoking. *Reproductive Toxicology*, **11**, 675–680.

Shesser, R., Jotte, R., & Olshaker, J. (1991). The contribution of impurities to the acute morbidity of illegal drug use. *American Journal of Emergency Medicine*, **9**, 336–342.

Shield, K.D., Rehm, M., Patra, J., Sornpaisarn, B., & Rehm, J. (2011). Global and country specific adult per capita consumption of alcohol, 2008. *SUCHT–Zeitschrift für Wissenschaft und Praxis/Journal of Addiction Research and Practice*, **57**, 99–117.

Shield, K.D., Gmel, G., Kehoe-Chan, T., Dawson, D.A., Grant, B.F., & Rehm, J. (2013). Mortality and potential years of life lost attributable to alcohol consumption by race and sex in the United States in 2005. *PloS ONE*, **8**(1), e51923.

Shuper, P.A., Joharchi, N., Irving, H., & Rehm, J. (2009). Alcohol as a correlate of unprotected sexual behavior among people living with HIV/AIDS: review and meta-analysis. *AIDS and Behavior*, **13**, 1021–1036.

Shuper, P.A., Neuman, M., Kanteres, F., Baliunas, D., Joharchi, N., & Rehm, J. (2010). Causal considerations on alcohol and HIV/AIDS—a systematic review. *Alcohol and Alcoholism*, **45**, 159–166.

Sierksma, A., Patel, H., Ouchi, N., et al. (2004). Effect of moderate alcohol consumption on adiponectin, tumor necrosis factor-alpha, and insulin sensitivity. *Diabetes Care*, **27**, 184–189.

Skog, O.J. (1996). Public health consequences of the J-curve hypothesis of alcohol problems. *Addiction*, **91**, 325–337.

Song, D.Y., Song, S., Song, Y., & Lee J.E. (2012). Alcohol intake and renal cell cancer risk: a meta-analysis. *British Journal of Cancer*, **106**, 1881–1890.

Sopori, M. (2002). Effects of cigarette smoke on the immune system. *Nature Reviews Immunology*, **2**, 372–377.

Sopori, M.L., Goud, N.S., & Kaplan, A.M. (1994). Effects of tobacco smoke on the immune system. In: *Immunotoxicology and Immunopharmacology* (ed. J.H. Dean, M.I. Luster, A.E. Munson, & I. Kimber), pp. 413–433. New York: Raven Press.

Spivack, S.D., Fasco, M.J., Walker, V.E., & Kaminsky, L.S. (1997). The molecular epidemiology of lung cancer. *Critical Reviews in Toxicology*, **27**, 319–365.

Stall, R. & Leigh, B. (1994). Understanding the relationship between drug or alcohol use and high risk sexual activity for HIV transmission: where do we go from here? *Addiction*, **89**, 131–134.

Stanbrook, M. (2012). Addiction is a disease: we must change our attitudes toward addicts. *Canadian Medical Association Journal*, **184**, 155.

Stewart, B.W. & Wild, C.P. (2014). *World Cancer Report 2014*. Geneva: International Agency for Research on Cancer.

Swadi, H. (1999). Individual risk factors for adolescent substance use. *Drug and Alcohol Dependence*, **55**, 209–224.

Szabo, G. & Mandrekar, P. (2009). A recent perspective on alcohol, immunity, and host defense. *Alcoholism: Clinical and Experimental Research*, **33**, 220–232.

Szabo, G., Mandrekar, P., & Catalano, D. (1995). Inhibition of superantigen-induced T-cell proliferation and monocyte IL-1a TNF and IL-6 production by acute ethanol. *Journal of Leukocyte Biology*, **58**, 342–350.

Talamini, G., Bassi, C., Falconi, M., et al. (1999). Alcohol and smoking as risk factors in chronic pancreatitis and pancreatic cancer. *Digestive Diseases and Sciences*, **44**, 1303–1311.

Tavares, L., Graça, P., Martins, O., & Asensio, M. (2005). *External and Independent Evaluation of the 'National Strategy for the Fight Against Drugs' and of the 'National Action Plan for the Fight Against Drugs and Drug Addiction –Horizon 2004'*. Lisbon: Portuguese National Institute of Public Administration.

Taylor, B., Irving, H.M., & Baliunas, D., et al. (2009). Alcohol and hypertension: gender differences in dose-response relationships determined through systematic review and meta-analysis. *Addiction*, **104**, 1981–1990.

Taylor, B., Irving, H.M., Kanteres, F., et al. (2010). The more you drink, the harder you fall: a systematic review and meta-analysis of how acute alcohol consumption and injury or collision risk increase together. *Drug and Alcohol Dependence*, **110**, 108–116.

Tomsen, S. (1997). A top night out—social protest, masculinity and the culture of drinking violence. *Journal of Criminology*, **37**, 990–1002.

Tramacere, I., Negri, E., Pelucchi, C., et al. (2012a). A meta-analysis on alcohol drinking and gastric cancer risk. *Annals of Oncology*, **23**, 28–36.

Tramacere, I., Pelucchi, C., Bonifazi, M., et al. (2012b). A meta-analysis on alcohol drinking and the risk of Hodgkin lymphoma. *European Journal of Cancer Prevention*, **21**, 268–273.

Tramacere, I., Pelucchi, C., Bonifazi, M., et al. (2012c). Alcohol drinking and non-Hodgkin lymphoma risk: a systematic review and a meta-analysis. *Annals of Oncology*, **23**, 2791–2798.

Tramacere, I., Pelucchi, C., Bonifazi, M., et al. (2012d). A meta-analysis on alcohol drinking and esophageal and gastric cardia adenocarcinoma risk. *Annals of Oncology*, **23**, 287–297.

Treno, A., Gruenewald, P., & Ponicki, W. (1997). The contribution of drinking patterns to the relative risk of injury in six communities: a self-report based probability approach. *Journal of Studies on Alcohol*, **58**, 372–381.

Treno, A. & Holder, H.D. (1997). Measurement of alcohol-involved injury in community prevention: the search for a surrogate III. *Alcoholism: Clinical and Experimental Research*, **21**, 1695–1703.

Tuma, D.J. & Casey, C.A. (2003). Dangerous by-products of alcohol breakdown—focus on addicts. *Alcohol Research and Health*, **27**, 285–290.

Tyas, S.L. (2001). Alcohol use and the risk of developing Alzheimer's disease. *Alcohol Research and Health*, **25**, 299–306.

USDHHS (2000). *Tenth Special Report to the US Congress on Alcohol and Health: Highlights from Current Research*. Rockville, MD: US Department of Health and Human Services, National Institute on Alcohol Abuse and Alcoholism.

van der Vaart H., Postma, D.S., Timens, W., et al. (2005). Acute effects of cigarette smoking on inflammation in healthy intermittent smokers. *Respiratory Research*, **6**, 22.

Vonlaufen, A., Wilson, J.S., Pirola, R.C., & Apte, M.V. (2007). Role of alcohol metabolism in chronic pancreatitis. *Alcohol Research and Health*, **30**, 48–54.

Wang, H., Dwyer-Lindgren, L., Lofgren, K.T., et al. (2012). Age-specific and sex-specific mortality in 187 countries, 1970–2010: a systematic analysis for the Global Burden of Disease Study 2010. *Lancet*, **380**, 2071–2094.

Wannamethee, S.G. & Shaper, A.G. (2003). Alcohol, body weight, and weight gain in middle-aged men. *American Journal of Clinical Nutrition*, **77**, 1312–1317.

Wannamethee, S.G., Camargo, C.A. Jr, Manson, J.E., et al. (2003). Alcohol drinking patterns and risk of type 2 diabetes mellitus among younger women. *Archives of Internal Medicine*, **163**, 1329–1336.

Washburne, C. (1956). Alcohol, self and the group. *Quarterly Journal of Studies on Alcohol*, **12**, 108–123.

Wells, S. & Graham, K. (1999). The frequency of third-party involvement in incidents of barroom aggression. *Contemporary Drug Problems*, **26**, 457–480.

Wells, S. & Graham, K. (2003). Aggression involving alcohol: relationship to drinking patterns and social context. *Addiction*, **98**, 33–42.

Wells, S., Graham, K., & West, P. (2000). Alcohol-related aggression in the general population. *Journal of Studies on Alcohol*, **61**, 626–632.

Wilkins, C. & Casswell, S. (2002). The cannabis black market and the case for the legalisation of cannabis in New Zealand. *Social Policy Journal of New Zealand*, **18**, 31–43.

Willi, C., Bodenmann, P., Ghali, W.A., Faris, P.D., & Cornuz, J. (2007). Active smoking and the risk of type 2 diabetes: a systematic review and meta-analysis. *Journal of the American Medical Association*, **298**, 2654–2664.

Wimalasena, J. (1994). Ethanol has direct effects on human choriocarcinoma cell steroid hormone secretion. *Alcoholism: Clinical and Experimental Research*, **18**, 369–374.

World Health Organization (2008). *The Global Burden of Disease: 2004 Update*. Geneva: World Health Organization.

World Health Organization (2010). *Equity, Social Determinants and Public Health Programmes*. Geneva: World Health Organization.

World Health Organization (2011). *Prevention and Control of NCDs: Priorities for Investment*. Geneva: World Health Organization.

World Health Organization (2013). *WHO Report on the Global Tobacco Epidemic 2013: Enforcing Bans on Tobacco Advertising, Promotion and Sponsorship*. Geneva: World Health Organization.

Xie, X.T., Liu, Q., Wu, J., & Wakui, M.(2009). Impact of cigarette smoking in type 2 diabetes development. *Acta Pharmacologica Sinica*, **30**, 784–787.

Zakhari, S. (1997). Alcohol and the cardiovascular system: molecular mechanisms for beneficial and harmful action. *Alcohol Health and Research World*, **21**, 21–29.

Zaridze, D., Lewington, S., Boroda, A., et al. (2014). Alcohol and mortality in Russia: prospective observational study of 151 000 adults. *Lancet*, **383**, 1465–1473.

Zhang, P., Bagby, G.J., Happel, K.I., et al. (2008). Alcohol abuse, immunosuppression, and pulmonary infection. *Current Drug Abuse Reviews*, **1**, 56–67.

Chapter 6

Drug and alcohol policy for European youth: current evidence and recommendations for integrated policies and research strategies

Patricia J. Conrod, Angelina Brotherhood, Harry Sumnall, Fabrizio Faggiano, and Reinout Wiers

6.1 Introduction: prevalence of substance use among adolescents

Adolescence is an important developmental period for the onset of substance use and related harm, with 50% of American high-school students reporting binge-drinking and up to 25% saying they have tried an illicit substance (Office of National Statistics, 2008). Canadian statistics show that more than 60% of users of illegal drugs are aged 15–24 years and that, depending on the province, 19–30% of 12–18-year-olds report binge-drinking in the past month and 17–32% have used cannabis in the past year (Young et al., 2011). Trends across European countries are similar, with 39% of 15–16-year-olds reporting binge-drinking in the past month and 17% having consumed cannabis in the past year (Hibell et al., 2012). Adolescent binge-drinking, alcohol intoxication, and illicit drug use appear to be on the rise worldwide (WHO, 2011). More troubling still are results showing that the age of onset of alcohol use has been decreasing globally over the last 35 years, with youngsters now beginning to drink at an average age of 12 years (Johnston et al., 2011), and 50% of all adult substance use disorders have their onset by 15 years of age (Merikangas et al., 2010). However, very recent trends in annual prevalence data from the United States and Europe suggest that the prevalence of illicit drug use might have declined in recent years (e.g. Hale and Viner, 2013).

6.2 **Consequences of adolescent substance use**

Early exposure to alcohol and illicit substances is associated with a plethora of short- and long-term negative consequences. These include school drop-out, higher risk for assault, suicide, homicide, alcohol poisoning, behavioural and mental-health problems, with alcohol-use and its consequences accounting for almost 4% of the global burden of health (World Health Organization, 2011). Onset of alcohol use before 14 years of age is strongly associated with increased risk of developing alcohol-use disorders, with rates of adult alcohol dependence in this early onset group estimated at 40% (Grant and Dawson, 1998). It should be noted that this relationship is mediated by early drunkenness, i.e. drinking small quantities of alcohol at an early age is in itself not related to averse outcomes, only when it leads to early drunkenness (Kuntsche et al., 2013). Similarly, earlier onset of cannabis use has been associated with elevated risk for addiction as well as additional cognitive and psychiatric problems (Meier et al., 2012).

Current theories of how early onset substance use impacts on future risk include: (1) early onset reflecting a marker for future problems, (2) early substance use having neurotoxic effects on the developing brain, which can induce functional and structural changes and neuropsychological deficits (Brown, et al., 2000; Tapert et al., 2005); and (3) intereference with the development of normal socialization processes (Botvin, 2000). Regarding the first mechanism, there is ample evidence that traits related to lack of behavioural control and impulsivity predict both an early onset of drinking and of future problems (Verdejo-Garcia et al., 2008; Castellanos-Ryan et al., 2013). Regarding the second mechanism, there is an emerging literature of animal (Crews and Boettinger, 2009; Nasrallah et al., 2009) and human research (Maurage et al., 2012, 2013; Thomson et al., 2012; Hermens et al., 2013) indicating brain damage after frequent heavy episodic drinking or binge-drinking with multiple detoxifications. Identifying those factors in childhood and adolescence that are related to early heavy use of substances, which can be targeted in early prevention strategies, is thus essential given the sensitivity of the adolescent brain to such substances, as well as the serious consequences and global burden that substance use entails.

6.3 **Risk factors for adolescent substance use and related harm**

Numerous risk and protective factors have been implicated in substance use and related harm of young people (Hawkins et al., 1992; Spooner et al., 1996; Swadi, 1999; Brook et al., 2003; Loxley et al., 2004; Stockwell et al., 2004; Frisher et al., 2007) and include: (1) genetic and familial factors (predispositions to drug use); (2) environmental/contextual factors (broad societal and cultural factors) (Hawkins et al., 1992; Spooner et al., 1996; Loxley et al., 2004; Stockwell et al., 2004; Frisher et al., 2007); and (3) individual factors (characteristics within individuals and their interpersonal environments).

Twin and adoption studies reveal a robust genetic component in alcohol, cannabis, opiate, cocaine, and tobacco addictions, suggesting that a genetic predisposition to substance use problems and addictions are probable (Hawkins et al., 1992; Spooner et al., 1996; Lynskey et al., 2002; Loxley et al., 2004; Volkow and Li 2007).

Environmental and contextual factors also play a role in influencing drug use by socially influencing initiation into drugs and certain drug practices (Bandura, 1977; Botvin, 2000). Accordingly, social acceptability and permissiveness are good predictors of prevalence of use (Tyas and Pederson, 1998) and explain why environmental factors such as peer influence (Oetting and Lynch, 2003; Kuntsche and Delgrande Jordon, 2006), family, and societal norms (Hawkins et al., 1992; Spooner et al., 1996; Loxley et al., 2004; Stockwell et al., 2004) are such strong predictors of drug and alcohol use and related harm in young people.

A number of individual-level factors have been identified which are often considered as intermediate risk factors within the context of genetic or environmental predisposition to alcohol- and drug-related harm. Although the onset of most problems relating to substance use is typically in late adolescence or early adulthood, there is consistent evidence that they have their developmental origins in childhood and/or early adolescence. Associations between substance-related harm and other mental health disorders have been reported in a number of large-scale epidemiological studies, and co-morbidity between substance-related harm and internalizing or externalizing problems is common. Many disorders have been shown to pre-date substance-related harm, and thus are considered to be risk factors. Externalizing problems in childhood are often associated with substance-related harm in adolescence (Giancola, 2007), with some studies suggesting a common underlying aetiology (Castellanos-Ryan and Conrod, 2011), including common genetic factors (Slutske et al., 1998). Of these externalizing problems in childhood, conduct disorder is the most consistent predictor of later substance-related harm (Pardini et al., 2007). Attention deficit/hyperactivity disorder has also been associated with adolescent substance use, although some suggest this is largely due to the co-occurrence of symptoms of conduct disorder or deficits in executive function (Dawes et al., 2000). On the internalizing spectrum, individuals who experience depressed mood and/or anxiety drink more, and more often. The few studies that have examined the prospective link between childhood depression and adolescent substance use show that children with high negative affect, depression, or symptoms of anxiety are more likely to experience problems with alcohol (Cooper et al., 2003).

6.3.1 **The four-factor model of personality, vulnerability to addiction, and co-occurring mental disorders**

Personality traits are related to the onset of substance-related harm, substance use disorders, and to some extent their co-occurring psychological disorders. Personality traits appear to be related to substance-related harm through different motivational processes, as well as to different patterns of substance use and related harm. Hopelessness and anxiety–sensitivity are associated with problems with substance use and alcohol, and individuals with elevated levels of these traits use substances in order to regulate a negative affective state, for example to cope with depression (Grant et al., 2007). Personality traits have been shown to moderate the association between psychopathology and alcohol use, with individuals having high levels of hopelessness and depressive symptoms, as well as those with high levels of anxiety–sensitivity and anxiety, showing a more rapid increase in alcohol use across adolescence (Mackie et al., 2011). Anxiety–sensitivity has been consistently associated with self-medication motivations for substance use and increased substance use in adults, and with telescoping to alcohol dependence, despite being associated with later onset and less heavy use in teenagers (Castellanos-Ryan et al., 2013). It is understood as a risk factor for a rapidly spiralling and difficult-to-treat form of substance-related harm that co-occurs with panic anxiety (see Stewart and Conrod, 2008).

Disinhibition/impulsivity has often been associated with the consumption of a range of different substances and, importantly, with early onset and experimentation (Castellanos-Ryan et al., 2013). Impulsivity is associated with increased emotional reactivity and conduct/externalizing problems in general, and may even account for a proportion of the co-morbidity between problems with substance use and conduct disorder (Castellanos-Ryan and Conrod, 2011, 2012). Sensation-seeking has also been frequently associated with adolescent alcohol use, binge-drinking, and, somewhat less consistently, with drug use (Krank et al., 2011). Individuals high in sensation-seeking generally use substances for enhancement motives (Cooper et al., 1995) and show a specific sensitivity to reward (Castellanos-Ryan et al., 2011), including drug-induced reward (Leyton et al., 2002), which often results in developing patterns of substance use to enhance psychostimulation (e.g. binge-drinking). This literature, recently reviewed by Castellanos-Ryan and Conrod (2012), suggests that there are four motivational pathways to substance-related harm that concurrently predispose to other mental health problems. This theoretical framework is helpful in understanding how vulnerability factors at the individual level interact with major developmental processes and specific pharmacological effects of substances of abuse to increase the risk for addiction. Note that while the emphasis in this approach is on pre-morbid personality risk factors for addiction, some risk factors may mediate others, such as genetic factors (e.g. Laucht et al., 2007) and environmental factors such as trauma or peer violence (e.g. Topper et al., 2011). Furthermore, these risk factors, such as impulsivity, may be further enhanced through early heavy drinking (Nasrallah et al., 2009; White et al., 2011). It is within the context of this framework that treatment and prevention approaches should be targeting underlying processes of risk for addiction and co-morbid mental health problems. This approach would also provide an opportunity to concurrently address vulnerability to substance-related harm and co-occurring mental health problems early in a youth's trajectory of risk.

6.4 Prevention and intervention approaches

It is not easy to develop a rational and evidence-based approach to addiction-related issues among young people. Many current drug policies have failed to understand the complexities of youth behaviours and addiction and the different and competing interests related to them, such as consumer choice, harm prevention, and regulatory alternatives. A series of activities were carried out between 2011 and 2013, including: an overview of EU policy documents relating to the four behaviours of interest; an online survey with policy experts in 20 European countries; the development of a framework of policies and interventions; a systematic review of reviews on the effectiveness of potential policies and interventions; a review of existing policy scales and indices; and the development of a policy evaluation framework (Brotherhood et al., 2013). A summary of findings from the policy mapping exercise and systematic review of reviews are presented in the following subsections.

6.4.1 Policy mapping and review

A structured online questionnaire was sent to policy experts in 32 European countries to identify components targeted at young people in Member State policies. Policy experts from 20 countries provided information on national or regional policy documents on alcohol, tobacco, illegal drugs, or gambling. Respondents included academics, civil servants, and individuals working with European Monitoring Centre for Drugs and Drug Addiction (EMCDDA) Focal Points. Findings from the survey suggested that few addiction policies specific to young people have been developed, and they generally form a subcomponent of addiction or substance use policies for the general population. Policy development was seen by experts as a process of negotiation between a variety of stakeholders, including industry representatives; but it appeared that young people were not usually involved in this process, although there were some exceptions where young people or advocacy groups had been consulted. Activities were delivered across multiple modalities, although prevention programmes and age restrictions on the access to goods were reported as the main approaches for addressing young people's addictive behaviours with regard to legal substances. For illegal drugs, the emphasis was on prevention and treatment, although specific programmes and approaches were rarely identified. The complexity of funding mechanisms made it difficult to determine the value of resources allocated to policies and programmes addressing young people's addictive behaviours, and it was often difficult to differentiate those approaches which specifically targeted addictive behaviours from those which aimed to support health and social development in general, although the two were often linked.

The effects of substance use policies were perceived positively by many respondents, even though evaluations of the impacts of policy on health and behaviour were rarely reported, either by experimental or statistical modelling techniques. Where identified, evaluations tended to focus on individual policy components, such as prevention programmes, rather than the combined effects of policy across multiple modalities and with important moderating contextual factors (Weiner et al., 2012). This was unsurprising, as methodologies for the evaluation of systems of policy activity are underdeveloped (Sussman et al., 2013) (see also Section 6.5.4). As responses to the determinants for and impact of young people's addictive behaviours are increasingly spread across a wide variety of policy areas (e.g. family, health, education, justice, business, social welfare) it is important that frameworks for modelling how they interact in mutually reinforcing ways are developed.

6.4.2 Review of reviews

A systematic review of reviews was also conducted to assess the effectiveness of policy options for addressing young people's addictive behaviours, with an emphasis on the approaches identified through policy mapping. *High-quality* systematic reviews of quantitative primary studies evaluating the effectiveness of policies or interventions were included if: they were written in English, reported separate data for young people aged 25 years or under, reviewed a policy or intervention approach addressing substance use (alcohol, tobacco, illegal drugs) or gambling, or related health and social harms, and reported behavioural outcomes (outcomes such as knowledge and attitudes) in young people related to substance use or gambling (gambling not reported here). Whist natural experiments were included, statistical modelling studies and epidemiological approaches were not. Searches were conducted using a number of electronic databases (MEDLINE, PsycINFO, Cochrane Library; for 2000–2012), and supplemented by hand searches up until March 2013. Of the 2960 unique publications identified through these searches, 65 high-quality reviews met the inclusion criteria. 'Quality' was determined through use of the A MeaSurement Tool to Assess systematic Reviews (AMSTAR) instrument (Shea et al., 2007). This tool assesses the methodological quality and completeness of reporting of a systematic review and supports assessment of publication bias. The quality threshold established by the tool is high, and may be considered analogous to the assessment of study quality used in Cochrane Reviews (Higgins and Green, 2011).

A bespoke framework of policies and interventions was developed using data from the surveys and a literature search to review and synthesize the evidence, comprising 11 broad approaches: (1) control and regulation of supply; (2) gambling/substance-free zones; (3) age limits; (4) taxation and pricing; (5) control and regulation of advertising, marketing and sponsorship; (6) warning labels; (7) prevention programmes; (8) treatment and social reintegration; (9) harm reduction; (10) general delivery structures and quality assurance measures; and (11) general approaches

The included review-level evidence concentrated on three areas: prevention, treatment, and harm reduction (mostly interventions to address the potential harms to children resulting from parental participation in addictive behaviours, rather than reduction of harm in young drug users). Despite the extensive research undertaken in these areas, there was little high-quality evidence (according to the AMSTAR tool) to conclude 'what works' to address young people's addictive behaviours. The conclusions of the review are briefly summarized in this chapter. Readers should note that the absence of a particular approach in this summary does not necessarily reflect a lack of high-quality individual studies in that area but a lack of high-quality review-level evidence. Furthermore, from this review-level body of evidence it was easier to identify ineffective approaches than effective ones.

6.4.3 **Prevention**

Mass media campaigns should only be delivered as part of multi-component programmes to support school-based prevention; standalone mass media campaigns on illegal drug use were at best ineffective and at worst associated with increased drug use. With regard to school-based prevention, the provision of information alone was not considered to be an effective strategy, but skills development programmes were found to prevent use of alcohol, tobacco, and some types of illegal drugs (we expand on these findings in Section 6.4).

6.4.4 **Treatment**

The evidence on the effectiveness of psychosocial treatment approaches for addictive behaviours in young people was inconclusive; some evidence suggested that cognitive behavioural therapy (CBT), when delivered in combination with other interventions and certain types of family-based therapy, may be effective in reducing substance use. Overall, there was insufficient evidence to judge the effectiveness of pharmacological treatment for the use of alcohol and illegal drugs; pharmacological approaches appeared to be ineffective for smoking cessation in young people.

6.4.5 **Harm reduction**

Non-pharmacological interventions for cessation of smoking in pregnancy were effective in improving birth weight and reducing the likelihood of pre-term birth. Server liability laws and graduated driver licensing may be effective in reducing motor vehicle crashes among young drivers, but the applicability of these findings to contemporary Europe is questionable.

6.4.6 **General approaches**

There was limited evidence to suggest that developmental interventions in pre-school can have beneficial effects on tobacco and cannabis use in adult life; and there was conflicting evidence regarding the effects of non-drug-specific home visits on child outcomes and the effects of developmental interventions in pre-school on alcohol use in adult life.

6.5 **Evidence-based psychosocial interventions**

6.5.1 **Universal prevention**

Most prevention approaches for substance-related harm that focus on individuals are universal in nature, with strategies targeting risk factors for drinking and drug use directly. Many universal approaches based on knowledge, social norms, or social competences have been shown to be ineffective (Faggiano et al., 2005; Foxcroft and Tsertsvadze, 2011). Nevertheless, a recent review of school-based universal prevention has identified a number of effective programmes, all of which incorporate a social influence and social competence approach to prevention (Foxcroft and Tsertsvadze, 2011). These include LifeSkills Training (Botvin et al. 2001, 2003), the Unplugged programme (Faggiano et al., 2005, 2008), the Climate Schools programme (Newton et al., 2009a,b, 2010; Vogl et al., 2009), and the Good Behaviour game (van Lier et al., 2009). Regardless of the approach, the effective components of school-based prevention programmes are the same.

Reviews have consistently established that school-based prevention can result in significant increases in knowledge about substances and improved attitudes towards substance use (Hansen, 1992; Tobler et al., 1999, 2000; Botvin, 2000; Roona et al., 2000; Midford et al., 2001; Soole et al., 2005; Botvin and Griffin, 2007; Faggiano et al., 2008). However, these programmes only appear to be able to consistently reduce actual substance when performed in a school-based setting. Recently, Newton et al. (2011) summarized the principles that have consistently been associated with effective drug prevention programmes in schools. They must: (1) be evidence-based and theory-driven; (2) target risk factors for substance use and psychopathology; (3) be developmentally appropriate; (4) be implemented prior to the onset of harmful patterns of use; (5) be integrated into a comprehensive health education curriculum; (6) includes content that incorporates a social influence approach (provides resistance skills training and normative education) and is developmentally and experientially appropriate for young people; (7) uses peer interaction, but retains the teacher in the central role; (8) is sensitive to cultural and local attitudes; (9) provides adequate initial coverage and continued follow-up in booster sessions; and (10) is delivered using interactive teaching approaches and within an overall framework of harm minimization. Newton et al. (2011) also argued that the main barriers to evidence-based prevention education in schools are coverage, fidelity, and quality when programmes are disseminated, issues which can all be addressed through the use of new web-based technologies.

Nevertheless, specific programme formats or approaches cannot predict effectiveness, since even theoretically sound and well-implemented interventions can be ineffective or even result in iatrogenic effects (Sloboda et al., 2009). The addition of other components does not usually improve the effectiveness of the programme (Faggiano et al., 2010), but once again there are exceptions: a Dutch trial found that a classroom-based general intervention only had effects on adolescents' alcohol use in the arm where information for parents was added (Koning et al., 2009). The combined intervention had long-term effects, mediated by self-control and parental rules and attitudes about alcohol use (Koning et al., 2011, 2012). Therefore, despite having identified effective and promising universal programmes, research has yet to identify the sociocultural and individual-level factors that moderate the effects of evidence-based interventions as they are more broadly disseminated and evaluated within transdisciplinary and cross-cultural research efforts.

6.5.2 **Targeted prevention**

The selective approach involves delivering programmes to specific populations, ideally those at greatest risk for developing substance use problems or those most likely to benefit from a particular approach. Selective interventions have the advantage of allowing the focus of limited resources to be used on those most at need and have the potential to better address the individual needs of homogeneous at-risk groups (Conrod et al., 2006, 2008, 2010). Selective prevention programmes are not widely used in the field of drug and alcohol education due to a number of limitations, including lack of understanding of how risk factors translate to harm, concerns that targeted interventions might stigmatize at-risk groups, and a lack of validated research tools to reliably and feasibly identify those individuals who are at greatest risk. However, in recent years we have seen the development of assessment tools and selective prevention programmes which are showing that these ethical and practical obstacles can be overcome.

One particular prevention programme that has shown promise in the field of prevention of adolescent drug and alcohol use is the Preventure Programme, which recommends targeting four personality risk factors for early onset drinking or illicit drug use: hopelessness, anxiety–sensitivity, impulsivity, and sensation-seeking. This school-based programme has now been shown to prevent alcohol- and substance-related harm in three separate trials across Canada (Conrod et al., 2006) and the UK (Conrod et al., 2008, 2010, 2011; O'Leary-Barrett et al., 2010), and is based on a cognitive behavioural and motivational approach. This intervention is associated with a 50–60% reduction in drinking and binge-drinking rates over 6 months (O'Leary-Barrett et al., 2010), as well as 2-year reductions in symptoms of problem drinking and illicit drug use in high-risk youth (Conrod et al., 2010, 2011). Beneficial effects are found after only two brief (90-minute) group-based sessions, making this a cost-effective and practical programme to implement. Another recent trial showed that the programme can be effectively delivered by trained school-staff (O'Leary-Barrett et al., 2010). A recent analysis of the 2-year outcomes of the Adventure Effectiveness Trial showed that this targeted prevention programme produced 'herd' effects, in that the interventions indirectly resulted in less drinking behaviour in low-risk youth who simply attended schools where interventions were delivered to high-risk youth (Conrod et al., 2013). Finally, secondary analyses of this trial have shown that personality-targeted interventions also have an effect on young people's mental health outcomes, such as depression, anxiety, and conduct problems over a 2-year period (O'Leary-Barrett et al., 2013).

The Preventure Programme has been highlighted in a number of large reviews (e.g. Strang et al., 2012) as a promising strategy and an alternative to universal approaches that yield small effects. However, few reviews have explored targeted prevention programmes, and so this type of approach could not be considered in the review of reviews mentioned earlier and other systematic reviews (e.g. Foxcroft and Tsertsvadze, 2011).

6.5.3 **Dissemination of evidence-based alcohol and drug prevention**

According to the Society for Prevention Research's Standards Committee for evaluating the evidence in support of prevention programmes (Flay et al., 2005), there are a number of prevention programmes that could be considered to have adequate to high levels of evidence in support of treatment efficacy and effectiveness. This is particularly the case for personality-targeted interventions. In fact, a recent review of evidence-based youth programmes for the UK Department for Education concluded that the evidence supporting the efficacy and effectiveness of the Preventure Programme is of the highest level (6/6). Yet, when evaluated by a US-based registry (SAMHSA, 2010) the programme was positively evaluated but yielded less than perfect scores, possibly reflecting cross-cultural differences in concepts of prevention, scoring standards for evaluating the evidence base, or biases for programmes that have been evaluated within the country hosting the registry.

Despite the demonstrated efficacy and effectiveness of certain alcohol and drug prevention programmes, little research has been conducted on their broader dissemination. According to recommended criteria for broad dissemination of an evidence-based programme, a programme must be evaluated for its 'system elements' which 'contribute to adoption and sustainable programme delivery and a smoothly functioning relationship between programme developers and those responsible for dissemination in the field' (Flay et al., 2005). The first recommended criterion is a standard of effectiveness to establish that the programme can be implemented with fidelity. Validated screening and outcome scales, as well as intervention manuals and instruments that reliably measure programme fidelity, must be made available by programme developers. The two evidence-based prevention programmes that have been most widely studied in Europe (the Unplugged and Preventure programmes) have been shown to effectively help teachers and school staff deliver the programme in the way that the programmes were originally validated with highly trained research psychologists or staff (Faggiano et al., 2010; O'Leary-Barrett et al., 2010; Conrod et al., 2013). The second 'going to scale' criterion highlights the need to make all necessary materials available and have a feasible and affordable system for providing intervention material, supervision, evaluation, and technical assistance when implementing the programme. This criterion is always provided in the context of a rigorous research study, but is rarely available to schools and communities outside the research context. 'Cost information' is another recommended criterion for evaluating broad dissemination, in which the programme must be evaluated in terms of clear financial and staff resources required for programme delivery, as well as the relative impact and benefits of these costs, to guide policy-makers and others involved in the promotion of the programme. The fourth criterion is 'ongoing monitoring and evaluation', so that broad implementation can be evaluated for its impact and the conditions under which implementation is more or less effective. Research on evidence-based prevention programmes in Europe is currently lacking in regards to these last three criteria. Large and integrated research efforts are required for these criteria to be met.

6.5.4 Systems approach to prevention

Recently researchers have moved towards a more 'systems' perspective for promoting prevention programmes for chronic diseases. In a recent report by Dubé (2010), the case was made not only for accumulating economic data and building more models for chronic disease prevention, but also for identifying and encouraging other agents for change in both health and non-health sectors to improve the health and economic impacts of prevention. These players can provide both barriers to change and solutions, and it is important to understand how individual-level vulnerability to addiction and the effects of targeted prevention interact with macro- and micro-level agents of change. What is needed in prevention is cross-cultural research initiatives to support the identification and understanding of potential agents of change, within and outside the health sector, and how they interact with each other to promote effective delivery of drug and alcohol prevention. Within this framework, biologically determined motivational factors at the individual level, such as impulsivity and reward sensitivity, are robustly implicated in the vulnerability to early onset substance-related harm (e.g. Castellanos-Ryan et al. 2011; Nees et al., 2011; Whelan et al., 2012). Motivational factors at the social and political level, for example implicit marketing strategies or laws restricting availability, are theorized as interacting with individual-level variables to either push those at risk towards substance use or to help such individuals to navigate their risk in healthier environments. However, little empirical research has been conducted across these levels of investigation.

A number of large, European-based cohort studies investigating risk factors for drug and alcohol related harm, for example the European Commission-funded IMAGEN study (Schumann et al., 2010; <http://www.imagen-europe.com/index.php>) and ALICE-RAP (<http://www.alicerap.eu/>) are providing important insights into the cultural, genetic, and neural factors underlying personality and cognitive risk factors for addiction (e.g. Castellanos-Ryan et al., 2011; Nees et al., 2011; Whelan et al., 2012). The findings from all these studies suggest that impulsivity is a multifaceted construct, regulated by several fronto-striatal regions of the brain, and is implicated in a number of externalizing behaviours, including substance-related harm in adolescence. They also suggest that certain regions of the brain may be more susceptible to the effects of early exposure to alcohol and drugs (e.g. Whelan et al., 2012). Many of these cohort studies are embedded within different sociopolitical systems that allow for analysis of how risk factors and brief interventions impact on risk for addiction in interaction with different social and political agents. For example, the focus of some of the ALICE-RAP youth-oriented studies will be to explore the impact of impulsivity and reward sensitivity on alcohol initiation across countries that have different legal drinking ages, or that have different policies regarding the targeting of advertising at young people. New targeted intervention strategies will also be explored which better address the sociocultural and political situation of a particular population. For example, impulsive youth might benefit from specific media training to better resist the influences of the media on their drinking in contexts where advertising laws or legal drinking ages are more liberal.

6.5.5 Cultural and biological influences on automatic attitudes to drugs and alcohol

Embedded within the European Commission FP7-funded ALICE-RAP project is a study which will assess over 500,000 young people using a web-based platform that reliably measures individual-level risk factors (e.g. personality and approach tendencies towards addiction-related stimuli). Using this platform, researchers will investigate how specific social and political agents that differ across European countries impact on young people's attitudes and behaviours. One exceptional feature of this study is that it will measure implicit or automatic attitudes, in addition to explicit attitudes, which have both been shown to robustly and independently predict future drug and alcohol-related behaviours (see Rooke et al. (2008) for a meta-analysis and Wiers et al. (2013) for a recent review). First, this exceptionally large study will examine how cross-cultural differences in the acceptability of drunkenness contribute to youth binge-drinking in interaction with individual-level variables such as impulsivity and sensation seeking. Specifically, this study will investigate how cultural differences in media portrayals of drunkenness influence implicit attitudes towards intoxicated behaviour and how impulsivity and sensation seeking might interact with these influences to exacerbate automatic approach tendencies towards intoxication cues. The second year of this project will examine how automatic attitudes around cannabis as a 'herb' or 'drug' influence drug-taking behaviour and how such processes are mediated or moderated by different national drug policies. One promising avenue for future research is that recent interventions which directly target implicit or automatic alcohol-related cognitions have shown great promise in alcohol-dependent adult patients—they have replicated a 10% reduction in the chance of relapse 1 year later (Wiers et al., 2011; Eberl et al., 2013; review in Wiers et al., 2013). These interventions will go on to be tested for the first time in adolescents.

6.5.6 Sociopolitical moderators of evidence-based prevention

Another programme of research is compiling data from several large-scale prevention trials with the aim of identifying the active ingredients of evidence-based programmes and the different social, economic, and political systems that moderate their effectiveness. Through this project and the many ongoing trials of universal and targeted skills-based prevention programmes around the world, there will be a unique opportunity to examine specific moderators of the efficacy of interventions which can be measured at the individual level (e.g. impulsivity), at the social level (e.g. number of antisocial peers, acceptability of drunkenness or underage drinking), and the political level (e.g. laws aimed at reducing antisocial behaviours, legal drinking age, local advertising laws).

6.6 Challenges to evidence-based addiction policy for young people

As shown through the mapping and systematic review of reviews conducted here, there is little review-level evidence to suggest that the approaches currently adopted and delivered by many EU Member States to address young people's addictive behaviours are supported by high-quality evidence. Although some individual policies and programmes show beneficial effects on some addictive behaviour outcomes, it is not currently possible to generalize beyond implementation of specific interventions to recommend any broad policy approaches based upon the underpinning principles of these programmes. Currently, recommendations with regard to effective approaches for addressing young people's addictive behaviours can only be made with reference to 'promising' approaches, rather than approaches that have been proven to be effective. A further challenge lies in the need to balance the development of the prevention evidence base in order to improve its quality, with popular, feasible, and desirable policy demands in the real world. For example, several influential studies and narrative reviews suggest that young people are sensitive to alcohol pricing (e.g. Chaloupka et al., 2002; Booth et al., 2008; Babor et al., 2010), and there is strong advocacy for these types of policies in several European countries, but recent high-quality systematic reviews of natural experiments or evaluations of policy initiatives are lacking (see Wagenaar et al. (2009) for an example of a recent high-quality meta-analysis in adult drinkers).

In our final section we present the some recommendations for beginning to address some of these challenges.

6.7 Recommendations for policy and decision makers

1 Ensure the availability of well-formulated policy documents (e.g. a national strategy, action plan) developed in line with evidence and international good practice recommendations. There is a need for dedicated policies for tobacco use and gambling in young people, and respective policies could be modelled on those already available for alcohol and illegal drugs.

2 In addition to identifying effective interventions and approaches there is also a need to develop the systems required for the successful *implementation* of effective prevention policies and interventions.

3 We must acknowledge that many current activities and proposals rely on an incomplete evidence base of effectiveness and implementation and that careful consideration must be given to the activities being implemented, including unintended effects and opportunity costs (e.g. if new investments are made in one activity, then how does this affect [the financial security of] other activities?).

4 Where evidence suggests that actions are ineffective or have iatrogenic effects, policy-makers should seek to understand whether modifying these programmes in line with good practice recommendations would lead to an increased likelihood of success (e.g. becoming more effective for a targeted group, or when delivered in combination with another intervention approach). All modifications should be accompanied by consideration of the ethics of intervention, and rigorous research into the effects of changing an activity. Policy-makers should disinvest in approaches which have been consistently shown to have no beneficial effect.

5 Where evidence of effectiveness is unclear, policies and interventions should be implemented only as part of sufficiently funded scientific research projects to evaluate the effectiveness of these actions using robust research methodologies.

In order to help the development of evidence-based addictions policies for young people, researchers should also consider the following recommendations:

1 Where primary studies are available but high-quality reviews are lacking, the available evidence should be synthesized in well-documented systematic reviews. Meta-analyses, in particular, should take into account the heterogeneity of interventions.

2 Where no or few primary studies are available and evidence is needed to inform policy-making, primary studies should be conducted using the most rigorous study designs possible, preferably under real-world conditions. Research trials should, where possible, adopt a realistic approach to identifying the effectiveness of an intervention, seeking to understand mechanisms of change, differential outcomes for subpopulations, and the effects of context and complex systems on outcomes.

3 In effectiveness trials, the focus should be on behavioural outcomes rather than process data or mediators. Although in some cases interventions may address factors that are distal, and so preclude measurement of final outcomes (i.e. behavioural outcomes in young people), in many studies data collection appears to focus on process data or mediators, although behavioural outcomes in young people could also be measured (e.g. success of restrictions on tobacco sales measured via test purchasing only; success of gambling interventions measured as changes in knowledge or attitudes). Careful consideration should also be made of the choice of primary and secondary outcomes for interventions research. Although some interventions aim to address important policy targets (e.g. lifetime use of substances), outcomes should be chosen because of a robust prediction of meaningful health or social outcomes rather than the political priority of the behaviour.

4 Researchers should invest in data-pooling exercises, either through meta-analysis or mega-analysis (e.g. pooling datasets) to examine how cross differences in drug and alcohol policies impact on programme effectiveness.

5 Consider (and report) the effects of policies and interventions on young people, including (as appropriate) children, adolescents, and young adults; not just when policies and interventions are specifically targeted at young people (e.g. how do changes to adult welfare systems affect young people's use of substances in affected families?).

Acknowledgements

This chapter has been produced with the financial support of the European Union through the Seventh Framework Programme (FP7/2007–2013), under grant agreement no. 266,813 [Addictions and Lifestyle in Contemporary Europe—Reframing Addictions Project (ALICE RAP)]. Participating organizations in ALICE RAP can be seen at <http://www.alicerap.eu/about-alicerap/partner-institutions.html>. The contents of this chapter are the sole responsibility of the authors and can in no way be taken to reflect the views of the European Union or the wider ALICE RAP partnership.

References

Babor, T.F., Caetano, R., Casswell, S., et al. (2010). *Alcohol: No Ordinary Commodity. Research and Public Policy.* Oxford: Oxford University Press.

Bandura, A. (1977). *Social Learning Theory.* Englewood Cliffs, NJ: Prentice Hall.

Booth, A., Stockwell, T., Sutton, A., et al. (2008). *Independent Review of the Effects of Alcohol Pricing and Promotion, Part A: Systematic Reviews.* Project Report for the Department of Health. University of Sheffield, UK. URL: <http://www.sheffield.ac.uk/polopoly_fs/1.95617!/file/PartA.pdf>

Botvin, G.J. (2000). Preventing drug abuse in schools: Social and competence enhancement approaches targeting individual-level etiologic factors. *Addictive Behaviors,* **25,** 887–897.

Botvin, G.J. & Griffin, K.W. (2007). School-based programmes to prevent alcohol, tobacco and other drug use. *International Review of Psychiatry,* **19,** 607–615.

Botvin, G.J., Griffin, K.W., Diaz, T., & Ifill-Williams, M. (2001). Preventing binge drinking during early adolescence: one- and two-year follow-up of a school-based preventive intervention. *Psychology of Addictive Behaviours,* **15,** 360–365.

Botvin, G.J., Griffin, K.W., Paul, E., & Macaulay, A.P. (2003). Preventing tobacco and alcohol use among elementary school students through life skills training. *Journal of Child and Adolescent Substance Abuse,* **12,** 1–17.

Brook, J.S., Brook, D.W., Richter, L., & Whiteman, M (2003). Risk and protective factors of adolescent drug use: Implications for prevention programs. In: *Handbook of Drug Abuse Prevention: Theory, Science and Practice* (ed. Z. Sloboda & W.J. Bukoski). New York: Kluwer Academic/Plenum Publishers, 265–282.

Brotherhood, A., Atkinson, A.M., Bates, G., & Sumnall, H.R. (2013). Adolescents as customers of addiction. ALICE RAP Deliverable 16.1, Work Package 16. Liverpool: Liverpool Centre for Public Health.

Brown, S.A., Tapert, S.F., Granholm, E., & Delis, D.C. (2000). Neurocognitive functioning of adolescents: effects of protracted alcohol use. *Alcoholism: Clinical and Experimental Research,* **24,** 164–171.

Castellanos-Ryan, N. & Conrod, P.J. (2011). Personality correlates of the common and unique variance across conduct disorder and substance related harm symptoms in adolescence. *Journal of Abnormal Child Psychology,* **39,** 536–576.

Castellanos-Ryan, N., Rubia, K., & Conrod, P.J. (2011). Response inhibition and reward response bias mediate the predictive relationships between impulsivity and sensation seeking and common and unique variance in conduct disorder and substance related harm. *Alcoholism, Clinical and Experimental Research,* **35,** 140–155.

Castellanos-Ryan, N., O'Leary-Barrett, M., Sully, L., & Conrod, P. (2013). Sensitivity and specific of a brief personality screening instrument in predicting future substance use, emotional and behavioral problems. 18-month predictive validity of the Substance Use Risk Profile Scale. *Alcoholism, Clinical and Experimental Research,* **37(Suppl. 1),** E281–E290.

Chaloupka, F.J., Grossman, M., & Saffer, H. (2002). The effects of price on alcohol consumption and alcohol-related problems. *Alcohol Research and Health,* **26,** 22–34.

Conrod, P., Stewart, S.H., Comeau, N., & Maclean, A.M. (2006). Preventative efficacy of cognitive behavioural strategies matched to the motivational bases of alcohol related harm in at-risk youth. *Journal of Clinical Child Adolescent Psychology,* **35,** 550–563.

Conrod, P.J., Castellanos, N., & Mackie, C. (2008). Personality-targeted interventions delay the growth of adolescent drinking and binge drinking. *Journal of Child Psychology and Psychiatry*, **49**, 181–190.

Conrod, P.J., Castellanos-Ryan, N., & Strang, J. (2010). Brief, personality-targeted coping skills interventions and survival as a non-drug user over a 2-year period during adolescence. *Archives of General Psychiatry*, **67**, 85–93.

Conrod, P.J., Castellanos-Ryan, N., & Mackie, C. (2011). Long-term effects of a personality-targeted intervention to reduce alcohol use in adolescents. *Journal of Consulting and Clinical Psychology*, **79**, 296–306.

Conrod, P.J., O'Leary-Barrett, M., Newton, N., et al. (2013). Effectiveness of a selective, personality-targeted prevention program for adolescent alcohol use and related harm: a cluster randomized controlled trial. *JAMA Psychiatry*, **70**, 334–342.

Cooper, M.L., Frone, M.R., Russell, M., & Mudar, P. (1995). Drinking to regulate positive and negative emotions: a motivational model of alcohol use. *Journal of Personality and Social Psychology*, **69**, 990–1005.

Cooper, M.L., Wood, P.K., Orcutt, H.K., & Albino, A. (2003). Personality and the predisposition to engage in risky or problem behaviours during adolescence. *Journal of Personality and Social Psychology*, **84**, 390–410.

Crews, F.T. & Boettiger, C.A. (2009). Impulsivity, frontal lobes and risk for addiction. *Pharmacology Biochemistry and Behavior*, **93**, 237–247.

Dawes, M.A., Antelman, S.M., Vanyukov, M.M., et al. (2000). Developmental sources of variation in liability to adolescent substance use disorders. *Drug and Alcohol Dependence*, **61**, 3–14.

Dubé, L. (2010). Introduction: on the brain-to-society model of motivated choice and the whole-of-society approach to obesity prevention. In: *Obesity Prevention: The Role of Brain and Society on Individual Behavior* (ed. L. Dubé, A. Bechara, A. Dagher, et al.), pp. xxiii–xxix. Amsterdam: Academic Press, Elsevier Inc.

Eberl, C., Wiers, R.W., Pawelczack, S., Rinck, M., Becker, E.S., & Lindenmeyer, J. (2013). Approach bias modification in alcohol dependence: Do clinical effects replicate and for whom does it work best? *Developmental Cognitive Neuroscience*, **4**, 38–51.

Faggiano, F., Vigna-Taglianti, F.D., Versino, E., Zambon, A., Borraccino, A., & Lemma, P. (2005). School-based prevention for illicit drugs' use. *Cochrane Database of Systematic Reviews*, **(2)**:CD003020.

Faggiano, F., Vigna-Taglianti, F.D., Versino, E., Zambon, A., Borraccino, A., & Lemma, P. (2008). School-based prevention for illicit drugs use: a systematic review. *Preventive Medicine*, **46**, 385–396.

Faggiano, F., Vigna-Taglianti, F., Burkhart, G., et al. (2010). The effectiveness of a school-based substance abuse prevention program: 18-month follow-up of the EU-Dap cluster randomized controlled trial. *Drug and Alcohol Dependence*, **108**, 56–64.

Flay, B.R., Biglan, A., Boruch, R.F., et al. (2005). Standards of evidence: criteria for efficacy, effectiveness and dissemination. *Prevention Science*, **6**, 151–175.

Foxcroft, D.R. & Tsertsvadze, A. (2011). Universal school-based prevention programs for alcohol related harm in young people. *Cochrane Database of Systematic Reviews*, **(5)**:CD009113.

Frisher, M., Crome, I. Macleod, J., Bloor, R., & Hickman, M. (2007). *Predictive Factors For Illicit Drug Use Among Young People: A Literature Review*. Home Office Online Report 05/07. URL: <http://dera.ioe.ac.uk/6903/1/rdsolr0507.pdf>

Giancola, P.R. (2007). The underlying role of aggressivity in the relation between executive functioning and alcohol consumption. *Addictive Behaviors*, **32**, 765–783.

Grant, B. F. & Dawson, D. A. (1998). Age of onset of drug use and its association with DSM-IV drug abuse and dependence: results from the national longitudinal alcohol epidemiologic survey. *Journal of Substance Abuse*, **10**, 163–173.

Grant, V.V., Stewart, S.H., Birch, C.D. (2007). Impact of positive and anxious mood on implicit alcohol-related cognitions in internally motivated undergraduate drinkers. *Addictive Behaviors*, **32**, 2226–2237.

Hale, D. & Viner,. R. (2013). Trends in the prevalence of multiple substance use in adolescents in England, 1998–2009. *Journal of Public Health (Oxford)*, **35**, 367–374.

Hansen, W.B. (1992). School-based substance abuse prevention: A review of the state of the art in curriculum, 1980-1990. *Health Education Research*, **7**, 403–430.

Hawkins, J.D., Catalano, R.F., & Miller, J.Y. (1992). Risk and protective factors for alcohol and other drug problems in adolescence and early adulthood: implications for substance abuse prevention. *Psychological Bulletin*, **112**, 64–105.

Hermens, D.F., Lagopoulos, J., Tobias-Webb, J., et al. (2013). Pathways to alcohol-induced brain impairment in young people: a review. *Cortex*, **49**(1), 3–17.

Hibell, B., Guttormsson, U., Ahlström, S., et al. (2012). *The 2011 ESPAD Report—Substance Use Among Students in 36 European Countries*. Stockholm: The Swedish Council for Information on Alcohol and Other Drugs (CAN).

Higgins, J.P.T. & Green, S. (eds). (2011). *Cochrane Handbook for Systematic Reviews of Interventions*, Version 5.1.0 [updated March 2011]. The Cochrane Collaboration. URL: <http://handbook.cochrane.org/>

Johnston, L.D., O'Malley, P.M., Bachman, J.G., & Schulenberg, J.E. (2011). *Monitoring the Future. National Results on Adolescent Drug Use. Overview of Key Findings, 2010*. Ann Arbor, MI: Institute for Social Research, The University of Michigan.

Koning, I.M., Vollebergh, W.A., Smit, F., et al. (2009). Preventing heavy alcohol use in adolescents (PAS): cluster randomized trial of a parent and student intervention offered separately and simultaneously. *Addiction*, **104**, 1669–1678.

Koning, I.M., van den Eijnden, R.J., Engels, R.C., Verdurmen, J.E., & Vollebergh, W.A. (2011). Why target early adolescents and parents in alcohol prevention? The mediating effects of self-control, rules and attitudes about alcohol use. *Addiction*, **106**, 538–546.

Koning, I.M., Verdurmen, J.E., Engels, R.C., van den Eijnden, R.J., & Vollebergh, W.A. (2012). Differential impact of a Dutch alcohol prevention program targeting adolescents and parents separately and simultaneously: low self-control and lenient parenting at baseline predict effectiveness. *Prevention Science*, **13**, 278–287.

Krank, M., Stewart, S.H., O'Connor, R., Woicik, P.B., Wall, A.M., & Conrod, P.J. (2011). Structural, concurrent, and predictive validity of the Substance Use Risk Profile Scale in early adolescence. *Addictive Behaviors*, **36**, 37–46.

Kuntsche, E. & Delgrande Jordon, M. (2006). Adolescent alcohol and cannabis use in relation to peer and school factors: results of multilevel analyses. *Drug and Alcohol Dependence*, **84**, 167–174.

Kuntsche, E., Rossow, I., Simons-Morton, B., Bogt, T.T., Kokkevi, A., & Godeau, E. (2013). Not early drinking but early drunkenness is a risk factor for problem behaviors among adolescents from 38 European and North American countries. *Alcoholism: Clinical and Experimental Research*, **37**, 308–314.

Laucht, M., Becker, K., Blomeyer, D., & Schmidt, M.H. (2007). Novelty seeking involved in mediating the association between the dopamine D4 receptor gene exon III polymorphism and heavy drinking in male adolescents: results from a high-risk community sample. *Biological Psychiatry,* **61**, 87–92.

Leyton, M., Boileau, I., Benkelfat, C., Diksic, M., Baker, G., & Dagher, A. (2002). Amphetamine-induced increases in extracellular dopamine, drug wanting, and novelty seeking: a PET/[11C]raclopride study in healthy men. *Neuropsychopharmacology,* **27**, 1027–1035.

van Lier, P.A., Huizink, A., & Crijnen, A. (2009). Impact of a preventive intervention targeting childhood disruptive behavior problems on tobacco and alcohol initiation from age 10 to 13 years. *Drug and Alcohol Dependence,* **100**, 228–233.

Loxley, W., Toumbouru, J.W., Stockwell, T., et al. (2004). *The Prevention of Substance Use, Risk and Harm in Australia: A Review of the Evidence.* Canberra: Ministerial Council on Drug Strategy.

Lynskey, M.T., Heath, A.C., Nelson, E.C., et al. (2002). Genetic and environmental contributions to cannabis dependence in a national young adult twin sample. *Psychological Medicine,* **32**, 195–207.

Mackie, C.J., Castellanos-Ryan, N., & Conrod, P.J. (2011). Personality moderates the longitudinal relationship between psychological symptoms and alcohol use in adolescents. *Alcoholism: Clinical and Experimental Research,* **35**, 703–716.

Maurage, P., Joassin, F., Speth, A., Modave, J., Philippot, P., & Campanella, S. (2012). Cerebral effects of binge drinking: respective influences of global alcohol intake and consumption pattern. *Clinical Neurophysiology,* **123**, 892–901.

Maurage, P., Petit, G., & Campanella, S. (2013). Pathways to alcohol-induced brain impairment in young people: a review by Hermens et al. 2013. *Cortex,* **49**, 1155–1159.

Meier, M.H., Caspi, A., Ambler, A., et al. (2012). Persistent cannabis users show neuropsychological decline from childhood to midlife. *Proceedings of the National Academy of Sciences of the United Staes of America,* **109**, E2657–E2664.

Merikangas, K.R., He, J.P., Burstein, M., et al. (2010). Lifetime prevalence of mental disorders in U.S. adolescents: results from the National Comorbidity Survey Replication—Adolescent Supplement (NCS-A). Journal of the American Academy of Child and Adolescent Psychiatry, **49**, 980–989.

Midford, R., Snow, P., & Lenton, S. (2001). *School-Based Illicit Drug Education Programs: A Critical Review and Analysis.* Melbourne: Department of Employment, Training and Youth Affairs, National Drug Research Institute.

Nasrallah, N.A., Yang, T.W., & Bernstein, I.L. (2009). Long-term risk preference and suboptimal decision making following adolescent alcohol use. *Proceedings of the National Academy of Sciences of the United States of America,* **106**, 17600–17604.

Nees, F., Tzschoppe, J., Patrick, C.J., et al. (2011). Determinants of early alcohol use in healthy adolescents: the differential contribution of neuroimaging and psychological factors. *Neuropsychopharmacology,* **37**, 986–995.

Newton, N.C., Andrews, G., Teesson, M., & Vogl, L.E. (2009a). Delivering prevention for alcohol and cannabis using the internet: a cluster randomised controlled trial. *Preventive Medicine,* **48**, 579–584.

Newton, N.C., Vogl, L.E., Teesson, M., & Andrews, G. (2009b). CLIMATE Schools: alcohol module: cross-validation of a school-based prevention programme for alcohol related harm. *Australian and New Zealand Journal of Psychiatry,* **43**, 201–207.

Newton, N.C., O'Leary-Barrett, M., & Conrod, P.J. (2011). Adolescent substance related harm: neurobiology and evidence based interventions. *Current Topics in Behavioural Neuroscience*, **13**, 685–708.

Oetting, E.R. & Lynch, R.S. (2003). Peers and the prevention of adolescent drug use. *Handbook of Drug Prevention: Theory, Science and Practice* (ed. Z. Sloboda & W.J. Bukoski), pp. 101–127. New York: Kluwer Academic/Plenum Publishers.

Office of National Statistics (2008). *Drug Use, Smoking and Drinking Among Young People in England in 2007*. NHS Health and Social Care Information Centre. URL: <http://www.hscic.gov.uk/pubs/sdd07fullreport>

O'Leary-Barrett, M., Mackie, C.J., Castellanos, N., et al. (2010). Personality-targeted interventions delay uptake of drinking and decrease risk of alcohol-related problems when delivered by teachers. *Journal of the American Academy of Child and Adolescent Psychiatry*, **49**, 954–963.

O'Leary-Barrett, M., Topper, L., Al-Khudhairy, N., et al. (2013). Two-year impact of personality-targeted, teacher-delivered interventions on youth internalizing and externalizing problems: a cluster-randomized trial. *Journal of the American Academy of Child and Adolescent Psychiatry*, **52**, 911–920.

Pardini, D., White, H.R., & Stouthamer-Loeber, M. (2007). Early adolescent psychopathology as a predictor of alcohol use disorders by young adulthood. *Drug and Alcohol Dependence*, **88(Suppl. 1)**, S38–S49.

Rooke, S.E., Hine, D.W., & Thorsteinsson, E.B. (2008). Implicit cognition and substance use: a meta-analysis. *Addictive Behaviors*, **33**, 1314–1328.

Roona, M.R., Streke, A.V., Ochshorn, P., Marshall, D., & Palmer, A. (2000). *Identifying Effective School-Based Substance Abuse Prevention Interventions: Background Paper for Prevention 2000 Summit*. URL: <http://www.silvergategroup.com/public/PREV2000/Roona.pdf>

SAMHSA (2010). *Results from the 2009 National Survey on Drug Use and Health: Volume I. Summary of National Findings*. NSDUH Series H-38A, HHS Publication No. SMA 10–4586 Findings. Rockville, MD, Office of Applied Studies.

Schumann, G., Loth, E., Banaschewski, T., et al. (2010). The IMAGEN study: reinforcement-related behaviour in normal brain function and psychopathology. *Molecular Psychiatry*, **15**, 1128–1139.

Shea, B., Grimshaw, J.M., Wells, G.A., et al. (2007). Development of AMSTAR: a measurement tool to assess the methodological quality of systematic reviews. *BMC Medical Research Methodology*, **7**, 10.

Sloboda, Z., Stephens, R.C., Stephens, P.C., et al. (2009). The Adolescent Substance Abuse Prevention Study: a randomized field trial of a universal substance abuse prevention program. *Drug and Alcohol Dependence*, **102**, 1–10.

Slutske, W.S., Heath, A.C., Dinwiddie, S.H., et al. (1998).Common genetic risk factors for conduct disorder and alcohol dependence. *Journal of Abnormal Psychology*, **107**, 363–374.

Soole, D.W., Mazerolle, L., & Rombouts, S. (2005). *Monograph No. 07: School Based Drug Prevention: a Systematic Review of the Effectiveness on Illicit Drug Use*. DPMP Monograph Series. Fitzroy: Turning Point Alcohol and Drug Centre.

Spooner, C., Mattick, R., & Howard, J. (1996). The nature and treatment of adolescent substance abuse. NDARC Monograph No. 26. Sydney: National Drug and Alcohol Research Centre.

Stewart, S.H. & Conrod, P.J. (2008). Anxiety disorder and substance use disorder co-morbidity: Common themes and future directions. In: *Anxiety and Substance Use Disorders: The Vicious Cycle of Comorbidity* (ed. S.H. Stewart & P.J. Conrod), pp. 239–257. New York: Springer.

Stockwell, T., Toumbourou, J.W., Letcher, P., Smart, D., Sanson, A., & Bond, L. (2004). Risk and protective factors for different intensities of adolescent substance use: when does the prevention paradox apply? *Drug and Alcohol Review*, **23**, 67–77.

Strang, J., Babor, T., Caulkins, J., Fischer, B., Foxcroft, D., & Humphreys, K. (2012) Drug policy and the public good: Evidence for effective interventions. *Lancet*, **379**, 71–83.

Sussman, S., Levy, D., Lich, K.H., et al. (2013). Comparing effects of tobacco use prevention modalities: need for complex system models. *Tobacco Induced Diseases*, **11**, 2.

Swadi, H. (1999). Individual risk factors for adolescent substance use. *Drug and Alcohol Dependence*, **55**, 209–224.

Tapert, S.F., Caldwell, L., & Burke, C. (2005). Alcohol and the adolescent brain: human studies. *Alcohol Research and Health*, **28**, 205–212.

Thomson, A.D., Guerrini, I., Bell, D., et al. (2012). Alcohol-related brain damage: report from a Medical Council on Alcohol Symposium, June 2010. *Alcohol and Alcoholism*, **47**, 84–91.

Tobler, N.S., Lassard, T., Marshall, D., Ochshorn, P., & Roona, M. (1999). Effectiveness of school-based drug prevention programs for marijuana use. *School Psychology International*, **20**, 105–137.

Tobler, N.S., Roona, M.R., Ochshorn, P., Marshall, D.G., Streke, A.V., & Stackpole, K.M. (2000). School-based adolescent drug prevention programs: 1998 meta-analysis. *Journal of Primary Prevention*, **20**, 275–336.

Topper, L.R., Castellanos-Ryan, N., Mackie, C., & Conrod, P.J.(2011). Adolescent bullying victimisation and alcohol-related problem behaviour mediated by coping drinking motives over a 12 month period. *Addictive Behaviors*, **36**, 6–13.

Tyas, S.L. & Pederson, L.L. (1998). Psychosocial factors related to adolescent smoking: a critical review of the literature. *Tobacco Control*, **7**, 409–420.

Verdejo-Garcia, A., Lawrence, A.J., & Clark, L. (2008). Impulsivity as a vulnerability marker for substance-use disorders: review of findings from high-risk research, problem gamblers and genetic association studies. *Neuroscience and Biobehavioral Reviews*, **32**, 777–810.

Vogl, L., Teesson, M., Andrews, G., Bird, K., Steadman, B., & Dillon, P. (2009). A computerised harm minimisation prevention program for alcohol related harm and related harms: randomised controlled trial. *Addiction*, **104**, 564–575.

Volkow, N.D. & Li, T.K. (2007). Drugs and alcohol: treating and preventing abuse, addiction, and their medical consequences. In: *Recognition and Prevention of Major Mental and Substance Use Disorders* (ed. M.Y. Tsuang, W.S. Stone, & M.J. Lyons), pp. 263–296. Washington, DC: American Psychiatric Publishing Inc.

Wagenaar, A.C., Salois, M.J., & Komro, K.A. (2009). Effects of beverage alcohol price and tax levels on drinking: a meta-analysis of 1003 estimates from 112 studies. *Addiction*, **104**, 179–190.

Weiner, B.J., Lewis, M.A., Clauser, S.B., & Stitzenberg, K.B. (2012). In search of synergy: strategies for combining interventions at multiple levels. *Journal of the National Cancer Institute Monographs*, **44**, 34–41.

Whelan, R., Conrod, P., Poline, J.-B., et al. and the IMAGEN Consortium (2012). Adolescent impulsivity phenotypes characterized by distinct brain networks. *Nature Neuroscience*, **15**, 920–925.

White, H.R., Marmorstein, N.R., Crews, F.T., Bates, M.E., Mun, E.Y., & Loeber, R. (2011). Associations between heavy drinking and changes in impulsive behavior among adolescent boys. *Alcoholism: Clinical and Experimental Research*, **35**, 295–303.

Wiers, R.W., Eberl, C., Rinck, M., Becker, E.S., & Lindenmeyer, J. (2011). Retraining automatic action tendencies changes alcoholic patients' approach bias for alcohol and improves treatment outcome. *Psychological Science*, **22**, 490–497.

Wiers, R.W., Gladwin, T.E., Hofmann, W., Salemink, E., & Ridderinkhof, K.R. (2013). Cognitive bias modification and cognitive control training in addiction and related psychopathology: mechanisms, clinical perspectives, and ways forward. *Clinical Psychological Science*, **1**, 192–212.

World Health Organization (2011). *Global Status Report on Alcohol and Health*. Geneva: World Health Organization.

Young, M.M., Saewyc, E., Boak, A., et al. (Student Drug Use Surveys Working Group) (2011). *Cross-Canada Report on Student Alcohol and Drug Use: Technical Report*. Ottawa: Canadian Centre on Substance Abuse.

Chapter 7

Addictive substances and behaviours and social justice

Jacek Moskalewicz and Justyna I. Klingemann

7.1 Introduction to concepts of social justice and inequality

The term 'social justice' first appeared in the mid-nineteenth century during the time of various European uprisings, sometimes known as the Spring of Nations, when the struggle for social emancipation was strongly associated with the fight for national liberation. Soon afterwards, John Stuart Mill (1879) defined social justice as equal treatment of all citizens. However, he made the important caveat that only virtuous citizens deserve equal treatment, i.e. social justice. This exception from the rule of equal treatment has survived for more than a century and served to justify policies and political structures that entrenched social injustice. As can be seen, from its early appearance the term had both political and moral dimensions. It was around the mid-nineteenth century that unrestricted access to alcohol paradoxically tended to both uphold existing inequalities and fuel social riots. At the same time attempts among under-privileged classes to abstain or to promote sobriety legitimized their demands for social and sometimes national emancipation. Since then, and up to very recent times, alcohol has been used in the fight for moral superiority by those struggling for social justice as well as by those who wish to discredit movements demanding social justice for people seen as not deserving it.

Towards the end of the nineteenth century 'social justice' meant attempts by the ruling classes to satisfy the basic needs of the rural and particularly the urban proletariat. Neglecting their rights would have been very likely to facilitate the development of revolutionary movements aimed at destroying the existing economic and political order and replacing it with a new system in which social justice would be secured by working people occupying the ruling positions. Calls for social justice went beyond the initial demands for equal rights or equal treatment of all citizens who 'deserved' it and demanded a fundamental redistribution of power and wealth. In the Marxist concept of social justice, the ruling classes, first of all capitalists, were made accountable for the lack of social justice and the suffering of the proletariat (Kołakowski, 2009). In that way, the moral postulate of social justice became a radical demand for class justice: this first materialized in Russia—a country where there was a very high level of social injustice and where the First World War even reinforced existing inequalities. In political systems, first in Soviet Russia and then in a large part of eastern Europe, social justice was strongly associated with class justice and covered the nationalization of large properties of the bourgeoisie and landlords and their apparent redistribution among the working classes. In fact, the nationalized wealth was controlled by the administration of the State and the bureaucratic apparatus of the ruling party. This form of State socialism soon degenerated because too much power was vested in a relatively small number of political bureaucrats (Đjilas, 1957), leading to numerous social conflicts and tensions and, in effect, after several decades, a decline in economic efficiency. Nevertheless, this 'real' or State socialism reduced the level of social inequality and built a more egalitarian society with free access to basic social services such as health and education as well affordable access to housing, cultural activities, and leisure. It also offered full employment.

In parallel, egalitarian values had also become more important in countries with free market economies and more pluralistic political systems. This was especially so in the welfare states of western Europe which had high levels of redistribution of national wealth and upheld such values as equal rights, including equal access to health and education. Even though such welfare systems seem to have had their best days behind them, and used to be blamed for lower productivity, a number of countries in Europe still successfully combine high productivity with a large amount of welfare and a relatively equal distribution of economic gains. Moreover, neoclassical theories rejecting the welfare state that were popular in the UK under the conservative government of Margaret Thatcher and in the United States during the presidency of Ronald Reagan are now being challenged by contemporary economic ideas which stress that a major rationale of economic activity is to provide well-being, and that the labour force cannot be treated as just another economic factor, like the means of production or raw materials. It is argued that productivity may suffer as inequality in the labour market leads to market failures. Thus, equality in the labour market between those who provide labour and those who buy it becomes a prerequisite of both social justice and productivity (Stiglitz, 2002).

Contemporary deliberations on social justice, like the economic theories developed by Stiglitz (2002), go a step beyond distributionary aspects of social justice and combine it with well-being. They argue that inequalities really matter to the extent they affect well-being. However, some inequalities do not necessarily reduce societal or individual well-being as long as those who have less do not feel disadvantaged by their material standard and consider it satisfactory. On the other hand, inequalities tend to accumulate and reinforce each other, often leading to social exclusion. Thus, inequalities may be justified and socially enforced by a lack of respect for and stigma imposed on those who 'deserve' to have lesser access to goods and services as well as to human rights.

Despite substantial efforts that have been made in the European Union (EU), the fundamental aims of which are to offer equal chances to all its citizens, to promote social inclusion, and to protect those who are the most vulnerable, huge discrepancies exist and have deepened within individual societies and across individual countries. Real per capita gross domestic products (GDPs) differ three-fold between member states, from US$15,000 in Romania and Bulgaria to over US$40,000 in Austria, the Netherlands, and Nordic member states (HFA-DB, 2013). The level of inequality is often inversely related to national wealth, with the Gini index being the lowest in rich Luxembourg (24.5) and the highest in Bulgaria (45.3) (HDR, 2010). (The Gini index measures the degree of inequality in the income distribution of residents in a country. The more nearly equal a country's income distribution the lower its Gini index.) The current recession has mostly affected the poorer segments of societies and more wealth has accumulated in the hands of the better-off (Stawicka, 2012). Income inequalities correspond to huge inequalities in health. Life expectancy within the EU varies from about 74 years in Bulgaria, Latvia, and Lithuania to over 82 in Sweden. This gap is even larger for men, ranging from less than 70 in Latvia and Lithuania to 78–80 in most other countries that joined the EU before 2004 (HFA-DB, 2013). As men drink several times more alcohol than women, and excess mortality due to alcohol mostly affects populations at their most productive ages, alcohol as well as other psychoactive substances of addictive potential still contribute to social injustice within and between individual countries.

In the following sections of this chapter we will reflect first how alcohol has been interwoven in the struggle of underprivileged classes for social justice, then how stigma associated with being an 'alcoholic' or 'drug addict' contributes to entrenchment of existing inequalities, obstructing access to basic rights and services and justifying the low priority given to management of addiction-related problems.

7.2 Historical lessons

As we have already noted, alcohol often served as a means to exploit the lower classes. A classic example is a privilege known as the right of *propination* given to landlords by Polish kings to exercise a monopoly of alcohol production and distribution on their lands. In practice, landlords often forced their serfs to drink in the landlord's inn and prohibited drinking in other inns (Bystroń, 1960). These practices were common, particularly in the nineteenth century when the feudal Polish agricultural system could not compete on the international markets and excess grain was used for the production of vodka. The peasants who were forced or tempted to drink in the landlord's inns increasingly perceived the pushing of alcohol as a form of exploitation and social injustice which deprived them of the little money that they possessed (Baranowski, 1979). Numerous riots erupted against this form of exploitation, the most well known of which occurred in the 1840s in western Galicia near Krakow. First, the peasants overran their local inn (inns were often run by a Jewish innkeeper but owned by the landlord). They celebrated their victory over this symbol of injustice and then the drunken mob moved to the landlord's manor house to set it on fire and kill the inhabitants. Much bloodshed followed and special laws restricting access to alcohol were adopted for Galicia and Bukowina, which was then part of the Austro-Hungarian empire (Eisenbach-Stangle, 1993).

The Industrial Revolution at the end of the eighteenth century triggered intense social mobility which pushed thousands of rural dwellers to the cities to provide industrial manpower; this consisted mostly of working class men employed in a new technical environment. Major technical advances increased productivity, including more sophisticated distilling technologies which offered the possibility of producing spirits from potatoes instead of grain throughout the spirit-drinking countries. As potato yield per hectare was several times higher than that of grain and did not differ much from year to year (being relatively independent of capricious weather), the cost of spirit production fell; vodka became very cheap and supplies more stable. Overproduction of vodka reduced its price to very low levels and increased its physical availability. Alcohol could be bought everywhere and at any time. Often a lump sum was enough to allow one to enter an inn and to drink as much as one could. Despite these low prices, the alcohol trade was hugely profitable. In the first half of the nineteenth century, revenues from alcohol constituted over 60% of the income of large Polish estates (Rożenowa, 1961). Moreover, in a number of countries, such as Prussia, alcohol was served at the inns located next to industrial plants where work contracts were signed and workers had to come to receive their wages (Vogt, 1982). Most of them were tempted to drink, often in excess, and to drink away their incomes. Nevertheless, they could drink on credit as their debts could easily be regained from their next wage packet. In that way, integration of alcohol capital within the more general industrial capital led to the recirculation of the income of the working class back to the pockets of capitalists. Heavy drinking could and did damage the health of the working classes. However, those affected could easily be replaced by crowds of others waiting in front of the factory gate. The low social position of the working class and their misery could be attributed to their intoxication which thus legitimized the existing social order. Workers apparently constituted a class of those who did not deserve social justice. On the other hand, socialist thinkers not only justified the drunkenness of the working class but argued that their heavy drinking was a result of the material conditions in which they had to live and work:

> Drunkenness has here ceased to be a vice, for which the vicious can be held responsible; it becomes a phenomenon, the necessary, inevitable effect of certain conditions upon an object possessed of no volition in relation to those conditions. They who have degraded the working-man to a mere object have the responsibility to bear. (Engels, 1892, p. 1779)

Engels and Marx both argued that drunkenness of the working class was an inherent feature of capitalism and could only be overcome by revolutionary change in the social system. In *The Communist Manifesto* they passionately attacked charitable organizations and temperance associations which tried to ameliorate various social ailments in order to uphold the existence of a capitalist society (Engels and Marx, 1888). This strong message found its way to the most radical communist movements. Nevertheless, temperance ideas were also present in less radical socialist movements throughout the next decades. As claimed at the first All-Russian Temperance Congress, the fight against alcoholism should be seen as a means to break one chain in the political oppression and capitalist exploitation of the working class (Snow, 1991). In some countries temperance activities served as a cover for conducting socialist meetings, especially in countries where socialist movements were prohibited, like Finland under Russian rule (Sulkunen, 1987). Paradoxically, in other settings, alcohol served as a lubricant for the foundation and existence of working class movements. In this context, temperance movements were seen as acting against the interests of the working class. In the late nineteenth century Karol Kautsky (1891) argued:

> If temperance movement achieves its objective and convinces German workers to spend their leisure time with family instead in a pub then we achieve what could not be achieved by the anti-socialist legislation. Solidarity of the proletariat will be destroyed, proletariat will be reduced to the mass of defenceless atoms.

Pubs became the major place where German activists in the working class movement could meet, in particular at times when anti-socialist legislation was in force. Strong ties between the socialist movement and pubs continued after the repeal of this legislation. Some pubs targeted a mainly socialist clientele and a number of publicans not only supported the socialist movement but were active members of it. Opponents of socialist movements keenly picked up the alcohol question to discredit them and show their moral superiority. It was claimed that a pub was the most powerful supporter of the social-democratic doctrine, as a decent worker could join it only under influence of alcohol. In the discussion on shortening working hours in factories, Emperor Wilhelm II expressed concern that workers would waste their time in pubs, exposed to drunkenness and radical political ideas (Roberts, 1985).

Links between alcohol, the struggle for social justice, and political domination did not disappear in more recent history. American prohibition could be seen as a technical measure to reduce the magnitude of alcohol-related problems, but may also be interpreted as an attempt by the traditional rural middle classes to morally legitimize their political domination over consecutive waves of migrants from countries known to represent heavy drinking cultures such as Germany, Ireland, Italy, or Poland (Gusfield, 1986). In that way, prohibition became a measure to maintain existing inequalities and was repealed after dozen or so years under strong pressure from the trade unions. Paradoxically, interwar prohibition in Finland was initially massively supported by the working class due to the history of involvement of workers in temperance movements (Sulkunen, 1987).

The utopian view that alcoholism would disappear in just, egalitarian socialist societies has never materialized. Prohibition of vodka imposed by the Tsar during the First World War continued in Soviet Russia for about 10 years. Its repeal was motivated officially by the needs of the working class, but in fact Stalin decided to reintroduce vodka for economic reasons to return to the State budget money paid to the rapidly growing working class. A similar disappointing scenario took place in all eastern European countries where the Soviet political and economic model was imposed after the Second World War. Similar to western Europe, alcohol consumption tended to grow from the early 1950s due to increasing levels of employment and growing purchasing power (Litmanowicz and Moskalewicz, 1986). However, the question of alcohol was not just reduced to economic matters but continued to have significant symbolic dimensions, in particular in Poland whose post-war history was interrupted every 10 years by serious confrontations between the ruling Polish United Workers Party and the working class. The demonstrations and bloody street riots that took place in Poznań in 1956 and in Gdańsk in 1970 were discredited by the State media as being provoked by drunken hooligans who used the opportunity for looting shops, including alcohol outlets (Moskalewicz and Sierosławski, 1985). In 1980, during the historic strikes which gave birth to the Solidarity movement, striking workers introduced alcohol prohibition in major factories including shipyards and oil refineries. In parallel, prohibition was announced in the coastal region by local authorities with the purpose of avoiding bloody confrontation. Prohibition was not only a technical measure to reduce the risk of violent developments but could also be interpreted as a gesture symbolizing peaceful intentions (Bielewicz and Moskalewicz, 1982). Soon afterwards, Solidarity blamed the State for pushing alcohol to maximize budget revenues and to manipulate a drunken society. The weapon of alcohol was thus used to gain moral superiority for the workers in their fight for social justice. After a dozen or so months of symbolic competition, both sides in the conflict agreed on a new alcohol law which introduced a highly centralized system of alcohol control based on the Nordic model (Moskalewicz and Wald, 1984).

A few years after that bottom-up alcohol reform, a top-down alcohol crusade was launched in the Soviet Union in parallel with the efforts to change the Soviet system, known as *perestroika*. The alcohol crusade that drastically reduced the affordability and availability of alcohol was meant as a symbolic message heralding the fundamental nature of change as much as the power of the State to interfere with the deeply rooted habits of individual citizens (Partanen, 1993). Despite its initial operational success, and a significant improvement in public health, the crusade was not welcome at all. In a couple of years moonshine replaced the State's monopoly. The failure of alcohol reform reflected an overall failure of the last attempt to reconstruct the Soviet State and society.

The collapse of the centrally planned economies in the Soviet Union and a number of its allies in eastern Europe witnessed a new chapter in the history of the relationship between alcohol and social justice. A radical jump into the market economy and rapid privatization of State property led to enormous redistribution of wealth and its high concentration. A significant segment of society, including industrial workers, were left behind and excluded from social and economic development. Prices of most consumer goods increased drastically, while the price of alcohol declined. For those excluded from the benefits of economic transformation, alcohol consumption became one of a few options for imitating the lifestyle of successful elites. Popular media often showed pictures of unemployed families or homeless people where heavy drinking and alcoholism seemed to be common. The message was clear—those unrestricted drinkers, immoral individuals, deserved their fate. Social injustice is in a way legitimized by stigmatizing the victims.

It is not only alcohol which has been used to legitimize social injustice and the superiority of the ruling classes. Drug prohibition has widely been used to control and subordinate poor segments of society, in particular migrants. The State on behalf of decent citizens applies legal measures and the power of law enforcement against those who dare to use so-called illicit drugs. The modern history of drug control, however, is not longer than 120 years. Towards the end of the nineteenth century opium was present in almost every home in the United States and Europe. After the American Civil War, laudanum was the major pain killer used without any prescription for those who suffered from injuries and had little or no access to medical care (Hartjen, 1977). Opium became an alien drug deserving prohibition as soon as it appeared to be a major drug of abuse of the Chinese migrant workers who were employed in construction works, particularly in building railroads. Extreme exploitation, low wages, and no protection by trade unions required a moral legitimization, an impression that they deserve their fate. Prohibiting opium, their favourite drug, was an ideal solution (Weinberg, 2005). As almost all of them smoked opium, its prohibition made the Chinese migrants criminals almost overnight. They deserved their low social position and economic discrimination. Their claims for social justice could easily be turned down as these immoral individuals did not merit it. On the contrary, they deserved continuous close control by the criminal justice system.

Since then drug laws, as well as international conventions, have often been used to uphold the inferior position of the lower classes and discredit their claims for more social justice. There is a well-documented history of drug scares in the United States which 'typically link a scapegoated drug to a troubling subordinate group – working class immigrants, racial or ethnic minorities, rebellious youth' (Reinarman and Levin, 1995, p. 148). One of the most extreme examples of a drug scare was the anti-crack campaign that lasted for about 6 years from 1986 to 1992. In that period, concepts such as 'drug epidemic' and 'plague' were present in the popular media, including the most important television networks, newspapers, journals, and magazines, which particularly focused on crack cocaine. The chemical composition of crack cocaine does not differ much from that of regular cocaine. What was new was its marketing, which consisted of the provision of expensive powdered cocaine in small cheap smokable units which were affordable to the urban poor and better suited their need for a short but strong effect. Crack was mainly used in the poor neighbourhoods of large cities populated by Latinos and African Americans. The drug was distributed among and used by the same category of deprived young people whose prospects for regular employment as well as purchasing power were very low (Reinarman and Levin, 1995). The war on crack constituted an important message for decent Americans, that those young people deserve their inferior position and do not merit social justice. In fact, they deserved a severe response from the criminal justice system. Penalties for crimes related to crack adopted in that period were several times higher than for similar crimes related to cocaine use (Beaver, 2010). Seventy per cent of the budget for the inner-city 'wars on drugs' was spent on the police and prisons in order to double the prison capacity. Over 90% of those arrested and imprisoned were either African Americans or Latinos (Reinarman and Levin, 1995).

7.3 **Addictions and stigma**

Health-related stigma, including stigma related to addictions, can be defined as a social process characterized by exclusion, rejection, blame, or devaluation that results from experience, perception, or reasonable anticipation of an adverse social judgement about a person or group on the basis of a socially discredited health condition (Weiss et al., 2006; Scambler, 2009; Livingston et al., 2011). There is no obvious relation between psychoactive substance use and stigma. Drinking is closely associated with many positively valued and prestigious activities or statuses, for example champagne for a wedding reception or complementary drinks for first-class passengers. This also holds true for some youth subcultures and for some forms of illicit substance use, for example ecstasy at a rave or cannabis at a student party (Room, 2005). At the same time, addiction-related stigma is considered to be most persistent and damaging for people suffering from problems related to substance use. It seems that social inequality, stigmatization, and marginalization linked to substance use interact in complex ways. Cross-cultural studies, both qualitative and quantitative, suggest that the consequences of stigma are remarkably similar for different health conditions and cultures. However, one should keep in mind that similar consequences of stigma may be a product of entirely different structural and cultural relations (Scambler, 2009). Therefore, this chapter continues by discussing research on stigma and its consequences from an international perspective.

7.3.1 **Individual consequences**

A central part of addiction-related stigma is negative stereotyping. Studies show that dependent people are perceived as lacking willpower and being dangerous and unpredictable (Schomerus et al., 2011). This social condemnation covers consumers of both licit and illicit drugs. Transgression of norms regulating the consumption of licit drugs is condemned as their abusers violate the status of our favourite drugs, such as alcohol and tobacco, whereas the use of illicit drugs is seen as challenging domestic values. Consequently, all abusers attract more irritation, anger, and repulsion from their social environment. They also experience less empathy, understanding, pity, and desire to help them than individuals suffering from other disorders. This leads to the social exclusion of addicted people, with drug addicts being rejected even more than alcohol addicts. Studies show that people suffering from addiction are rejected more strongly than someone with schizophrenia or depression and more than travelling populations or right-wing extremists (Link et al., 1999; Hallman, 2001; Schomerus et al., 2011). The picture becomes even more complex when we consider the phenomenon of self-stigma, which can be described as a subjective process characterized by negative feelings (about oneself), maladaptive behaviour, identity transformation, or endorsement of stereotype resulting from an individual's experiences, perceptions, or anticipation of negative social reactions on the basis of a stigmatized health condition (Livingston and Boyd, 2010; Livingston et al., 2011). From the perspective of the sociology of deviance this is a process in which deviant behaviour becomes the 'master status' of an individual: the person accepts the socially assigned status of 'being an addict' and starts complying with societal expectations regarding the role of the addict (Goffman, 1963).

Both social stigma and self-stigma contribute to a delayed recovery and diminish prospects for reintegration. Stigma impedes the process of seeking professional and lay help for addiction problems. It increases the tendency to hide away, and, in this way, prolongs and aggravates the course of disease (Buchanan and Young, 2000; Brewer, 2006; van Olphen et al., 2009; Livingston et al. 2011). Self-change studies identified stigma as one of the most important reasons for not seeking professional help because people fear being labelled as 'addicts' and subsequently experiencing loss of status and discrimination (Klingemann, 1991, 2010; Tucker and Vuchinich, 1994; Room, 2005; Schomerus et al., 2011).

7.3.2 Structural discrimination

The majority of studies on stigma used Goffman's classical framework (Goffman, 1963) and consequently focused mainly on individual suffering as a consequence of stigmatization. Subsequent studies provided evidence that people suffering from addiction are at particular risk of being *structurally* discriminated against. Marginalization of those defined as having alcohol or drug problems is a process which includes both personal and interactional elements on institutional and structural levels (Room, 2005). One example is the lower coverage of addiction treatment by private and public health insurance schemes, which suggests that addicted patients are considered to be less well-off and less welcomed. It is also argued that people with lower social status suffer worse treatment outcomes for their addictive behaviour than those with higher social status (Hanson, 1998; Room, 2005). Along similar lines, the 'deviance paradigm' was recently complemented by an 'oppression paradigm' (Thomas, 2007), shifting the focus from the labelled to the labellers. Scambler (2009) suggests that Young's (1990) five modes of oppression are especially useful for the empirical analysis of the dynamic dyad of shame and blame with their impact on the lives of some individuals and not others (i.e. 'exploitation', 'marginalization', 'powerlessness', 'cultural imperialism', and 'violence').

Structural stigma can manifest itself in many different ways in health care and addiction treatment. Studies show that health professionals in North America, Europe, and Australia have more negative attitudes towards patients with substance use problems than those with depression (Ding et al., 2005; Brener et al., 2007; van Boekel et al., 2013) or even diabetes, which is partially related to sugar abuse (Gilchrist et al., 2011). Negative attitudes of health professionals towards people suffering from addiction lead to poor communication, sub-optimal therapeutic alliances, and diagnostic overshadowing (the misattribution of physical symptoms to substance use problems) (Thornicroft et al., 2007; Palmer et al., 2009; van Boekel et al., 2013). At the same time, studies have also shown that those who more frequently work with or who have more contact with patients with substance use disorders expressed more *positive* attitudes (Ding et al., 2005; Brener et al., 2007; van Boekel et al., 2013). This is in line with the contact hypothesis, which states that people who have more contact with or more experience of a stigmatized condition are more tolerant and have more positive attitudes towards this group (Penn et al., 1994; Corrigan et al., 2001a,b). There is some evidence that in the absence of personal or professional experience with addiction, health professionals tend to have similar perceptions of people with substance use disorders as the general population. An American survey showed high support for compulsory treatment of alcoholism: 39% of respondents approved of compulsory outpatient treatment, 25% endorsed compulsory medication, and 41% supported compulsory in-patient treatment (Pescosolido et al., 1999, 2000). A study among general practitioners concluded that patients who abuse drugs are perceived as manipulative, aggressive, rude, and poorly motivated. It is believed that care for these people should be provided solely by addiction specialists, other health professionals feeling unable or unwilling to empathize with substance-abusing patients (Mc Gillion et al., 2000; van Boekel et al., 2013). This is not surprising, because many professions are associated with a particular field of action and competence. Doctors deal with illness, police and judges with crime, social workers with disability or destitution, priests with sin. However, problems from alcohol or drugs commonly fall into areas of shared jurisdiction (Room, 2005).

7.3.3 **Targeting stigma**

The process of medicalization of addictions, which was reinvigorated in the mid-twentieth century, was crafted as a measure of counteracting addiction-related stigma. It was argued that being ill is less stigmatizing then being immoral. However, in the minds of a majority in the general population these conditions are not seen as mutually exclusive: those who subscribe to a disease model of alcoholism may at the same time also be inclined to think of it as a vice or moral weakness. The concept of dependence as mental illness never succeeded in replacing the moral model, but complemented it with new elements such as the chronic nature of this condition or the institution of coercive treatment (Room, 1977, 1983, 2005; Schneider, 1978; Conrad, 1992, 2005; Rouse and Unnithan, 1993; Schomerus et al., 2011). Studies show that the substance-dependent individual is held to be much more responsible for her/his condition than people suffering from depression, schizophrenia, or other mental disorders unrelated to substance use (Albrecht et al., 1982; Corrigan et al., 2009; Livingston et al., 2011; Schomerus et al., 2011).

The reason for the partial failure of the process of medicalization is that the use of psychoactive substances occurs in a highly charged field of moral forces (Room, 2005). However, it is not seen as negative by everybody. It is sometimes argued that the major function of stigmatization is the enforcement of social norms and that reducing the stigma may produce negative effects, for example higher rates of substance use among young people and lower rates of help-seeking behaviour (Satel, 2007; Adlaf et al., 2009; Livingston et al., 2011). Stigma is seen a tool to discourage unhealthy behaviours such as problematic substance use, but has a collateral consequence of marginalizing and devaluing people suffering from addiction problems. Stigmatizing attitudes regarding certain contexts of substance use (substance use during pregnancy, drink driving, intravenous drug injection) are not only accepted in contemporary culture but are also formally endorsed in policy or criminal law. Outlawing a drug and punishing those caught using it may be intended to 'send a message' about standards of behaviour (Room, 2005; Phelan et al., 2008; Livingston et al., 2011; Schomerus et al., 2011), yet criminalization of substance-using behaviours exacerbates stigma and produces exclusionary processes that deepen the marginalization of people who use illegal substances (Ahern et al., 2007; Livingston et al., 2011). Consequently, the social processes and institutions that are created to control substance use may, in actuality, contribute to its persistence (Erikson, 1962; Livingston et al., 2011).

Therefore, governments and professional organizations are increasingly mobilizing resources towards preventing and managing health-related stigma. Interventions are addressing self-stigma, social stigma, and also structural stigma. Some attempts have been made to reduce self-stigma: studies show that interventions like skills training, vocational counselling, or a surgical procedure to remove needle track-marks from injecting drug users have some positive outcomes (Livingston et al., 2011).

These social stigma interventions are mainly focused on societal attitudes towards people suffering from addiction and are mostly educational in nature, attempting to depict positive stories of recovered addicts. So the major focus of those interventions is to address addiction-related stereotypes (Livingston et al., 2011). Stereotypes are generalizations by definitions—even if they do apply in individual cases, their cultural application to the majority is unjust. The fact that stereotypes about addicts have a small degree of accuracy creates challenges for counteracting stigma (Corrigan et al., 2005; Livingston et al., 2011). The goal of combating stigma should not be to create a 'better', positive, but similarly stereotypical, image of an addict; campaigns should be less focused on 'how they really are' but more on 'what they really need'. And what addicts need is empowerment and help from others—stigma is contrary to these needs (Schomerus et al., 2011).

Some policies also target *structural* stigma: interventions have been designed to decrease stigmatizing attitudes of medical students, police officers, and substance use counsellors and to increase comfort levels for those working with those populations by providing information on issues related to substance use and direct contact with addicts. This seems to be a reasonable course of action: studies show that health professionals have low levels of knowledge about substance use disorders, and have the feeling they lack specific knowledge and skills in caring for this particular patient group (McGillion et al., 2000; Giannetti et al., 2002; Deans and Soar, 2005; McLaughlin et al., 2006). All studies on the effectiveness of such interventions have reported some positive results; however, most of them assessed reduction of stigma-related outcomes immediately during the post-intervention period and the medium- to long-term effects remain unknown (Livingston et al., 2011).

7.4 **Conclusion**

Against the background of humanity's long history, the concepts of social justice as much as social injustice appeared relatively recently, no more than 150 years ago. Surprisingly, both concepts preserved their initial connotations as equal treatment of all individuals. Reservations such as those expressed by John Stuart Mill, that social justice is not a privilege for all but should be applied only to those who deserve it, are still found and are often used to restrict the benefits of social justice to obedient, decent citizens and to deprive equal treatment to those who transgress an arbitrary definition of abuse or dependence. Throughout history, those who manifested addictive behaviour were stigmatized as deviants and deprived of their social rights. On the other hand, abstaining from addictive substances or their controlled use became a symbol of moral superiority, legitimizing either the superior position of the ruling classes or the claims of the apparently inferior classes for more social justice.

Attempts at removing the moral stigma of addictions by their medicalization proved to be only partially successful. People suffering from addictions still experience discrimination in the labour market as much as in their access to appropriate health services. Medical stigmatization is often cumulative: addicted individuals are perceived not only as mentally incapable but also as sinful criminals. In particular, consumers of drugs declared as illicit suffer discrimination not just in health and social services—their discrimination is reinforced by the criminal justice system. After being criminalized due to their use of illicit psychoactive substances they are persistently marginalized, socially excluded, and deprived of the prospects of being treated equally to their fellow citizens.

In parallel with these manifestations of individual injustice, addictive behaviour may be used to justify social injustice collectively affecting a significant segment of the society, i.e. underprivileged classes and ethnic minorities.

References

Adlaf, E.M., Hamilton, H.A., Wu, F., & Noh, S. (2009). Adolescent stigma towards drug addiction: effects of age and drug use behaviour. *Addictive Behaviours*, **34**, 360–364.

Ahern, J., Stuber, J., & Galea, S. (2007). Stigma, discrimination and the health of illicit drug users. *Drug and Alcohol Dependence*, **88**, 188–196.

Albrecht, G.L., Walker, V.G., & Levy, J.A. (1982). Social distance from the stigmatized. A test of two theories. *Social Science and Medicine*, **16**, 1319–1327.

Baranowski, B. (1979). *Polska karczma. Restauracje. Kawiarnia*. Warsaw: Ossolineum.

Beaver, A.L. (2010). Getting a fix on cocaine sentencing policy: reforming the sentencing scheme of the Anti-Drug Abuse Act of 1986. *Fordham Law Review*, **78**, 2531–2575.

Bielewicz A. & Moskalewicz J. (1982). Temporary prohibition: the Gdańsk experience. *Contemporary Drug Problems*, Fall, 367–381.

van Boekel, L.C., Brouwers, E.P.M., van Weeghel, J., & Garretsen, H.F.L. (2013). Stigma among health professionals towards patients with substance use disorders and its consequences for healthcare delivery: systematic review. *Drug and Alcohol Dependence*, **131**, 23–35.

Brener, L., von Hippel, W., & Kippax, S. (2007). Prejudice among health care workers toward injecting drug users with hepatitis C: does greater contact lead to less prejudice? *International Journal of Drug Policy*, **18**, 381–387.

Brewer, M.K. (2006). The contextual factors that foster and hinder the process of recovery for alcohol dependent women. *Journal of Addictions Nursing*, **17**, 175–180.

Buchanan, J. & Young, L. (2000). The war on drugs—a war on drug users. *Drugs: Education, Prevention Policy*, **7**, 409–422.

Bystroń, J. (1960). *Dzieje Obyczajów w Dawnej Polsce. Wiek XVI-XVIII*. Warsaw: Państwowy Instytut Wydawniczy.

Conrad, P. (1992). Medicalization and social control. *Annual Review of Sociology*, **18**, 209–232.

Conrad, P. (2005). The shifting engines of medicalization. *Journal of Health and Social Behavior*, **46**, 3–14.

Corrigan, P.W., Edwards, A.B., Green, A., Diwan, S.L., & Penn, D.L. (2001a). Prejudice, social distance, and familiarity with mental illness. *Schizophrenia Bulletin*, **27**, 219–225.

Corrigan, P.W., Green, A., Lundin, R., Kubiak, M.A., & Penn, D.L. (2001b). Familiarity with and social distance from people who have serious mental illness. *Psychiatric Services*, **52**, 953–958.

Corrigan, P.W., Watson, A.C., Byrne, P., & Davis, K.E. (2005). Mental illness stigma: problem of public health or social justice? *Social Work*, **50**, 363–368.

Corrigan, P.W., Kuwabara, S.A., & O'Shaughnessy, J. (2009). The public stigma of mental illness and drug addiction: findings from a stratified random sample. *Journal of Social Work*, **9**, 139–147.

Deans, C. & Soar, R. (2005). Caring for clients with dual diagnosis in rural communities in Australia: the experience of mental health professionals. *Journal of Psychiatric and Mental Health Nursing*, **12**, 268–274.

Ding, L., Landon, B.E., Wilson, I.B., Wong, M.D., Shapiro, M.F., & Cleary, P.D. (2005). Predictors and consequences of negative physician attitudes toward HIV-infected injection drug users. *Archives of Internal Medicine*, **165**, 618–623.

Djilas, M. (1957). *The New Class: An Analysis of the Communist System* [1983 edition]. San Diego: Harvest/HBJ Publishers.

Eisenbach-Stangl, I. (1993). The beginnings of Galician and Austrian Alcohol Policy: a common discourse on Dependence. *Contemporary Drug Problems*, **20**, 705–718.

Engels, F. (1892). *The Condition of the Working-Class in England in 1844 with a Preface written in 1892*. Reprinted from George Allen & Unwin edition. Kindle Edition, loc. 1779.

Engels, F. & Marx, K. (1888). *The Communist Manifesto*. Reprinted from the English edition of 1888, edited by Friedrich Engels. Kindle Edition.

Erikson, K.T. (1962). Notes on the sociology of deviance. *Social Problems*, **9**, 307–314.

Giannetti, V.J., Sieppert, J.D., & Holosko, M.J. (2002). Attitudes and knowledge concerning alcohol abuse: curriculum implications. *Journal of Health and Social Policy*, **15**, 45–58.

Gilchrist, G., Moskalewicz, J., Slezakova, S., et al. (2011). Staff regard towards working with substance users: a European multi-centre study. *Addiction*, **106**, 1114–1125.

Goffman, E. (1963). *Stigma: The Management of Spoiled Identity*. Harmondsworth: Penguin.

Gusfield, J.R. (1986). *Symbolic Crusade. Status Politics and the American Temperance Movement*, 2nd edn. Urbana, IL: University of Illinois Press.

Halman, L. (2001). *The European Values Study: A Third Wave. Source Book of the 1999/2000 European Values Study Surveys*. Tilburg: WORC, Tilburg University.

Hanson, K.W. (1998). Public opinion and the mental health parity debate: lessons from the survey literature. *Psychiatric Services*, **49**, 1059–1066.

Hartjen, C.A. (1977). *Possible Trouble. An Analysis of Social Problems*. New York: Praeger Publishers.

HDR (2010). *Human Development Report 2010. 20th Anniversary Edition. The Real Wealth of Nations: Pathways to Human Development*. New York; United Nations Development Programme (UNDP).

HFA-DB (2013). *European Health for All Database* (July 2013 version). [Current versions available at: <http://www.euro.who.int/en/data-and-evidence/databases/european-health-for-all-database-hfa-db>.]

Kautsky, K. (1891). Noch einmal die Alkoholfrage: Schlusswort. Die neue Zeit: Revue des geistigen und öffentlichen Lebens, pp. 344–354. [In: Moskalewicz, J. & Sierosławski, J. (ed.) (1985). Alkohol i Robotnicy. Spojrzenie z perspektywy społecznej. In: *Położenie Klasy Robotniczej w Polsce. Tom IV: Problemy Patologii i Przestępczości* (ed. P. Wójcik), pp. 257–343. Warsaw: Akademia Nauk Społecznych, Instytut Badań Klasy Robotniczej.]

Klingemann, H.K.H. (1991). The motivation for change from problem alcohol and heroin use. *British Journal of Addiction*, **86**, 727–744.

Klingemann, J.I. (2010). *Horyzonty Zmiany Zachowania Nałogowego w Polsce*. Warsaw: Uniwersytet Warszawski, IPSiR.

Kołakowski, L. (2009). *Główne Nurty Marksizmu. Powstanie, Rozwój, Rozkład* [*Main Currents of Marxism: The Founders—The Golden Age—The Breakdown*]. Warsaw: Wydawnictwo Naukowe PWN. (First edition Paris, 1976–1978.)

Link, B., Phelan, J., Bresnahan, M., Stueve, A., & Pescosolido, B. (1999). Public conceptions of mental illness: labels, causes, dangerousness and social distance. *American Journal of Public Health*, **89**, 1328–1333.

Litmanowicz, M. & Moskalewicz, J. (1986). Wielkość i struktura spożycia alkoholu w różnych krajach. In: *Alkohol i Związane z nim Problemy Zdrowotne i Społeczne* (ed. I. Wald), pp. 63–78. Warsaw: Państwowe Wydawnictwo Naukowe.

Livingston, J.D. & Boyd, J.E. (2010). Correlates and consequences of internalized stigma for people living with mental illness: a systematic review and meta-analysis. *Social Science and Medicine*, **71**, 2150–2161.

Livingston, J.D., Milne, T., Fang, M.L., & Amari, E. (2011). The effectiveness of interventions for reducing stigma related to substance use disorders: a systematic review. *Addiction*, **107**, 39–50.

McGillion, J., Wanigaratne, S., Feinmann, C., Godden, T., & Byrne, A. (2000). GPs' attitudes towards the treatment of drug misusers. *British Journal of General Practice*, **50**, 385–386.

McLaughlin, D., McKenna, H., Leslie, J., Moore, K., & Robinson, J. (2006). Illicit drug users in Northern Ireland: perceptions and experiences of health and social care professionals. *Journal of Psychiatric and Mental Health Nursing*, **13**, 682–686.

Mill, J.S. (1879). Utilitarianism. Reprinted from Fraser's Magazine, 7th edn. London: Longmans, Green, & Co. Kindle edition, loc. 1057–1061.

Moskalewicz, J. & Sierosławski, J. (1985). Alkohol i Robotnicy. Spojrzenie z perspektywy społecznej. In: *Położenie Klasy Robotniczej w Polsce. Tom IV: Problemy Patologii i Przestępczości* (ed. P. Wójcik), pp. 257–343. Warsaw: Akademia Nauk Społecznych, Instytut Badań Klasy Robotniczej.

Moskalewicz, J. & Wald, I. (1984). Alcohol policy in a crisis situation. *British Journal of Addiction*, **79**, 331–335.

Olphen van, J., Eliason, M.J., Freudenberg, N., & Barnes, M. (2009). Nowhere to go: how stigma limits the options of female drug users after release from jail. *Substance Abuse Treatment, Prevention, and Policy*, **4**, 10.

Palmer, R.S., Murphy, M.K., Piselli, A., & Ball, S.A. (2009). Substance user treatment dropout from client and clinician perspectives: a pilot study. *Substance Use and Misuse*, **44**, 1021–1038.

Partanen, J. (1993). Failures in alcohol policy—lessons from Russia, Kenya, Truk and history. *Addiction,* **88,** S129–S134.

Penn, D.L., Guynan, K., Daily, T., Spaulding, W.D., Garbin, C.P., & Sullivan, M. (1994). Dispelling the stigma of schizophrenia—what sort of information is best. *Schizophrenia Bulletin,* **20,** 567–568.

Pescosolido, B.A., Monahan, J., Link, B.G., Stueve, A., & Kikuzawa, S. (1999). The public's view of the competence, dangerousness, and need for legal coercion of persons with mental health problems. *American Journal of Public Health,* **89,** 1339–1345.

Pescosolido, B.A., Martin, J.K., Link, B.G., et al. (2000). *American's Views of Mental Health and Illness at Century's End: Continuity and Change.* Bloomington, IN: Indiana Consortium for Mental Health Service Research and Joseph P. Mailman School of Public Health, Columbia University. URL: <http://www.indiana.edu/~icmhsr/docs/Americans%27%20 Views%20of%20Mental%20Health.pdf> (last accessed 20 December 2013).

Phelan, J.C., Link, B.G., & Dovidio, J.F. (2008). Stigma and prejudice: one animal or two? *Social Science and Medicine,* **67,** 358–367.

Reinarman, C. & Levine, H.G. (1995). The crack attack: America's latest drug scare, 1986–1992. In: *Images of Issues. Typifying Contemporary Social Problems* (ed. J. Best), pp. 147–186. New York: Aldine de Gruyter.

Roberts, J.S. (1985). Alcohol, public policy, and the Left: the socialist debate in early twentieth century Europe. *Contemporary Drug Problems,* Summer, 309–330.

Room, R. (1977). Measurement and distribution of drinking patterns and problems in general populations. In: *Alcohol-Related Disabilities* (ed. G. Edwards, M.M. Gross, M. Keller, J. Moser, & R. Room), pp. 61–87. Geneva: World Health Organization.

Room, R. (1983). Sociological aspects of the disease concept of alcoholism. In: *Recent Advances in Alcohol and Drug Problems* (ed. R. Smart, F.B. Glaser, Y. Israel, H. Kalant, R.E. Popham, & W. Schmidt), pp. 47–91. New York: Plenum.

Room, R. (2005). Stigma, social inequality and alcohol and drug use. *Drug and Alcohol Review,* **24,** 143–155.

Rouse, T.P. & Unnithan, N.P. (1993). Comparative ideologies and alcoholism: the protestant and proletarian ethics. *Social Problems,* **40,** 213–227.

Rożenowa, H. (1961). *Produkcja Wódki i Sprawa Pijaństwa w Królestwie Polskim 1815–1863.* Warsaw: Państwowe Wydawnictwo Naukowe.

Satel, S. (2007). In praise of stigma. In: *Addiction Treatment: Science and Police for the Twenty-First Century* (ed. J.E. Henningfield, P.B. Santora, & W.K. Bickel), pp. 147–151. Baltimore, MD: Johns Hopkins University Press.

Scambler, G. (2009). Health-related stigma. *Sociology of Health and Illness,* **31,** 441–455.

Schneider, J.W. (1978). Deviant drinking and disease: alcoholism as a social accomplishment. *Social Problems,* **25,** 361–372.

Schomerus, G., Lucht, M., Holzinger, A., Matschinger, H., Carta, M.G., & Angermeyer, M.C. (2011). The stigma of alcohol dependence compared with other mental disorders: a review of population studies. *Alcohol and Alcoholism,* **46,** 105–112.

Snow, G. (1991). Socialism, alcoholism and the working classes before 1917. In: *Drinking. Behavior and Belief in Modern History* (ed. S. Barrows & R. Room), pp. 243–264. Berkeley, CA: University of California Press.

Stawicka, M.K. (2012). Ekonomiczne rozwarstwienie społeczeństwa Unii Europejskiej po światowym kryzysie gospodarczym. In: *Nierówności Społeczne a Wzrost Gospodarczy.*

Modernizacja dla Spójności Społeczno-Ekonomicznej w Czasach Kryzysu. Zeszyt nr 24 (ed. M.G. Woźniak), pp. 125–135. Rzeszów: Wydawnictwo Uniwersytetu Rzeszowskiego.

Stiglitz, J.E. (2002). Employment, social justice and societal well-being. *International Labour Review*, **141**, 9–29.

Sulkunen, I. (1987). Temperance as a 'civic religion': the cultural foundation of the Finnish working class temperance ideology. In: *The Social History of Alcohol: Drinking and Culture in Modern Society* (ed. S. Barrows, R. Room, & J. Verhey), pp. 90–91. Berkeley, CA: Alcohol Research Group.

Thomas, C. (2007). *Sociologies of Disability and Illness. Contested Ideas in Disability Studies and Medical Sociology.* London: Palgrave Macmillan.

Thornicroft, G., Rose, D., & Kassam, A. (2007). Discrimination in health care against people with mental illness. *International Review of Psychiatry*, **19**, 113–122.

Tucker, J.A. & Vuchinich, R.E. (1994). Environmental events surrounding natural recovery from alcohol-related problems. *Journal of Studies on Alcohol*, **55**, 401–411.

Vogt, I. (1982). Einige Fragen zum Alkoholkonsum der Arbeiter. *Geschichte und Gesellschaft*, **8**, 134–140.

Weinberg, D. (2005). *Of Others Inside. Insanity, Addiction and Belonging in America.* Philadelphia, PA: Temple University Press.

Weiss, M.G., Ramakrishna, J., & Somma, D. (2006). Health-related stigma: rethinking concepts and interventions. *Psychology, Health and Medicine*, **11**, 277–287.

Young, M. (1990). *Justice and the Politics of Difference.* Princeton, NJ: Princeton University Press.

Chapter 8

Impact of the economic recession on addiction-prone behaviours

Aleksandra Dubanowicz and Paul Lemmens

8.1 Introduction to the impact of the recession on addiction-prone behaviours

In 2008, the world faced a financial crisis that plunged western economies into an economic recession, the effects of which are still being felt (2014). The current long-lasting downturn raises questions about the impact it may have on addiction-prone behaviours. This chapter focuses on research on the impact of macro-economic changes on smoking and the use of alcohol and illicit drugs, as well as gambling. Of course, economic factors identified at the macro-level take effect through mechanisms at the individual level. Yet it has been shown that research into macro-level factors leads to additional insights into the dynamics of addiction-prone behaviours in society (Arkes, 2011).

The US National Bureau of Economic Research defines an economic crisis as 'a significant decline in economic activity spread across the economy, lasting more than few months, normally visible in real gross domestic product (GDP), real income, employment, industrial production, and wholesale-retail sales. A recession begins just after the economy reaches a peak of activity and ends as the economy reaches its trough' (Johnson et al., 2007). In Europe the recession led to tightened private sector credits, declines in trade, and the collapse of financial institutions (Suhrcke and Stuckler, 2012). Figures from the statistics office of the European Union (EU) show significant losses in GDP in European countries since 2008. Every country (except Poland) suffered from a decrease in GDP and economic downturn. Five EU states appear to be the most severely affected by the crisis, namely Greece, Spain, Portugal, Italy, and Ireland (Koba, 2012).

Loss of income, loss of buying power, price increases, tax increases, job insecurity and unemployment, social exclusion, and budget cuts in social welfare and health care are among the effects that an economic downturn may have on people that in turn may affect substance use or other addiction-related behaviours. The evidence presented in this chapter focuses on findings from aggregate-level studies, as well as on responses to the day-to-day life crises of people losing their jobs, who face reduced access to health services, or who feel excluded from certain areas of social life.

8.2 The credit crunch of 2008 and the resulting economic recession

Economic development can be characterized by many indicators. Figures 8.1 and 8.2 present GDP and purchasing power for the EU (GDP since 2008 and purchasing power from 1999 to 2011). In 2008 several European banks, including some of the most important such as Barclays, Deutsche Bank, and Credit Suisse, faced a serious threat of bankruptcy (Kostohryz, 2011), and some were nationalized. Public debts increased as national interest rates went up dramatically (e.g. in Greece and Spain), and markets became affected by insufficient resources. Austerity measures had an impact on income and purchasing power.

More relevant in connection to substance use is job and financial security. Figure 8.3 shows patterns in the rates of unemployment for a selection of Eurozone countries since 2000. The unemployment rates increased dramatically in response to the weakening of the labour market in the second half of 2008. Total unemployment rates in the EU increased from 6.7% in 2008 to 9.1% in August 2009 (EC, 2009) and rose even more in 2010. In November

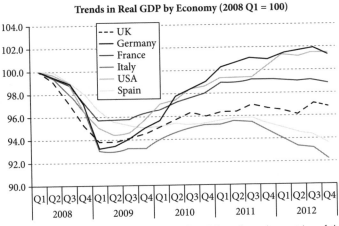

Fig. 8.1 Trends in real gross domestic product (GDP) for selected countries of the European Union (EU) (first quarter of 2008 is reference, =100).
Reproduced with permission from Market®Economics, Copyright © 2014 Markit Group Limited, available from http://www.markit.com/

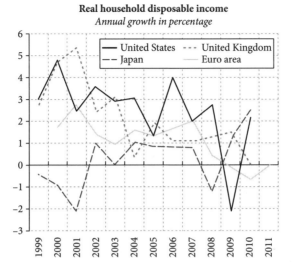

Fig. 8.2 Annual percentage growth of real household disposable income, 1999–2011.
Reproduced with permission from OECD (2013), *OECD Factbook 2013: Economic, Environmental and Social Statistics*, OECD Publishing. http://dx.doi.org/10.1787/factbook-2013-en

2012, 11.2% of Europeans, over 18.8 million people, were unemployed. Studies provide strong evidence that higher unemployment rates lead to poorer mental health, a higher suicide rate, and severe depressions in the population, and these facts may be considered as examples of possible adverse effects of the crisis (Kentikelenis, 2011).

In order to prevent budget deficits from increasing, governments are forced to introduce austerity measures affecting economic growth in general, and public investments, health, and social services in particular (EC, 2009). In the EU, the health-care sector has suffered greatly, and a decreased supply of resources together with cost-saving plans have resulted in the closing of branches and clinics and a reduction in the number of beds or patients admitted. Health prevention programmes have been cut, delayed, or underfunded and fewer resources are available for research, primary care, or health innovations. As a consequence, access to care may have become more limited. As the measures affect institutions, people with addiction problems increasingly face obstacles with receiving care. For example, in the Netherlands, where addiction care is funded from the mental health budget, across-the-board cuts of about 30% are expected to lead to a sizeable reduction in the number of residential beds and rehabilitation services (Dutch Ministry of Health, response to parliamentary questions, 26 September 2012). Fears were expressed by the heads of addiction care institutions that the successful measures to reduce homelessness, which in

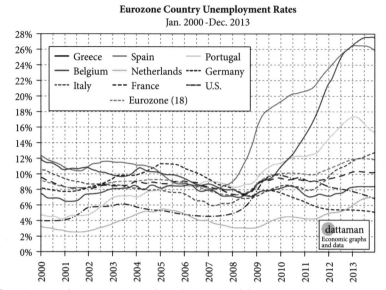

Fig. 8.3 Unemployment rates in selected countries of the Eurozone and the United States from 2000–2013.

Reproduced with permission from dattaman, Eurozone Country Unemployment Rates, available from http://dattaman.com/?p = 1330, Copyright © 2014 John Csellak. Source: data from Eurostat European Statistics Office, Statistic database, available from http://epp.eurostat. ec.europa.eu/portal/page/portal/eurostat/home, Copyright © European Union 2013.

the larger cities had resulted in reductions of up to 50% in crime and drug use, would be offset by the suggested budget cuts. Hundreds of homeless and addicted people would be cut off from the care they received at the time. This would lead to estimated increases in costs related to crime and degradation (Czyzewski, 2011).

Between 2009 and 2010 the budget cuts in Greece led to a loss of a third of the street-work programmes. In October 2010, more than 85% of the drug users in Athens were not covered by any drug rehabilitation programme (Kentikelenis et al., 2011). In general, countries that face the most severe public budget cuts and where increases in unemployment are highest are the countries where people are the most vulnerable to adverse consequences of the crisis. On the other hand, countries such as Iceland that decided not to make cuts to health care and rejected austerity measures did not report significant impacts due to economic troubles in the health sector (Karanikolos et al., 2013).

Budget cuts and decreased access to care are also closely linked with the issue of the exclusion of those with addiction problems. This could be a double-edged sword. Not only do people lose current facilities, but 'those socially excluded or vulnerable, experience even more exclusion and less support during the crisis times' (Betcherman et al., 2001). 'Social exclusion' is a relevant and a central theme in current discussions about European inequalities and social policy and includes the situation that addicts find themselves in (European Commission, n.d.). Hence it is highly possible that this concept gains even more importance when the situation of vulnerable groups worsens due to the economic crisis.

8.3 Ascertaining the impact of economic fluctuations on addiction-related behaviours

In the following section, the results of a literature review into two main research questions are presented, primarily related to substance use and its consequences. Gambling will be dealt with in a separate section. The first question is whether unemployment, social exclusion, and budget cuts, as the effects of the crisis, influence changes in addictive behaviour. The second question relates to the kinds of mechanisms responsible for the behavioural changes and which mechanisms tend to dominate?

For this review, articles published between 2000 and 2013 in PubMed, Google Scholar, and Science Direct were used. The databases differed in the type of topic covered by the articles. In all, 44 articles were selected for analysis (for a more detailed description of the selection process, see Dubanowicz, 2013).

8.3.1 Pro-cyclical versus counter-cyclical

Generally, there are two contrasting assumptions made in the literature about the type of relationship between the economy and substance use and problems related to addictive behaviours. Pro-cyclical means that the relationship is positive and the value of the service, the good, or the indicator tends to move in the same direction as the economy: declining with an economic decline and rising when the economy improves. In contrast, counter-cyclical relationships occur when indicators go in opposite ways—one declines when the second increases and vice versa.

The counter-cyclical assumption asserts that economic slowdowns cause an increased use of addictive substances. This popular assumption is repeatedly explained in several studies, mostly by the following factors: dealing with the distress of losing one's job and redistribution of leisure time due to unemployment or shortened working hours. Additionally, some researchers associate increases in alcohol, tobacco, and drug consumption with insufficient or inadequate social benefits for addicts and the unemployed as well as with poverty and government budget cuts and austerities (Ritter and Chalmers, 2011). Previous research also suggests that while an individual is safely employed, with a stable income and receiving wages above the poverty line, he or she is less likely to engage in risky or unhealthy behaviours (Stuckler et al., 2010). By analogy, unemployment, underemployment, or income problems would be expected to trigger an increase in the number of those who drink, smoke, or experiment with drugs.

Other studies with a more economic perspective that take aspects such as personal income, the opportunity costs of leisure time, and the prices of goods into consideration come to different conclusions (Pacula, 2011). For example, the income effect theory assumes that during times of recession disposable income may drop significantly. Having fewer resources will lead to reduced expenditure on goods that are not considered vital or necessary. Along these lines, evidence is brought forward that the use of addictive substances is not that different from the use of non-addictive ones, when an increase in income will lead to an increase in use, and vice versa. Studies indeed have shown that addicted users show income-elastic behaviour (Ritter and Chalmers, 2011). Pacula (2011) concludes that the effects of the economic cycles and macro-economic changes on addictive behaviours vary among different groups and patterns of problematic use, and that the results depend greatly on the measures taken.

8.3.2 **Alcohol**

The nature of the relationship between the aggregate unemployment rate and the use of alcohol has been much debated. Ruhm (2000) found proof of a pro-cyclical relationship between state-level unemployment rates and the employment-to-population ratio and four alcohol-related measures, i.e. chronic liver disease, major cardiovascular disease, traffic accidents, and homicides. When unemployment goes up, these indicators drop. On the other hand, results at the individual level for the self-reported number of drinks in the past month were counter-cyclical, though not statistically conclusive. However, smoking did follow the pro-cyclical path (a reduction when employment indicators drop).

In a later study, Ruhm and Black (2002) extended their measures to include drink driving, number of drinks, and drinking participation in the last 30 days, and found proof of a pro-cyclical relationship for the first two factors. Several other authors ended up with similar findings. Neumayer (2004) found a pro-cyclical relationship for traffic accidents and major cardiovascular diseases, but not for unemployment and alcohol use, homicide, or chronic liver disease. A Spanish study indicated a positive association between economic decline and fatalities in motor vehicle accidents (Granados, 2005), as did Stuckler et al. (2009) who identified a similar pro-cyclical relationship in a Europe-wide analysis. These last authors also reported positive associations with cirrhosis, homicide, mortality rates from cardiovascular disease, and unemployment, yet they did not appear to be statistically significant. Studies from Australia with data from 1999 to 2007 found that Australians generally reduce their alcohol consumption in times of an economic downturn, with unemployment and consequential loss of as personal income being probable mechanisms (Chalmers and Ritter, 2011).

Most reviewed results indicate that there is strong evidence for a pro-cyclical relationship between heavy drinking and macro-economic development, meaning that heavy drinkers tend to consume less alcohol in times of recession. This suggests that reduced financial means have a larger impact on heavy drinking than the psychological mechanisms of stress. An Estonian study found a drop in rates of alcohol consumption after the last economic recession. This counteracted the enormous rise (>100%) in per capita consumption in the decade before the recession (Lai, 2011).

Despite the numerous studies, the relationship between drinking and economic conditions is still confusing. While some authors find a pro-cyclical relationship, some provide evidence for the opposite, a counter-cyclical relation. The biggest contradictions to findings of pro-cyclical relationships are seen in the studies of Dee (2001). He estimated fixed-effect models and concluded that although there was proof of a pro-cyclical relationship between unemployment and alcohol consumption, binge-drinking and the unemployment rate seem to be counter-cyclically linked (Dee, 2001). Given this and other exceptions, Ritter and Chalmers (2011) concluded that most evidence tends to lean towards the positive, pro-cyclical relationship between macro-economic development and alcohol use.

A recent review of the impact of the economic crisis on alcohol use in Europe was conducted by de Goeij and Kunst (2013). Their approach along the lines of a so-called 'realist review' (Pawson et al., 2005) was context-specific and assessed mechanisms explaining the changes observed. They mostly found proof for counter-cyclical changes in alcohol consumption. Consumption among middle-aged men declined, because of loss of income and unemployment and higher prices. Drinking problems increased because of stress (insecure future) and budget cuts in health care. They also found evidence for increases in consumption and drinking problems as a result of loss of social status.

8.3.3 Tobacco and illegal drugs

Probably the strongest evidence for a positive, pro-cyclical variation has been found between tobacco use and economic downturns, especially with unemployment as a mediating factor. All of the reviewed studies found that overall smoking decreases in worsening economic times (McClure et al., 2012). For example, an Icelandic prospective cohort study found a significant reduction (of about 3%) in the number of smokers during the recent economic recession. In this example, decrease in smoking was explained by the weakened purchasing power of Icelandic citizens and lowered affordability. The income effect seems to predominate over social aspects or stress-coping strategies (McClure et al., 2012). Interestingly, the risk of smoking relapse decreased as well, regardless of gender, mostly in the older age group (40–59 and over 60). While adjusting for changes in individuals' economic status and income, McClure et al. (2012) found that men who move from a high-income group to a lower one are at less risk of relapse than those moving up. In contrast, Arkes (2011) argued that in times when economies are weaker, teenagers tend to smoke more because a recession induces more stress and depression among young people, causing uncertainty about their future prospects. Cigarette smoking may become the way to deal with emotions and a method of adding to the excitement of life. The results of that study stand in contrast to the general findings of McClure et al. (2012) and Ruhm (2000), yet they could hint at differential effects among age categories.

Fewer studies are available on illicit drug use and recessions. In a literature review, Arkes (2011) found most evidence for a counter-cyclical link between drug use in the young and economic development. Arkes presents a conceptual model in which drug is use is placed within Beckers' theory of crime. Unemployment, fewer future prospects, lower legal sanctions (opportunity costs), and stress relief would be the mechanisms by which adolescents' drug use would increase. Moreover, a significant outcome of this study was the suggestion of a positive correlation between unemployment and the participation of younger people in black markets. This could be explained by the opportunity of a quick profit and need to ensure financial supplies during bad times. However, evidence of this is relatively scarce. Bretteville-Jensen (2011) notes that a recession may affect the illegal drug market differently from legal markets in tobacco and alcohol. Decreasing buying power may affect the prices of illegal drugs, but also cause a shift, for example from expensive cocaine to less expensive amphetamines. This makes it difficult to assess to what extent such changes are associated with the direct outcomes of an economic crisis. For example, the available evidence suggests that if the price of drugs declines during the recession, consumption and the number of users would increase. However, reduced purchasing power would lead to the reverse effect. A combination of these influences decides which of the two effects will manifest and have a more significant impact on users' behaviour (see Table 8.1) (Ritter and Chalmers, 2011).

Table 8.1 Review of studies on the relationship between economic recession and addictive behaviours

Substance	Country	Study	Type of data	Statistically significant findings
Alcohol	USA	Ruhm (2000)	From 1972 to 1991, aggregate state-level data. Data from 1987 to 1995 on microlevel from BRFSS	Pro-cyclical relationship between unemployment rate and alcohol consumption
	USA	Dee (2001)	1984 to 1995 data from microlevel, BRFSS	Pro-cyclical relationship for number of drinks in past month. Counter-cyclical relation with binge-drinking
	USA	Ruhm and Black (2002)	Data on microlevel from 1987–1999 from BRFSS	Pro-cyclical relationship for drink driving and number of drinks
	Germany	Neumayer (2004)	From 1980 to 2000, aggregate state-level data	Pro-cyclical relation for driving fatalities and CVD
	Spain	Tapia Granados (2005)	From 1980 to 1997, aggregate data	Pro-cyclical relationship for traffic accidents only
	USA	Ruhm (2000)	1960–1997 aggregate data on a country level from the OECD	Pro-cyclical results for liver disease, vehicle accidents, and CVD
	26 EU Member States	Stuckler et al. (2009)	From 1971–2006 aggregate data	Pro-cyclical (traffic accidents, unemployment, liver cirrhosis)
	Netherlands	Knibbe et al. (1987)		Relationship between less structured social life and harmful consumption
	Australia	Chalmers and Ritter (2011)	Aggregate data on substance use, EMCDDA, annual report for 2010, individual level (NDSHS)	Pro-cyclical relationship for number of drinks
	Australia	Ritter and Chalmers (2011)	Individual-level data (NDSHS) from 1991–2007	Pro-cyclical evidence

Table 8.1 (continued) Review of studies on the relationship between economic recession and addictive behaviours

Substance	Country	Study	Type of data	Statistically significant findings
	Estonia	Lai (2011)	Review of pertinent legislation and publications, aggregate data from Bank of Estonia, Estonian Institute of Economic Research, and Statistics Estonia	Positive relationship between affordability and alcohol consumption during times of crisis
	USA	Richman et al. (2013)	663 responses from mail survey on life-related stressors of Great Recession	Significant link between LCCGR and drinking, more clearly related to problematic drinking
Smoking	Iceland	McClure et al. (2012)	Population-based, prospective cohort study based on a mail survey (health and well-being, assessed in 2007 and 2009)	Positive (pro-cyclical) relationship between economic recession and smoking for unemployment as a mediator; positive correlation between income increase and smoking relapse
	USA	Arkes (2011)	Data from the 1997 National Longitudinal Survey of Youth (teenagers 15–19 years) and young adults (20–24 years) with repeated measures over the period 1997–2006	Counter-cyclical relationship for cigarette use and weak economy among youth
Illicit drugs	Norway	Bretteville-Jensen (2011)	Review of the existing literature	Established price responsiveness in times of recessions, assumption for a pro-cyclical relationship between economy and drug use
	Australia	Chalmers and Ritter (2011)	Individual-level data (NDSHS) from 1991–2007	Counter cyclical findings for cannabis use and unemployment
	USA	Arkes (2011)	Conceptual framework and review of empirical literature on impact of recessions on youth drug use and selling and a strength of association between economy and such behaviours	Counter-cyclical relationship found for drug use and the economic recession among youth; increase in drug market involvement and engagement in dealing

BRFSS, Behavioral Risk Factor Surveillance System; CVD, cardiovascular disease; EMCDDA, European Monitoring Centre for Drugs and Drug Addiction; NDSHS, National Drug Strategy Household Survey; LCCGR, life change consequences of the Great Recession.

8.3.4 **Gambling and recession**

The scope of gambling and gaming activities is broad and involves card games, roulette, sport bets, slot machines in casinos or online, blackjack, keno, lotteries, bingo, or dice and coin-based games. Gambling is no longer considered to be an innocent activity but to possess addictive potential. The fourth edition of the *Diagnostic and Statistical Manual of Mental Disorders* (DSM-IV) classified problematic or compulsory gambling as an impulse-control disorder rather than an addiction. However, in the fifth edition (DSM-5) pathological gambling is defined as an addictive disorder. Excessive gambling can have severe disruptive effects on an individual's life, health, family, and society (Petry, 2006). Excessive gamblers often face debts, bankruptcy, work problems, unemployment, and commit property crime (Parsons and Webster, 2000; Vorvick and Rogge, 2013).

Gambling in society has become a large multimillion-dollar leisure industry (Parsons and Websters, 2000). In the United States alone, the revenues from gambling increased between 2011 and 2012 by almost 5%, up to more than US$37 billion (American Gaming Association, 2013), and the business is expanding worldwide. The industry is attractive to administrations because it contributes to the economy and offers additional employment, and gambling revenues contribute to the national budget without the need to increase general taxation (Walker, 2007).

However, introduction of gambling into a country is always controversial as there appears to be a lack of good research on its potential benefits and harms (Walker, 2007). It is argued that losses for problematic gamblers may overturn the benefits of playing.

Although a direct link between recession and gambling is difficult to establish, some sources claim that gambling is recession proof. Such resilience would indicate a counter-cyclical development. Studies from the UK indicated an increase in casino gaming during the recent European economic crisis (O'Donnell, 2012). In the first half of 2010, Paddy Power, the biggest online betting company in Ireland and the third largest in the UK, reported a 50% rise in profits. Next to economic indicators, it is also important to look at the number of people engaging in gambling. According to the Gambling Commission, the percentage of adults engaging in gambling activities increased by 5% (from 68% in 2007 to 73% in 2010). The absolute numbers, however, do not reveal the causes of such an increase. On the one hand it is sometimes assumed that gambling is an appealing option for quick financial gains, particularly during hard times when other options are low. On top of that, as Mikesell (1994) suggested, during a recession people may value tiny chances of winning as more attractive than in times of economic stability. As unemployment in times of recession is a major reason for declines in household income, gambling may provide opportunity and prospect. Lotteries or (online) gambling may provide excitement, hope, and chances for easy profits in times of need. The increasing popularity of on-line gambling activities, however, may not be related to recession as such but could be the result of the improved ease of access to gambling opportunities.

Proof of a pro-cyclical link may be found in data from the United States for 2008. The American Gaming Association reported a decline in casino gambling revenues between 2007 and 2008 by almost 5.5% in seven out twelve states. Similarly, Conner (2009) reported a decrease in the performance of Indian ca-sinos after 2007. Horvath and Paap (2012) investigated the effects of recessions on gambling expenditures in the United States between 1950 and 2010, using aggregated monthly per capita US consumption measures in comparison with consumption of other services. This study revealed that out of parimutuel wa-gering, lottery, and casino gambling, only the lottery business was recession-proof, the others showing signs of pro-cyclical change.

No individual-level studies have been found that assess the effects of eco-nomic recessions. As for mechanisms, Mikesell (1994) reported evidence of a positive relationship between increases in income and lottery sales. Horvath and Paap (2012) reported a positive association between individual loss of income and lower expenditure on gambling activity. The permanent-income hypothesis (PIH) assumes that the consumption of households is determined by long-term changes in income rather than short-lived, temporary changes, suggesting that stable changes in income would result in changes in gambling activity. Counter to this rational model is the finding that stress and anxiety due to fears of losing one's job or becoming unemployed in times of crisis ap-pear to be positively correlated with gambling (Lightsey and Husley, 2002). Another aspect brought about by unemployment is an increase in leisure time and boredom. Mercer and Eastwood (2010) and Blaszczynski et al. (2004) support the view that self-reported boredom induces engagement in gambling activities.

8.4 Mechanisms by which economic recession has an effect on addictive behaviours

Davalos (2011) presented an overview of possible explanatory mechanisms by which a macro-economic recession could impact on addictive behaviours. Some of the mechanisms in that empirical overview have been mentioned al-ready. It is worth discussing Davalos' ideas in a comprehensive fashion. In this section we give an overview of the possible mechanisms explained by the Dava-los model (Fig. 8.4). Table 8.2 gives a summary of the findings.

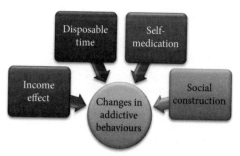

Fig. 8.4 Four main factors explaining changes in addictive behaviours in times of recession.

Source: data from Davalos, M., Easing the pain of economic downturn: macroeconomic conditions and alcohol consumption, *Health Economics*, Volume 21, Issue 11, pp.1318–1335, Copyright © 2011 John Wiley & Sons, Ltd.

Davalos (2011) introduced an income effect theory which assumes that consumption decreases with disposable income or buying power. In line with Davalos' argument, Skog (1986) assumed that drinking behaviour can be manipulated by changes in the price of beverages and disposable income. Using time-series analysis, Skog produced evidence for a positive relationship between changes in income and changes in consumption (Skog, 1986). These results are in line with those of most of the other studies (Ruhm, 2000; Ruhm and Black, 2002; Neumayer, 2004; Tapia Granados, 2005; Stuckler et al., 2009). Davalos pointed out that alcohol constitutes a particular economic good, as it also has addictive and mood-altering effects which may produce different effects for different types of drinkers during recessions. He suggested that individual income determines the type of drink and pattern of consumption. He further argued that the changes differ among different groups: proportionally, light and moderate drinkers may experience a greater change in drinking behaviour during an economic recession than established heavy drinkers. It differs for those who are already consuming alcohol regularly and those who use it occasionally and make a voluntary decision to drink. Alcoholics may not encounter very significant changes in their choices; however, according to supporting studies, they tend to respond to income effect and decrease their overall consumption (Skog, 1986).

The second mechanism in the Davalos model is the distribution of leisure time. It posits that in times of recession, workers gain more disposable time due to layoffs, a reduction in their working hours, or, in the worst case, loss of their job. Davalos claimed that such distortion of the day may lead to more time devoted to activities such as parties, watching TV or playing video games, social meetings, etc., which favour alcohol consumption. In their study of social roles

Table 8.2 Summary of finding into mechanisms by which a recession could affect use of addictive substances

Study	Main findings	Dominating factor
Skog (1986)	Buying power has an impact on over-consumption	Buying power: income effect, price changes
Anderson and Baumberg (2006)	Higher alcohol-related deaths rates among people of lower socioeconomic status	Income effect
Arkes (2007)	Employed people may have more opportunities to drink	Social coordination
Knibbe et al. (1987)	Partnership, parenthood, and paid labour decreases the risk of becoming a regular heavy drinker	Social roles and positions; reorganized leisure time
Kuntsche et al. (2009)	Unemployment together with higher prices of alcohol, lower income, and narrowed access to health care have an impact on addictive behaviours	Changes in employment status; income; prices
Rehm et al. (2009)	With the same consumption of alcohol, people from lower-income regions suffer from more disability-adjusted life years and alcohol-related fatalities	Income effect; social status
Davalos (2011)	Four possible mechanism that stimulate changes in addictive substance use: income, restructuring of daily life, self-medication, social coordination	Economic distress; reorganized leisure time
Richman et al. (2013)	Economy-related stressors significantly affect drinking behaviour (problematic and binge-drinking increased in men)	Economy-related stressors; self-medication

and drinking, Knibbe et al. (1987) found that the unemployed have a different structure of everyday life, and drink more often in relatively 'dry' situations, defined by time of day, location, and activity. Interestingly, when controlled for level of consumption, the unemployed experienced more negative consequences of their drinking.

A third explanation for the changes in behaviour as a response to the crisis is that alcohol or other substances may be used as a self-medication strategy against distress, work-related, or unemployment-related struggles, a getaway from day-to-day problems, or a way to deal with financial hardship. Richman et al. (2013) suggested that work-related and personal problems caused by economic hardship may have an effect on feelings of stress, hopelessness, and powerlessness. These, in turn, tend to lead to a need for self-medication with alcohol and other drugs. Richman et al. (2013) examined the life change consequences of the Great Recession (LCCGR). They found that there is clear evidence that economy-related stressors significantly affect drinking behaviour, especially problematic and binge-drinking.

Fourthly, social coordination plays an important role, and research suggests that the way the work itself is organized and the fact that it normally provides social and alcohol-related activities for employees may influence overall consumption as well. For instance, if the workplace organizes frequent parties, trips, holidays, or happy hours, those who are unemployed may drink less simply because of a lack of additional occasions for drinking (Arkes, 2011). Knibbe et al. (1987) make a distinction between situational and positional roles which in part determine drinking levels and practice. Positional roles, which, for example, come with a job, are also associated with proscriptive norms (having to get up early in the morning, proscribing drinking late at night).

Davalos (2011) hypothesized two possible outcomes. First, he affirmed the counter-cyclical association with binge-drinking and lack of a job, showing that a 1% increase in unemployment leads to an increase of 1.5% in the monthly prevalence of binge-drinking and higher odds for driving after drinking alcohol (ratio of 1.35). He concluded that for binge-drinking the income and social coordination effects are less important than the combined effects of economic distress and the changed structure of everyday life.

Classic role theory assumes that being involved in several social or positional roles, i.e. partnership, parenthood, and paid labour, decreases a person's possibilities to drink heavily (Knibbe et al., 1987). Such theory, as well as ecological models of the determinants of behaviour, could be used as an explanatory tool while identifying changes in lifestyle as a consequence of, for instance, unemployment. In summary, it could be hypothesized that in economic recession social exclusion and the loss of structure, as defined by social roles, tend to increase the opportunities to engage in risky or addictive behaviours.

It is important to consider when looking at the effect of economic factors that the impact of drinking-related harm is moderated by income. When alcohol consumption is held constant, people who live in regions of the world with lower incomes have higher alcohol-related deaths and disability-adjusted life years than people who live in higher-income regions of the world (Rehm et al., 2009). The same applies within countries. For the same amount of alcohol consumed, people with lower incomes have higher alcohol-related death rates than people with higher incomes (Anderson and Baumberg, 2006). Socioeconomic variables act at the collective as well as the individual level (Blomgren et al., 2004).

8.5 **Counterbalancing the effects of economic recession**

Stuckler et al. (2010) focused on social welfare expenditure and its possible influence on health outcomes in societies. Social welfare expenditure is defined by the Organisation for Economic Co-operation and Development (OECD) as the provision by public and private institutions of benefits to people in order to provide support during circumstances which adversely affect their welfare. Evidence suggests that all-cause mortality rates decrease by about 1.19% for each additional $100 spent per capita on social welfare (Stuckler et al., 2010). It is also proven that collective arrangements, as in governmental spending on social welfare, may lead to improved health outcomes in addition to the effects related to personal income. Furthermore, social spending has been found to be statistically associated with mortality caused by social factors, such as deaths related to alcohol use, whereas spending on health care as such is not. This has been interpreted as implying that investing in social welfare programmes could potentially lead to better outcomes (less harm from addictive behaviours) than investments in the health-care sector as such.

References

American Gaming Association (2013). *State of the States. The AGA Survey on Casino Entertainment.* Washington, DC: AGA.

Anderson, P. & Baumberg, B. (2006). *Alcohol in Europe.* London: Institute of Alcohol Studies.

Arkes, J. (2011). Recessions and the participation of youth in the selling and use of illicit drugs. *International Journal of Drug Policy,* **22**, 335–340.

Betcherman, G., Luinstra, A., & Ogawa, M. (2001). *Labor Market Regulation: International Experience in Promoting Employment and Social Protection.* The World Bank Social Protection Discussion Paper Series SP 0128. Washington, DC: World Bank.

Blaszczynski, A., Ladouceur, R., & Shaffer, H. (2004). A science-based framework for responsible gambling: the Reno model. *Journal of Gambling Studies,* **20**: 301–317.

Blomgren, J., Martikainen, P., Mäkelä, P., & Valkonen, T. (2004). The effects of regional characteristics on alcohol-related mortality; a register-based multilevel analysis of 1.1 million men. *Social Science and Medicine,* **58**, 2523–2535.

Bretteville-Jensen, A. (2011). Illegal drug use and the economic recession. What can we learn from the existing research? *International Journal of Drug Policy,* **22**, 353–359.

Chalmers, J. & Ritter, A. (2011). The business cycle and drug use in Australia: evidence from cross-sections of individual level data. *International Journal of Drug Policy*, **22**, 341–352.

Conner, T. (2009). A research note on the impact of the economic recession on Indian gaming in Connecticut. *Indigenous Policy Journal*, **XX**(3).

Czyzewski, E. (2011). *Consequenties bezuinigingen voor (de omvang van) de zorgverlening* [Consequences of the budget cuts for the size of the addiction care]. Open letter to the council of Rotterdam.

Davalos, M. (2011). Easing the pain of economic downturn: macroeconomic conditions and alcohol consumption. *Health Economics*, **21**, 1318–1335.

Dee, T. (2001). Alcohol abuse and economic conditions: evidence from repeated cross sections of individual-level data. *Health Economics*, **10**, 257–270.

Dubanowicz, A. (2013). *Impact of the Economic Downturns on Addictive Behaviour. Literature Review and Experts Opinion Survey Analysis*. Thesis. Maastricht: Maastricht University.

de Goeij, M.C.M. & Kunst, A.E. (2013). *Impact van de economische crisis op alcoholconsumptie in Europa* [Impact of the economic crisis on alcohol consumption in Europe]. Presentation at 23ste Forum Alcohol en Drugs Onderzoek (FADO), 12 November 2013.

European Commission (n.d.). *Poverty and social exclusion*. URL: <http://www.ec.europa.eu> (accessed March 2013; continually updated).

Horvath, C. & Paap, R. (2012). The effect of recession on gambling expenditures. *Gambling Studies*, **28**, 703–717.

Johnson, R., Kantor, S., & Fishback, P. (2007). Striking at the roots of crime: the impact of social welfare spending on crime during the Great Depression. *National Bureau of Economic Research Working Paper No. 12825*. Cambridge, MA: National Bureau of Economic Research.

Karanikolos, M., Mladovsky, P., Cylus, J., et al. (2013). Financial crisis, austerity, and health in Europe. *Lancet*, **381**, 1323–1331

Kentikelenis, A., Karanikolos, M., Papanicolas, I., & Basu, S. (2011). Health effects of financial crisis: omens of a Greek tragedy. *Lancet*, **378**, 1457–1458.

Knibbe, R.A., Drop, M.J., & Muytjens, A. (1987). Correlated of stages in the progression from everyday drinking to problem drinking. *Social Science and Medicine*, **24**, 463–473.

Koba, M. (2012). Europe's economic crisis: what you need to know. URL: <http://www.cnbc.com/id/47689157#> (accessed 22 October 2014).

Kostohryz, J. (2011). *European crisis only postponed*. URL: <http://www1.realclearmarkets.com/2011/10/27/european_crisis_only_postponed_119810.html> (accessed February 2012).

Kuntsche, S., Knibbe, R.A., & Gmel, G. (2009). Social roles and alcohol consumption: a study of 10 industrialized countries. *Social Science and Medicine*, **68**, 1263–1270.

Lai, T. (2011). Decline in alcohol consumption in Estonia: combined effects of strengthened alcohol policy and economic downturn. *Alcohol and Alcoholism*, **46**, 200–203.

Lightsey, O.R. Jr & Hulsey, D. (2002). Impulsivity, coping, stress, and problem gambling among university students. *Journal of Counseling Psychology*, **49**, 202–211.

McClure, C.B., Valdimarsdóttir, U.A., Hauksdóttir, A., et al. (2012). Economic crisis and smoking behavior: prospective cohort study in Iceland. *BMJ Open*, **2**, e001386. doi: 10.1136/bmjopen-2012-00138

Mercer, K. & Eastwood, J. (2010). Is boredom associated with problem gambling behaviour? It depends on what you mean by 'boredom'. *International Gambling Studies*, **10**, 91–104.

Mikesell, J. (1994). State lottery sales and economic activity. *National Tax Journal*, **47**, 165–171.

Neumayer, E. (2004). Recessions lower (some) mortality rates: evidence from Germany. *Social Science and Medicine*, **58**, 1037–1047.

O'Donnell, M. (2012). Has gambling been recession-proof? *Calvinayre.com Gambling News*. URL: <http://calvinayre.com/2012/11/20/business/has-gambling-business-been-recession-proof/>

Pacula, R. (2011). Substance use and recessions: what can be learned from economic analyses of alcohol? *International Journal of Drug Policy*, **22**, 326–334.

Parsons, K. & Webster, D. (2000). The consumption of gambling in everyday life. *Journal of Consumer Studies and Home Economics*, **24**, 263–271.

Pawson, R., Greenhalgh, T., Harvey, G., & Walshe, K. (2005). Realist review—a new method of systematic review designed for complex policy interventions. *Journal of Health Services Research and Policy*, **10**(Suppl. 1), 21–34.

Petry, N. (2006). Should the scope of addictive behaviors be broadened to include pathological gambling?. *Addiction*, **101**(Suppl. 1), 152–160.

Rehm, J., Anderson, P., Kanteres, F., Parry, C.D., Samokhvalov, A.V., & Patra, J. (2009). *Alcohol, Social Development and Infectious Disease*. Toronto, ON: Centre for Addiction and Mental Health.

Richman, J.P., Rospenda, K., & Johnson, T. (2013). Drinking in the age of the great recession. *Journal of Addictive Diseases*, **31**, 158–172.

Ritter, A. & Chalmers, J. (2011). The relationship between economic conditions and substance use and harm. *Drug and Alcohol Review*, **30**, 1–3.

Ruhm, C. (2000). Are recessions good for your health? *Quarterly Journal of Economics*, **115**, 617–650.

Ruhm, C. & Black, W.E. (2002). Does drinking really decrease in bad times? *Journal of Health Economics*, **21**, 659–678.

Skog, O.J. (1986). An analysis of divergent trends in alcohol consumption and economic development. *Journal of Studies in Alcohol*, **47**, 19–25.

Stuckler, D., Basu, S., & McKee, M. (2010). Budget crises, health, and social welfare programmes. *British Medical Journal*, **340**, c3311.

Stuckler, D., Basu, S., Suhrcke, M., Coutts, A., & McKee, M. (2009). The public health effect of economic crises and alternative policy responses in Europe: an empirical analysis. *Lancet*, **374**, 315–323.

Suhrcke, M. & Stuckler, D. (2012). Will the recession be bad for our health? It depends. *Social Science and Medicine*, **74**, 647–653.

Tapia Granados, J. (2005). Recessions and mortality in Spain, 1980–1997. *European Journal of Population*, **21**, 393–422.

Vorvick, L. & Rogge, T. (2013). *Pathological gambling*. University of Maryland Medical Center Online Medical Encyclopedia. URL: <http://umm.edu/health/medical/ency/articles/pathological-gambling>

Walker, D. (2007). *The Economics of Casino Gambling*. Heidelberg: Springer-Verlag.

Chapter 9

Social costs of addiction in Europe

Kevin D. Shield, Maximilien X. Rehm, and Jürgen Rehm

9.1 Introduction to the social costs of addiction in Europe

Alcohol consumption, tobacco smoking, illicit drug use, and gambling create substantial social costs for Europe. The most common way to estimate such costs is via a cost of illness (COI) study. COIs (typically defined as the value of the resources that are expended or foregone as a result of a health problem) as applied to substance use include health sector costs, workplace and productivity losses, crime and public disorder costs, costs to the drug user/gambler, their family, other people within their social network, and strangers, and prevention and research (see Fig. 9.1). Furthermore, the social costs attributable to drug use and gambling can be divided into tangible costs (those that can be directly calculated as having a monetary value, such as property damage and loss of productivity) and intangible costs (those that cannot be directly calculated, such as pain and suffering), and into direct costs (those that have a monetary value due to an object, such as costs related to property damage) and indirect costs (those that have a monetary value that are not related to an object, such as productivity loss). Due to the wide spectrum of costs attributable to drug use and gambling, the social costs are large and affect a significant segment of the economy, health systems, and population.

Following the seminal work of Rice and colleagues in the late 1980s and early 1990s (e.g. Rice et al., 1990), there has been a tradition of expanding COI studies to look at costs related to risk factors, especially in the areas of alcohol, tobacco, and illicit drugs (for more information about the rationale for this and guidelines see Single et al. (1996, 2003) and Single and Easton (2001)). With this expansion other costs became included, most notably costs related to the legal sector (policing, courts, prison), which are not typically included in COIs.

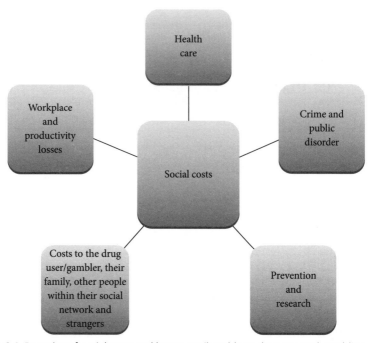

Fig. 9.1 Domains of social costs and harms attributable to drug use and gambling.

Some recent examples of comprehensive cost studies for substance use risk factors would be the Canadian or Australian studies on the costs of substance abuse by Rehm et al. (2007), Collins and Lapsley (2008), and Manning et al. (2013). The term 'abuse' in cost studies has a different meaning from that in psychiatric classifications such as the American Psychiatric Association's *Diagnostic and Statistical Manual of Mental Disorders* (DSM). For Europe, the most prominent cost study of the past decade concerning substance use was the study of Anderson and Baumberg (2006) on the costs of alcohol (see Fig. 9.2 for an overview of the relative impact of different cost categories). However, what is often lost in these analyses of the social costs of alcohol/substance use is the specific impact of addiction, however defined (for a discussion of definitions see Rehm et al., 2013a,b). There are comparatively fewer studies on addiction than on alcohol/substance use as a whole.

Any quantification of the social costs of substance use includes the costs incurred by addiction but also costs due to factors unrelated to addiction. For example, the costs of alcohol or cannabis use include costs associated with damage or injury due to alcohol- or cannabis-attributable traffic accidents caused by drivers who have consumed too much in that particular situation (affecting

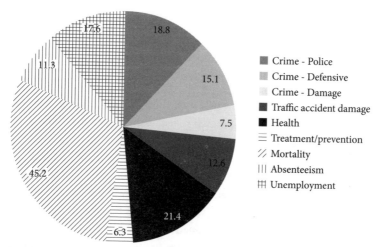

Fig. 9.2 Social cost of alcohol use in Europe, 2010, in €billion. Calculations for 2010 (see Rehm et al., 2012) are based on data from Anderson and Baumberg (2006). Total tangible costs to the European Union are €155.8 billion, equivalent to 1.3% (0.9–2.4%) of GDP.

Source: data from Rehm J., Cost of illness studies for alcohol consumption—Why are they still in demand?, *Nordisk Alkohol Nark*, Volume 29, Issue 4, pp.345–347, Copyright © 2012; and Anderson P., and Baumberg B., Alcohol in Europe: a public health perspective: A report of the European Commission, Institute of Alcohol Studies, London, UK, Copyright © 2006.

their psycho-motor coordination, their risk-taking, or their reaction time) but who do not have a substance use disorder or addiction (Taylor et al., 2010; Asbridge et al., 2012).

To quantify the costs due to addiction separately it is necessary to assess the burden specifically due to addiction; once this portion of the overall costs has been created one may potentially introduce particular responses to the issues surrounding addiction (as opposed to substance use/gambling as a whole). Therefore, we will give an overview of the literature on social costs relating to addiction, broken down into the categories of alcohol, tobacco, illicit drugs, and gambling. In addition, the implications of these costs will be assessed.

9.2 **Social costs of alcohol addiction**

There are two recent studies relevant to the social costs of alcohol dependence in Europe. Mohapatra et al. (2010) based their estimates on heavy drinkers, assuming that all people drinking above a certain threshold over time would be addicted (see Rehm et al. (2013c) for an elaboration of that assumption). These studies found that 0.96% of the total gross domestic product (GDP) of the European Union was due to alcohol dependence; 60.7% of all social costs attributable to alcohol use were caused by alcohol dependence. Based on the total social costs of alcohol (see Fig. 9.1), the cost of alcohol dependence amounted to €94.6 billion in 2010; when based on GDP the cost of alcohol dependence is €115.1 billion in Europe.

The most recent European study on the costs of addiction in Europe was made by the European Brain Council (Gustavsson et al., 2011; Olesen et al., 2012). They estimated that the overall costs related to addiction amounted to €65.7 billion. This figure is much lower than the estimates of Mohapatra et al. (2010), especially considering that it included not only alcohol addiction but also opioid dependence. However, the comparability of the two figures is difficult to assess: the Mohapatra et al. (2010) figure is based on a full cost study including indirect costs (e.g. lost productivity; see Fig. 9.1). These costs, which take into consideration lost productivity due to premature mortality and absenteeism, make up more than 50% of the total.

Overall, it clear that there are immense social costs associated with alcohol consumption in general and alcohol addiction in particular. While the numbers often conflict (due to different methodologies), any of the presented costs pose a serious challenge to European economies. A conservative estimate of the total yearly social costs of alcohol dependence in Europe for 2010 would be between €50 billion and €120 billion.

9.3 Social costs of tobacco dependence

The total social costs of smoking (taken as equal to tobacco use) in Europe are usually estimated to be even higher than those of alcohol. However, it is difficult to estimate the social costs of addiction to tobacco, primarily because it is hard to quantify how many people who use tobacco are actually addicted (Rehm et al., 2013b). A consistent definition of tobacco addiction (e.g. ten or more cigarettes per day on average) is necessary in this regard. However, based on the immense overall social costs of tobacco use, estimated to be close to €100 billion in 2000 (Aspect Consortium, 2004), the social cost burden for 2010 is likely to exceed €100 billion for Europe as a whole.

9.4 Social costs of illicit drugs

The social costs of illicit drugs, let alone drug addiction, are difficult to estimate, primarily due to the nature of these substances. The European Monitoring Centre for Drugs and Drug Addiction (EMCDDA) has made a number of laudable efforts to quantify public expenditure on illegal drugs (EMCDDA, 2008). Again, public expenditure covers only a part of all social costs attributable to drugs, and indirect costs, most notably the costs due to drug overdosing, are not covered, resulting in a severe underestimate. On the other hand, not all public expenses due to illegal drugs are necessarily a result of addiction. Consider the example of expenses due to cannabis use: although only a minority of cannabis users will become addicted, public expenditure would include all costs related to cannabis use per se.

Table 9.1 Total government expenditure attributable to illicit drugs for 2005 for selected European countries

Country	Amount (€ million)	Amount as a proportion of total public expenditure (%)
Ireland	176.8	0.32
Malta	4.9	0.23
United Kingdom	1463.8	0.18
Denmark	119.1	0.11
Poland	107.0	0.10
Portugal	69.1	0.10
Luxembourg	9.8	0.08
Greece	53.4	0.06
Slovenia	7.5	0.06
Estonia	1.9	0.05
Cyprus	3.2	0.05
Lithuania	3.5	0.05
Romania	13.5	0.04
Czech Republic	16.9	0.04
France	315.4	0.03
Slovakia	1.9	0.01
Finland	8.0	0.01
Germany	35.5	0.003
Austria*	4.0	0.003
Hungary	1.0	0.002
Croatia	7.2	n.a.

*Most of the expenditure in Austria is in regional and local budgets and was therefore not collected as part of this exercise.

Table 9.1 shows total government expenditure attributable to illicit drugs for 2005 in a selection of European countries as part of the most comprehensive assessment to date (EMCDDA, 2008). An update of these figures for 2008 revealed no marked changes (<http://www.emcdda.europa.eu/stats10/ppptab10>). While it is clear that the total social costs for Europe attributable to illegal drugs are of the order of billions of Euros, as for alcohol and tobacco, the lack of data makes it difficult to produce a breakdown of where those costs lie (see the various tables in EMCDDA (2008), which reveal a patchwork of data availability by country).

9.5 **Social costs of gambling**

There are no overall data on the social costs due to gambling available to date, making a specific estimate based on gambling addiction impossible. In the future, the ALICE RAP project will define the data essential for estimating the social costs of gambling and gambling addiction, as well as describing the methodologies needed to collect these data (<http://www.alicerap.eu/>).

9.6 **Discussion**

Since they were first published, social cost studies have been severely criticized (e.g. Shiell et al., 1987; for a recent summary see Mäkelä, 2012). However, they must fulfil some need as otherwise they would neither be published nor cited in increasing numbers (Rehm, 2012). The main problem at this point is the lack of standardization and underlying rationale for carrying out such studies in different countries. As long as various countries in Europe continue to produce their own studies with different methodologies we will be far from being able to clarify the costs of substance use or addiction in Europe. Moreover, it is not clear how addiction should be defined in order to make such studies most useful. However, there are good reasons to conduct such studies in a way consistent with the ALICE RAP definition of addiction as heavy use over time (Rehm et al., 2012, 2013b).

In Europe it is clear that the social costs of addiction are immense. However, it is also apparent that there is a gap in the literature on the subject. Even where research has been conducted, inconsistent methodologies and definitions make it difficult to give accurate estimates or draw conclusions. Social costs due to addiction are in theory fully avoidable, and in practice at least partially so (Collins et al., 2006; Rehm et al., 2006). It is therefore recommended that a European study with clear objectives, a consistent and unified methodology, and standardized procedures is launched. A detailed cost study is vital because policy decisions need to be informed by data on what portion of the current burden and costs could be avoided and how.

References

Anderson, P. & Baumberg, B. (2006). *Alcohol in Europe: A Public Health Perspective. A Report of the European Commission*. London: Institute of Alcohol Studies.

Asbridge, M., Hayden, J.A., & Cartwright, J.L. (2012). Acute cannabis consumption and motor vehicle collision risk: systematic review of observational studies and meta-analysis. *British Medical Journal*, **344**, e536.

Aspect Consortium (2004). *Tobacco or Health in the European Union. Past, Present, and Future*. Luxembourg: European Commission Office for Official Publications of the European Communities.

Collins, D.J. & Lapsley, H.M. (2008). *The Costs of Tobacco, Alcohol and Illicit Drug Abuse to Australian Society in 2004/05: Summary Version*. Canberra: Department of Health and Ageing.

Collins, D., Lapsley, H., Brochu, S., et al. (2006). *International Guidelines for the Estimation of the Avoidable Costs of Substance Abuse*. Ottawa, ON: Health Canada.

EMCDDA (2008). *Towards a Better Understanding of Drug-Related Public Expenditure in Europe*. Luxembourg: Publications Office of the European Union.

Gustavsson, A., Svensson, M., Jacobi, F., et al. (2011). Cost of disorders of the brain in Europe 2010. *European Neuropsychopharmacology*, **21**, 718–779.

Mäkelä, K. (2012). Cost-of-alcohol studies as a research programme. *Nordisk Alkohol och Narkotikatidskrift*, **29**, 321–343.

Manning, M., Smith, C., & Mazerolle P. (2013). The societal costs of alcohol misuse in Australia. *Trends and Issues in Crime and Criminal Justice*, **2013**, 454-1–454-6.

Mohapatra, S., Patra, J., Popova, S., Duhig, A., & Rehm J. (2010). Social cost of heavy drinking and alcohol dependence in high-income countries. *International Journal of Public Health*, **55**, 149–157.

Olesen, J., Gustavsson, A., Svensson, M., et al. (2012). The economic cost of brain disorders in Europe. *European Journal of Neurology*, **19**, 155–162.

Rehm, J. (2012). Cost of illness studies for alcohol consumption—Why are they still in demand?. *Nordisk Alkohol och Narkotikatidskrift*, **29**, 345–347.

Rehm, J., Taylor, B., Patra, J., & Gmel, G. (2006). Avoidable burden of disease: conceptual and methodological issues in substance abuse epidemiology. *International Journal of Methods in Psychiatric Research*, **15**, 181–191.

Rehm, J., Gnam, W., Popova, S., et al. (2007). The social costs of alcohol, illegal drugs and tobacco in Canada 2002. *Journal of Studies on Alcohol and Drugs*, **68**, 886–895.

Rehm, J., Shield, K.D., Rehm, M.X., Gmel, G. Jr., & Frick, U. (2012). *Alcohol Consumption, Alcohol Dependence, and Attributable Burden of Disease in Europe: Potential Gains From Effective Interventions for Alcohol Dependence*. Toronto, ON: Centre for Addiction and Mental Health.

Rehm, J., Anderson, P., Gual, A., et al. (2013a). The tangible common denominator of substance use disorders: a reply to commentaries to Rehm et al. *Alcohol and Alcoholism*, **49**, 118–122.

Rehm, J., Marmet, S., Anderson, P., et al. (2013b). Defining substance use disorders: do we really need more than heavy use?. *Alcohol and Alcoholism*, **48**, 633–640.

Rehm, J., Shield, K.D., Rehm, M.X., Gmel, G., & Frick, U. (2013c). Modelling the impact of alcohol dependence on mortality burden and the effect of available treatment interventions in the European Union. *European Neuropsychopharmacology*, **23**, 89–97.

Rice, D., Kelman, S., & Miller, L. (1990). *The Economic Costs of Alcohol and Drug Abuse and Mental Illness: 1985*. DHHS Publication No. (ADM) 90–1694. Washington, DC: Department of Health and Human Services.

Shiell, A., Gerard, K., & Donaldson C. (1987). Cost of illness studies: an aid to decision making? *Health Policy*, **8**, 317–323.

Single, E., Collins, D., Easton, B., Harwood, H., Lapsley, H., & Maynard, A. (1996). *International Guidelines for Estimating the Costs of Substance Abuse*. Ottawa, ON: Canadian Centre on Substance Abuse.

Single, E., Collins, D., Easton, B., et al. (2003). *International Guidelines for Estimating the Costs of Substance Abuse*, 2nd edn. Geneva: World Health Organization.

Single, E. & Easton, B. (ed.) (2001). Estimating the economic costs of alcohol misuse: why we should do it even though we shouldn't pay too much attention to the bottom line results. Paper presented at the annual meeting of the Kettil Bruun Society for Social and Epidemiological Research on Alcohol. Kettil Bruun Society Annual Meeting, May 2001, Toronto, Canada. Available at: <http://www.eastonbh.ac.nz/2001/05/estimating_the_economic_costs_of_alcohol_misuse/>

Taylor, B., Irving, H.M., Kanteres, F., et al. (2010). The more you drink, the harder you fall: a systematic review and meta-analysis of how acute alcohol consumption and injury or collision risk increase together. *Drug and Alcohol Dependence*, **110**, 108–116.

Chapter 10

Addictive substances and socioeconomic development

Robin Room, Sujatha Sankaran, Laura A. Schmidt, Pia Mäkelä, and Jürgen Rehm

10.1 Introduction to the relationship between addictive substances and behaviours and socioeconomic development

This chapter considers the interplay of socioeconomic factors with a set of habit-forming behaviours, and the social and health problems that may result from them. The behaviours for consideration, as in the rest of this book, include the use of alcohol, tobacco, and other psychoactive substances. While the patterns we discuss are also often applicable to gambling and other behavioural addictions, the main focus of this chapter will be on psychoactive substances, for which population-based research findings are globally available and robust. The socioeconomic factors to be considered include the relative penury or affluence of a society, and the socioeconomic status of people and families within a given society. These factors are set in a context of consideration of socioeconomic development at a global level—of rising though unevenly distributed standards of living globally—and the implications for addictive behaviours and for population rates of social and health problems arising from those behaviours.

Rising affluence has many positive impacts on the health and well-being of populations. Through improved sanitation, public health infrastructures, and access to education, economic development brings populations across the 'epidemiological transition' towards declining rates of prevalence of and mortality from infectious diseases (Wilkinson, 1996). However, development typically increases disposable income, and people often use that income to consume more alcohol, drugs, tobacco, and highly processed 'hyper-palatable' foods, as well as to gain digital access to potential sources of 'process disorders', such as internet gambling, gaming, and pornography. The growing prosperity of societies around the globe is, from the perspective of addictive substances and experiences, a double-edged sword. Under global trade regimes, commercial interests are often free to promote consumption and nullify market restrictions sought by nations and communities. Producers today have a virtually unfettered capacity to market many pleasure-inducing substances and experiences globally—but particularly in the 'emerging markets' of the developing world. Thus, development puts populations at risk for chronic, non-communicable 'diseases of affluence' that have afflicted the West for generations. Put differently, addictions may in their own right warrant the designation, 'diseases of development'.

In this chapter we review what is known about how socioeconomic variations in development are affecting the uneven burden of alcohol, illicit drugs, tobacco, and other habitual behaviours between and within societies around the globe. First, we define development and its functions in the production of addiction-related health risks and inequities. Secondly, we examine how, as societies undergo the process of development, the concentration and commercialized production of addictive products promotes their widespread use and growth in social inequities in health-related harms. Thirdly, we review socioeconomic variation in patterns of use and related problems, within and between societies, for the most common, best-researched addictive substances. We conclude with a brief discussion of those movements of thought and action that can counter the trends towards rising rates of use and social inequities in addictive disorders.

10.2 Harm from use of psychoactive substances and addictive behaviours

There have been a number of comparative ratings of the intrinsic harmfulness of different psychoactive substances (e.g. Hilts, 1994; Hall et al., 1999; Roques, 1999; Gable 2004; Strategy Unit, 2005; Nutt et al., 2007, 2010). While the ratings often consider various dimensions of harm separately, they tend to be summarized in terms of a single overall dimension. Often there is substantial unease and controversy over these ratings because the rank order of harmfulness clearly differs from both popular conceptions of relative harmfulness and from the legal standing and classifications of the substances in international and national laws (Room, 2006b). In particular, cannabis has tended to be rated as relatively less harmful than its legal status assumes, and alcohol as more harmful. In recent years, as more attention has been paid to harm from substance use to others around the user (e.g. Room et al., 2010; Melberg et al., 2011; Borch, 2012), alcohol's rank has moved higher; indeed it was ranked as the most intrinsically harmful substance in the most recent such ranking (Nutt et al., 2010). In a separate literature, issues concerning the intrinsic harmfulness of different forms of and settings for gambling have also been given consideration (e.g. Blaszczynski et al., 2001).

There are of course factors other than the substance or behaviour itself that contribute to the potential risk at a particular occasion or setting. The mode of use (oral, nasal, by intravenous injection, etc.) is one such factor, with injection drug use (IDU) generally being the most hazardous mode, at least in terms of potential overdose. Such considerations are brought into play in objections to the rankings (e.g. Caulkins et al., 2011), although such objections ignore the fact that the legal classifications of the substances, with fateful consequences for those arrested under the laws, are on a single dimension of presumed danger (Room, 2011). Thinking in terms of overall population harm from a substance or behaviour, the prevalence and intensity of use or the behaviour is of course potentially as important as intrinsic harmfulness, and factors such as mode, set, and setting of use are also important. Most obviously in the occurrence and se-quelae of social problems, but also for health harms, the extent of harm also often reflects the reactions of others to the behaviour (Room, 2005).

As further discussed later, the harms from addictive behaviours often differ according to socioeconomic status, whether we are considering the status of society as a whole or an individual. All the factors we have mentioned as affect-ing the occurrence of harm are potentially in play for different levels of socio-economic status.

10.3 **Defining development, inequity, and related concepts**

Economic development generally refers to sustained actions that promote im-provement in the standard of living and economic health of a specific area. The scope of development includes the process and policies by which a nation im-proves the economic, political, and social well-being of its people (World Bank, 2012). In the absence of counteracting policies, development typically leads to an uneven distribution of wealth and social benefits—including those between so-called 'developed' and 'developing' societies, as well as among socioeco-nomic groups or classes within a country's borders. Economic inequities tend to foster health inequities, with the latter referring to inequalities in health sta-tus or functioning between members of different social categories. One socio-economic differentiation is in terms of the development status of the society in which a person lives—does the person live in a rich, a middle-income or a poor society? It is well recognized that there is a strong but not perfect relationship between this and general life expectancy in the society, as in the World Health Organization's differentiations of countries in terms of levels of infant mortality and adult life expectancies. We will use these differentiations as a surrogate for development status (Wilkinson and Marmot, 2003).

A second kind of social differentiation occurs within a given society, particularly for differentiations that are socially recognized and affect social standing as well as access to resources. These include social class and socioeconomic status, but also such differentiations as gender, age, family status, and ethnic affiliation.

Socioeconomic differentiations between and within societies are often related to the patterns and intensity of substance use and addictive behaviours, although these are also affected by history and cultural and political factors. A separate issue is variation in the risks that a given pattern and intensity of consumption behaviour will result in adverse health and social effects. Such risks are usually greater for poorer than for richer people and populations. Thus, for a given level or pattern of population-wide use, addiction-related harms will generally be greater in poorer societies than in more affluent societies. However, *within* any given society, differentiations between rich and poor will produce further health inequities, often leading to a disproportionate burden of harm falling on the most poorly resourced groups. For chronic effects of heavy drinking such as liver cirrhosis, for instance, there will often be a worse outcome because of the existence of cofactors such as nutritional deficiencies or liver infections (Room et al., 2002). Where there is unequal treatment or access to resources, the health and injury consequences of a given level or pattern of substance use are also likely to be more severe for those with fewer resources.

The more serious consequences for poorer people and populations with heavy substance use or addictive behaviour are often a direct result of their restricted circumstances. An older, less well maintained car may offer less protection in a drink-driving crash, family members may have less private space to avoid a drunken relative, in a poorer society the social safety-nets financed by governments will generally be weaker. The consequences for the poor are also particularly affected by factors that are socially defined and enforced.

Stigma and marginalization are two concepts that are closely linked to discourses on addiction and usually differentially applied to poorer heavy users in a particular society (Room, 2005). In every society studied so far, addictive behaviours are to a greater or lesser degree moralized, meaning that those affected by severe addictions suffer from social dislocation and disenfranchisement. Thus in many languages there are stigmatizing terms for someone who is seen as habitually transgressing the boundaries (e.g. 'un ivrogne' or 'clochard' in French, 'a drunkard' or 'drunk' in English), and these terms may become a master status in terms of which the person is primarily defined (see Hughes, 1945). In a fourteen-country WHO cross-cultural study of disabilities, key informants assigned 'alcoholism' an average rank of fourth out of eighteen conditions in terms of the degree of social disapproval or stigma in the society—greater disapproval in most societies than for being 'dirty or unkempt' or for 'chronic mental disorder'. The key informants also ranked second out of ten conditions 'someone who is visibly drunk' in terms of adverse public reactions to appearing in public—consistently more adverse than for someone with a chronic mental disorder who 'acts out', or for someone who is dirty and unkempt (Room et al., 2001).

A lower socioeconomic status may also render obvious manifestations of addiction more visible, and make those affected even more vulnerable to marginalization and stigma (Goffman, 1967; Chambliss, 1973). People with a low income, because of their lack of resources, are often less able to avoid public scrutiny, while the more affluent can purchase social or spatial buffering of their behaviour. The end result, perhaps particularly in affluent societies, is that there is a strong overlap between the most marginalized population and those defined as having serious addiction problems. Thus, 77% of those entering treatment for alcohol problems in Stockholm were not in the workforce and 67% did not have fully stable living arrangements (Storbjörk and Room, 2008).

10.4 **Addictive disorders and the process of development: alcohol as an example**

Experience with alcohol provides an opportunity to see into the dynamics by which the *process* of development impacts upon patterns of consumption, and thereby related problems (see Schmidt and Room, 2012). Other authors have published similar accounts for the cases of sugar (Mintz, 1985), tobacco (Brooks, 1952), and other substances of abuse (Schivelbusch, 1992; Courtwright, 2001).

The use of alcoholic beverages was very widespread in tribal and village societies prior to the modern era. Fermented alcoholic beverages were known in all cultures except in Australia, Oceania, and North America (roughly, north of Mexico). In societies without alcohol aboriginally, the encounter with alcoholic beverages after European contact was often abrupt and highly problematic. Where alcohol was traditionally consumed, production of alcoholic beverages was common on a small scale as a household or artisanal activity, particularly when and where agricultural surpluses were available. Fermented beverages produced in such circumstances could not be stored indefinitely nor transported far, and often spoiled quickly if not consumed. Drinking was thus often an occasional and communal activity, associated with particular communal festivals (Room et al., 2002).

There are many places in the world where versions of these traditional patterns originating from tribal and village societies persist today. But superimposed on them, and often replacing them, are patterns of production and consumption that have developed over the last 500 years or so. These involved new beverages, new modes of production, distribution, and promotion, and new drinking customs and institutions. Distilled spirits, coming to Europe by way of Arabia, made it possible to produce alcoholic beverages which did not spoil, and thus could be transported across the world. By the 1500s, as European empire-building got under way, distilled spirits had escaped from the medicine cabinet and were becoming an everyday drink. In the long period of colonial expansion, distilled spirits and fortified wines were a major tool through which native people were subjugated and exploited (Room et al., 2002, pp. 23–27). As the Industrial Revolution got under way, an early stage was industrial production of alcoholic beverages, particularly beer and spirits. As transportation improved, alcoholic beverages became a market commodity that was available in all seasons of the year, and at any time during the week. In Europe in particular the result was a flood of alcoholic beverages washing over one country after another, producing scenes of disorder, illness, and death (e.g. Coffey, 1966). Elsewhere in the world, the result was also often catastrophic. The American statesman Benjamin Franklin, for instance, noted in the late 1700s that rum had 'already annihilated all the tribes who formerly inhabited the seacoast' of eastern North America (Room et al., 2002, p. 153).

In the countries with early industrialization, alcohol played a two-sided role. On the one hand it was an early instrument of industrialization. On the other hand the greatly increased supply and often the widespread availability of alcohol proved disastrous for much of the population. By the nineteenth century, leaders of industry came to see it also as a major impediment to industrial life, which demanded a sober and attentive workforce. Eventually, and with great difficulty, industrializing societies in Europe and elsewhere came to see the flood of alcohol as a substantial social and health problem. In a number of countries, popular social movements to limit drinking and even to prohibit it gained broad membership and eventually political strength. Typically, after a century or more of popular movements and political activity, a new and fairly stable alcohol control structure was put in place. In the latter part of the nineteenth century, European colonial powers to a greater or lesser extent also imposed restrictions on the availability of alcohol in their colonies on other continents, particularly for the indigenous populations (Room et al., 2002).

We live today with the legacies of this history, but also with the results of new developments in the last half-century. The dissolution of the colonial empires also meant the removal of many of the restrictions on drinking in all non-Islamic parts of the world. Industrialized alcoholic beverages, such as European-style beer, became prestige commodities in many places; a bottle of Heineken or Carlsberg in one's hand became a cheap way of staking a claim to be cosmopolitan, part of the modern world.

In the meantime, developments in brewing, distilling, and packaging methods, and in transportation networks, increased the availability of alcoholic beverages everywhere. In the modern world, alcohol production has largely lost its old function as an early driver of industrialization, since production of industrialized products is now increasingly in the hands of multinational corporations headquartered in the developed world, and the beverages are produced in imported turn-key plants by a small production staff, presided over by expatriate brewers or distillers (Room and Jernigan, 2000). Trade agreements and disputes and structural adjustment plans imposed by international development agencies, in treating alcohol as an ordinary commodity, have contributed to dismantling arrangements which often limited the alcohol market. Meanwhile, global alcohol producers and distributors are able to call in each local market on the full range of advertising and other promotional techniques which have been developed and honed in recent decades (e.g. Jernigan, 1997, 2010).

With respect to economic development, alcohol still has a two-sided role, but the balance has shifted. Production of alcohol brings less benefit to the local economy of a developing country, since only a small labour force is involved in producing beer or spirits. Production will in any case be primarily directed to the domestic market—this is true for 95% of alcohol production worldwide. The largest exporters of alcohol are in Europe, and there are few examples of successful exports of alcohol from a developing country. The main examples of success are Mexico, with a large market next door, and Chile and South Africa, with their long-standing winegrowing traditions. Other exports from developing countries are mostly limited to niche markets.

One alcohol-related contribution to the local economy, particularly for favourably located island countries, comes from tourism. Given the multinational organization of the tourist trade, again the primary benefit in terms of local employment is relatively low-skilled and low-paying jobs.

Against these benefits must be set the costs (Cisneros Örnberg and Room, 2014). In a Caribbean town oriented heavily to tourism, Padilla et al. (2012) write that:

> Binge drinking by tourists was described as having a profound impact on alcohol and illicit drug use among local residents, and especially those employed by businesses catering to foreigners. These environments normalized excessive drinking and made it nearly impossible to conceive of a life without alcohol. Thus, even though alcohol was associated with 'fun', participants also mentioned the consequences of excessive alcohol consumption, which were often described with morally laden terms such as *vicio* (vice).

In some cultural contexts, the encouragement of a heavy-drinking environment may in the end be self-defeating. As an elder on Lamu, an island off the coast of Kenya, noted, tourists come to see a different way of life. However, they also bring money and different customs, such as drinking alcohol, both of which are very difficult for the island's young inhabitants to resist. Lamu needs the tourist trade—but, in the end, the tourists' influences may destroy what they come to see (Caputo, 2001, p. 110). In the case of successful economic development, alcohol consumption is likely to rise—as can be seen in China, South Korea, Thailand, and other growing Asian economies today—in the absence of religious proscriptions or public health-oriented alcohol controls. Often, because of their prestige value, imported beverages lead the trend. Thus, in the context of the oil boom in Venezuela, Diageo reported that its sales of Scotch whisky rose by 60% in 2005, despite the disapproval of the president (Romero, 2006). Generally speaking, with a rise in alcohol consumption, rates of alcohol-related problems will also rise. Thus the World Health Organization (WHO) studies of the contribution of alcohol to the Global Burden of Disease show that alcohol becomes increasingly important as a source of disability and death in countries with a higher standard of living.

10.5 Socioeconomic variations in patterns of use and problems

10.5.1 Alcohol

We first turn to the question of variations between richer and poorer countries in alcohol consumption and the problems it causes. Figure 10.1 shows the variation in the rate of abstention from alcohol by men in a country by the level of affluence of that country, measured in terms of gross domestic product (GDP) (US dollars at purchasing power parity, PPP) in 2002 (Schmidt et al., 2010). It will be seen that it is mainly in countries with a GDP below $US5000 per year that the majority of adult men abstain from alcohol. In the absence of public health counter-measures, it seems very likely that success in raising the GDP of

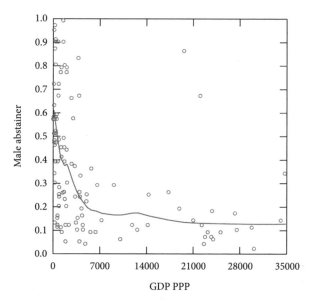

Fig. 10.1 The relation of gross domestic product (GDP) (at purchasing power parity, PPP) and the male abstention rate from alcohol in 2002.

Reproduced with permission from Schmidt, L.A., Mäkelä, P., Rehm, J., and Room, R., Alcohol: equity and social determinants, pp.11–30, in Blas, E. and Kurup, A.S. (Eds.), Equity, Social Determinants, and Public Health Programmes, World Health Organization, Geneva, Switzerland, Copyright © 2010, http://whqlibdoc.who.int/publications/2010/9789241563970_eng.pdf

the poorest countries will bring large numbers of people into the global drinking population. Figure 10.2 shows the relation between a country's affluence and the consumption of alcoholic beverages per adult. While the relationship is not so strong above a per capita GDP of $US9000, again there is a strong relationship between societal affluence and per capita alcohol consumption below a GDP of $US9000.

There are various ways of measuring the health burden from risk factors such as alcohol, but a commonly used one is disability-adjusted life years (DALYs), which reflects a combination of number of years lost from early deaths and fractional years lost when a person is disabled by an illness or injury. The proportions attributable to alcohol of all DALYs lost are higher in the middle- and high-income categories than in the low-income categories (Rehm et al., 2006). However, this partly reflects the much greater burden of disease in poorer regions of the world. If we consider the alcohol-attributable burden in absolute terms (DALYs per 1000 adults), then eastern Europe and Central Asia has the highest burden globally, with 36.48 DALYs per thousand adults. The second-highest toll is in the higher-consumption low-income countries, with 18.70

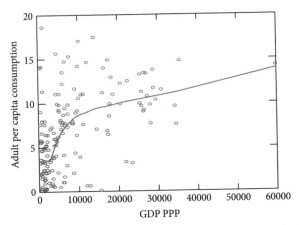

Fig. 10.2 Relationship between per capita purchasing power parity (PPP)-adjusted gross domestic product (GDP) and adult consumption (in litres) of alcohol per year, for 2002.
Reproduced with permission from Schmidt, L.A., Mäkelä, P., Rehm, J., and Room, R., Alcohol: equity and social determinants, pp.11–30, in Blas, E. and Kurup, A.S. (Eds.), Equity, Social Determinants, and Public Health Programmes, World Health Organization, Geneva, Switzerland, Copyright © 2010, http://whqlibdoc.who.int/publications/2010/9789241563970_eng.pdf

DALYs per thousand. At the bottom of the range is the low-consumption, low-income category, with 6.99 DALYs per thousand. The next lowest is the 'western' developed country category, at 11.75; the middle-income country category is in the middle, at 15.54.

We may tentatively conclude, taking into account the distribution of consumption by national income in Fig. 10.2, that it seems likely that adverse health consequences of drinking will rise with increasing income, particularly in countries at the poorer end of the global income distribution, but that a tendency for the rate of health problems per litre of alcohol to fall with increasing affluence may to some extent mitigate the relationship between the problems and societal affluence at higher levels of national income.

Next we turn to differences in how drinking-related patterns and problems contribute to differences between social groups within a given country. The proportion of drinking occasions that involve binge-drinking is typically larger for drinkers with a low socioeconomic status (Knupfer, 1989; Mäkelä et al., 2003). However, this is not only due to a higher number of binge-drinking occasions among drinkers of a low socioeconomic status but also to the higher number of non-binge-drinking occasions among high-socioeconomic-status drinkers, who can afford to drink on more varying types of occasions, including occasions where the primary aim is not intoxication (Mäkelä, 1983). Overall, income seems to have a special role with respect to alcohol use and heavy drinking, increasing their likelihood when other factors are held constant (McKee et al., 2000; Hradilova Selin, 2004).

The few existing studies from the developing world tend to show diverging results depending on the country in question. A positive social class gradient was observed for frequent drunkenness among both men and women in Bahia, Brazil (Almeida-Filho et al. 2005) and in Bloomfield et al.'s (2006) study of some European countries. In contrast, national results from India (Subramanian et al., 2005) implied a negative gradient between alcohol use and income and alcohol use and education among men; similar results were also obtained for the connection between education, income, and alcohol use in a study in a Delhi slum (Saxena et al., 2003). It is also clear that those who are less well off access non-beverage and other low-quality alcohol. In empirical studies, the use of non-beverage alcohol has been observed to be more common in Russia among those with a low level of education (Lachenmeier et al., 2007; Leon et al., 2007).

Evidence about differences in alcohol-attributable mortality according to socioeconomic status comes mainly from developed countries. These studies—with very few exceptions—have shown that deaths from alcohol-attributable causes are more common in positions with a lower than a higher socioeconomic status. The observed alcohol-attributable mortality ratios between the lowest and highest educational, occupational, and income groups in Finland range between 3.3 and 6.1 for men and 2.8 and 3.5 for women (Mäkelä, 1999). For manual versus upper non-manual groups in Sweden the alcohol-attributable mortality ratios were 3.2 for men and 2.4 for women (Hemström, 2002). In the UK, Harrison and Gardiner (1999) found mortality ratios of 15 between the lowest and highest occupational categories among UK men aged 25–39, of 3.2 among men aged 55–64, of 1.5 among women aged 25–39, and of 0.3 among women aged 55–64. In Russia, Shkolnikov et al. (1998) quoted mortality ratios of 3.5 for men and 4.6 for women between groups with low and high levels of education. Similar mortality ratios of 1.2–2.6 for cirrhosis of the liver between lower and higher educational groups among men aged 45–59 were found in the Czech Republic, Hungary, Estonia, the United States, Norway, and Finland by Kunst (1997). In the United States, Singh and Hoyert (2000) found mortality ratios of 2.4–5.1 among men and 1.8–4.8 among women between the lowest and highest educational, occupational, and family income groups. A mortality ratio of approximately 2.5 for cirrhosis of the liver was found in Australia for manual versus non-manual male workers (Najman et al., 2007). It has further been found that each new dimension of socioeconomic status has an additive effect on top of the others, reflecting the dimension of marginalization. In Finland, education, occupational class, personal income, household net income, and housing tenure each remained statistically significant predictors of alcohol-attributable mortality after adjusting for the other dimensions of socioeconomic status, each showing a negative gradient (Mäkelä, 1999).

There are few studies of self-reported alcohol problems and socioeconomic position in developing countries, but the existing ones point to a relatively strong negative gradient. In Nepal, using the CAGE questionnaire as the measure of problems, 36% of respondents with no education met the criteria for having alcohol problems (two or more positive answers out of four), whereas only 17% of respondents with 11 years of education did (Jhingan et al., 2003). In southern Brazil, the prevalence of Alcohol Use Disorders Identification Test (AUDIT) cases (with 8+ points as the cut-off point) was 2.7% in the highest socioeconomic status category (based on years of schooling and utilities in the household) and 13.7% in the lowest (Mendoza-Sassi and Béria, 2003).

Thus, although abstention is generally more common among poorer people in a given society, among those who drink at all health-related problems from drinking tend to be more common among poorer than richer drinkers in low- and middle-income societies. While this may in part reflect class differences in patterns of drinking, it usually primarily reflects the differential vulnerability of poorer people to alcohol problems from a given level and pattern of drinking.

10.5.2 Psychoactive substances controlled by international treaties

A wide variety of psychoactive substances are subject to control by three international drug treaties, which attempt on the one hand to ensure supplies of such substances for medicinal use while on the other hand prohibiting their availability for non-medical human consumption (Babor et al., 2010).

Globally, the use of substances produced and distributed (and often promoted) through legal channels for medical purposes is highly concentrated in high-income countries (HICs). This is demonstrated dramatically by data collected by the International Narcotics Control Board (INCB) for the medicinal use of opioids (INCB, 2014). The medicinal use of opioids is more than an order of magnitude higher in Europe and Oceania, dominated by HICs, and several times greater again in North America (the United States and Canada), than in other parts of the world. In HICs, there is now considerable worry about overuse of medically prescribed opioids (e.g. Manchikanti et al., 2012). At the other end of the availability continuum, the World Health Organization has estimated that about 80% of the world's population lacks access to effective medications for moderate and severe pain (Scholten et al., 2007).

The same general pattern of greater use with greater economic affluence is shown for use of psychotropic medications such as tranquillizers, anti-depressants, sedatives and hypnotics, anti-psychotics, and psychostimulants. Annual dosage units for these drugs per capita are several times higher in HICs than in low- to middle-income countries (LMICs; Rose, 2007). Data from commercial sources on the use of such psychoactive medications for selected countries is shown in Table 10.1.

At a global level, the most widely available estimates of illegal drug use are for lifetime or current use (in the last year). Use rates set an upper limit to the potential harm from substance use, but do not give much indication in themselves of the extent of health or social harm.

The use of illegal drugs is reported in almost every country of the world, but different types of drugs and levels of use are found in different regions (Degenhardt and Hall, 2012). Table 10.2 shows the estimated rates of use in 2009 for four main classes of illegal drugs in each continent, and also for high-income regions within two continents (Oceania is a third such region, with the figures dominated by Australia and New Zealand). Cannabis is by far the most commonly used controlled drug, with over five times the rate of current users in the population as for any other class of illegal drugs. Rates of use of cannabis are generally lower in Asia than in other regions. Rates of non-medical use of amphetamines and opioids are roughly equal overall, although one is dominant in particular regions: amphetamines in Africa and Asia, opioids in the Americas and eastern Europe. The use of illegal drugs is generally more prevalent in HICs. Particular regions stand out for some drug classes among LMICs: Africa for amphetamines, the Americas for cocaine, and poorer regions of Europe for

Table 10.1 Prescriptions for psychiatric drugs in 2001, in standard dosage units per 1000 population

	USA	Europe	Japan	South America	South Africa	Pakistan
Tranquillizers	20,361	22,630	28,211	4781	2266	3802
Antidepressants	33,768	19,010	9202	1835	2330	919
Sedatives and hypnotics	7362	15,562	14,721	1299	1701	387
Antipsychotics	6954	8373	14,437	1062	1490	754
Psychostimulants	6488	364	184	47	105	7
Total	74,934	65,940	66,755	9023	7892	5868

Reproduced with permission from Martin Knapp et al., *Mental Health Policy and Practice across Europe: The future direction of mental health care*, Copenhagen, WHO Regional Office for Europe, p. 152, Copyright © 2006, available from http://www.euro.who.int/en/publications/abstracts/mental-health-policy-and-practice-across-europe.-the-future-direction-of-mental-health-care.

Source: data from IMS Health First Study, *World FactBook 2001*, Central Intelligence Agency (CIA), Washington, DC, USA, 2001, available from https://www.cia.gov/library/publications/the-world-factbook/index.html

Table 10.2 Estimated 1-year prevalence of non-medical users of different drug classes by global region, percentage of adults aged 15–64

Region (selected subregions)	Cannabis	Amphetamines	Opioids	Cocaine
Africa	3.3	0.9	0.33	0.4
Americas	7.9	1.0	2.1	1.3
(North America)	(10.7)	(1.3)	(3.9)	(1.5)
Asia	1.9	0.7	0.4	0.05
Europe	5.6	0.5	0.7	0.8
(west and central Europe)	(7.6)	(0.7)	(0.4)	(1.2)
Oceania	10.9	2.1	3.0	1.5
Global	3.9	0.7	0.7	0.4

Source: data from *The Lancet*, Volume 379, Number 9810, Louisa Degenhardt and Wayne Hall, Extent of illicit drug use and dependence, and their contribution to the global burden of disease, pp. 55–70, Copyright © 2012 Elsevier Limited and United Nations Office on Drugs and Crime, *World Drug Report 2011*, United Nations, New York, USA, Copyright © United Nations, available from https://www.unodc.org/documents/data-and-analysis/WDR2011/World_Drug_Report_2011_ebook.pdf

opioids. Among HICs, fewer people in western and central Europe use amphetamines and opioids than in North America and Oceania.

Global estimates of population rates of harm from the use of illegal drugs are also approximations. One indicator is the proportion of people among the population aged 15–64 who inject drugs, since IDU involves a heightened risk of overdose and (particularly where sterile needles are not available) of HIV and other infections. The IDU rate is estimated to be over 0.5% in eastern Europe, Central Asia, the Caribbean, Latin and North America, and Australia and New Zealand—a mixture of HICs and LMICs—and 0.06% or lower in South Asia, the Middle East, and North Africa (Degenhardt and Hall, 2012). Again, the pattern emerges of rates of harm which seem to reflect the influence both of extent of use and of a lower level of economic resources.

In terms of variation by socioeconomic status within national populations, most studies have been carried out in HICs. A common finding is that, at least for youthful experimentation or regular use of illegal drugs, socioeconomic status is not an important source of variation (see Humensky (2010) for the United States and Challier et al. (2000) for France). More generally, a systematic review covering both alcohol and illegal drug use, and drawing on studies primarily from the United States but also from Canada, the UK, the Netherlands, and Finland, concluded that there was no clear relation between living in a disadvantaged neighbourhood and levels of drug use or heavy use (Karriker-Jaffe, 2011).

For one form of harm from drugs, arrest and prosecution for illegal selling or possession, there is clear evidence, again primarily from HICs, that the poor are more likely to get the blame, with arrest rates often being especially high for visible minority populations (e.g. Johnson et al., 1977; Room, 2005; Levine et al., 2010). There is also clear evidence that low socioeconomic status predicts more adverse health outcomes among drug users (Galea and Vlahov, 2002; Wood et al., 2002; Galea et al., 2003).

Whether through legal or illegal channels, the use of psychoactive substances is to a considerable degree a function of living in a relatively affluent society. Within particular societies, the patterning of substance use (whether legally or illegally) by socioeconomic status varies, with relatively little variation among youth cohorts in some societies. But the harms from a particular pattern of substance use are almost invariably more severe for those having a lower status in a society than for those of higher status. For many harms the same is likely to be true in comparing lower-income societies with higher-income societies.

10.5.3 **Tobacco**

Tobacco was well known as a psychoactive substance to indigenous cultures in much of the Americas, with some form of smoking being the usual mode of use (Robicsek, 1978). Brought to Europe from the New World, the custom of tobacco smoking, mostly in a pipe or as a cigar, spread widely and quickly, although there was also use without combustion by nasal inhalation of snuff.

The tobacco market and habits of tobacco smoking were transformed in the course of the twentieth century by the development of machines for the industrial production of cigarettes and the concomitant development of advertising and other promotional methods. Becoming widespread among men in the armies of the First World War, the cigarette habit was initially primarily a male prerogative, but it also spread among women in industrialized societies, particularly after the Second World War (Ferrence, 1989). While addiction doctors had already been concerned about tobacco smoking in the early 1900s (e.g. Towns, 1915), and several US states briefly prohibited cigarette sales in that era, cigarette sales quickly became a free and open market in much of the world, and to this day tobacco products are commonly treated in trade agreements and disputes as just another market commodity (Shaffer et al., 2005).

Meanwhile, beginning in the 1950s with the establishment of a firm basis for the harms to health from tobacco smoking, a public health effort to reduce tobacco smoking by regulations and restrictions as well as public information and persuasion has gathered force. Initially this was primarily in HICs, but now it has a global reach through such instruments as the Framework Convention on Tobacco Control (FCTC), an international treaty which came into force in 2005 (World Health Organization, 2013). In HICs the rate of smoking has considerably decreased, with a much greater decrease among those of a higher than of a lower socioeconomic status. Meanwhile, the global tobacco companies, which control much of the world cigarette market, have turned to the rapidly develop-ing LMICs, which they hope will grow as a market in the way that HIC markets grew during the twentieth century.

Thus the present time is one of transition, and mostly because of this there are a diversity of socioeconomic patterns of smoking and heavy smoking. Typically, heavy smoking in HICs now has a strong inverse relationship to social class, with heavy smokers most commonly found among those below the national median income. In LMICs this pattern may often be reversed. In terms of com-parisons between societies, the trends at the societal level look quite different in HICs, where cigarette smoking is stable or has considerably declined (in Aus-tralia, for instance, cigarette consumption per capita for the whole population has halved since 1980), while cigarette consumption is still rising with rising incomes in many LMICs.

Most of what we know about current global patterns of tobacco use comes from the Global Adult Tobacco Survey, a comprehensive system created by the World Health Organization in order to quantify tobacco use in each country and provide data about the patterns of use in different countries (World Health Organization, 2007). It tells us that nearly 80% of tobacco smokers live in devel-oping countries, which also have the highest burden of tobacco-related disease. However, regions of the world with the highest rates of death from tobacco use are the Americas and Europe, and, worldwide, men have higher mortality rates from tobacco use than women. However, because of the lead-time between to-bacco use and tobacco-related deaths, rates of death from tobacco use in women may skyrocket in the next several years. As noted, there are disparities between tobacco use and tobacco-related mortality for people in LMICs versus individ-uals in more affluent countries, as well as between individuals of a different so-cioeconomic status within countries. Worldwide, tobacco use causes approximately 7% of all deaths from tuberculosis, 12% of deaths from lower respiratory infections, 10% of deaths from cardiovascular diseases, 22% of deaths from cancer, and 36% of deaths from any respiratory system disease. Seventy-one per cent of all lung cancer deaths are due to tobacco use (Centers for Disease Control and Prevention, 2012).

Among developing countries, China is the largest cigarette-producing and cigarette-consuming nation in the world, with approximately 350 million smokers. China produces 42% of the world's cigarettes, and the Chinese Na-tional Tobacco Corporation is the largest manufacturer of tobacco products in the world. In 2010, 28.1% of the Chinese population smoked tobacco (World Health Organization, 2007). Other countries, however, have higher percentages of smokers, though their absolute numbers are lower. Approximately 39% of the Russian population used tobacco in 2009 (60% of men and 21% of women).

And in Turkey 31% of the population used tobacco in 2008 (48% of men and 15% of women) (World Health Organization, 2007).

India is the world's second-largest market for tobacco, and in 2011 approximately 275 million Indians, almost 35% of the Indian population, used tobacco in some form. Unlike much of the rest of the world, manufactured cigarettes do not constitute the majority of tobacco consumed in India. In India, higher-income populations primarily use manufactured cigarettes while lower-income segments of the population use bidis and smokeless tobacco (World Health Organization, 2007).

Other developing countries have patterns of tobacco use and problems closer to those observed in the West. The 2009 Global Adult Tobacco Survey showed that 15.9% of Mexicans are smokers but only 7.6% of the total population smokes daily. Almost 25% of Mexican men and 8% of Mexican women smoke cigarettes. In Brazil, approximately 17.2% of the total Brazilian population smoked tobacco: 21% of men and 13% of women smoke cigarettes and 24.4% of adults are exposed to tobacco smoke in the workplace. Sub-Saharan Africa has lower rates of tobacco use than other regions of the world. However, there is a notable paucity of data about rates of tobacco use in Africa, as no WHO Global Adult Tobacco Surveys were conducted in Africa until the first one in 2013, in Nigeria. This survey revealed that 10.0% of men, 1.1% of women, and 5.6% overall used tobacco products (World Health Organization, 2013).

Regarding within-society socioeconomic variations, in the United States in 2012, 29% of adults who were below the poverty line smoked, compared with 17.9% of adults who were at or above the poverty line. Approximately 25.5% of adults who have not graduated from high school smoke, compared with just 9.3% of those with a college education and 5% of those with a graduate degree. Among non-college-bound high-school seniors, the smoking rate is 27.9%, compared with 14.7% of college-bound seniors (Campaign for Tobacco-Free Kids, 2013).

Within-society variation is also evident in less developed countries. There is a relationship between annual household income and smoking; for example, individuals living below the poverty line in Thailand are more likely to smoke cigarettes than those with a higher income. The 2009 Global Adult Tobacco Survey showed that 0.9% of men and 5.6% of women in Thailand are daily users of smokeless tobacco. Conversely, in Mexico, higher education is associated with higher rates of smoking among Mexican women, and women in both rural and urban households with greater assets have higher rates of smoking. In contrast, higher education is associated with lower smoking rates among Mexican men in both urban and rural areas (World Health Organization, 2007).

In general, poorer and rural segments of populations in developing countries tend to use local and hand-rolled forms of tobacco, while wealthier urban individuals use manufactured cigarettes. These patterns vary greatly depending on region and cultural factors. In most societies, men tend to have higher rates of tobacco use than women. Wealth, education, and class have a complex relationship with rates of tobacco use. As individuals become wealthier and more educated there is often an increase in rates of tobacco use corresponding to class advancement that affords prestige to tobacco use. However, as wealth and education increase further, rates of tobacco use decrease because more importance is placed on the health consequences. Again, these are broad generalizations and the specific situation in each country varies based on particular cultural factors.

10.6 Conclusion: addictive behaviours, market forces, and public health

From the perspective of public health and addictive behaviours we are currently at a crossroads between elements both old and new. There is much that is redolent of the past, for example the strength of market forces in pushing for ever more open markets, unfettered by public health restrictions. In its imperial past, Britain fought two wars to enforce the opening of the Chinese market to opium grown in India as a major financial prop for its Indian empire. Tobacco companies using bilateral trade agreements to fight off minor impediments, such as the Australian legislation on plain packaging for cigarettes, can be seen as pursuing similar ambitions using current means. Ironically, the Australian government could be seen as operating a double standard in a budding dispute with Thailand where Australia is one of the countries opposing proposed graphic warning labels on alcoholic beverages in Thailand (O'Brien, 2013). Whereas drugs were the 'glue' of global political empires in past centuries (Courtwright, 2001), it is now global commercial empires that push for open markets, building demand with promotional efforts well beyond the capacity of the old empires, and resisting any market controls while working steadily toward 'regulatory capture', where regulatory control is neutralized.

Looking at the history of northern and western Europe and its settler offshoots, we see another potential turning point in a Hegelian dialectic which, for some addictive substances, has already taken several turns. A seven-society collaborative project studying the rise in alcohol consumption between 1950 and 1980 noted a pattern of 'long waves of alcohol consumption' (Mäkelä et al., 1981) with upsurges about every 70 years. Rising rates of consumption and problems may reach a pivot point, after which social activism takes over in the absence of government action. Thus the counterparts to tidal waves of alcohol consumption have been waves of spontaneously arising temperance movements and agitation, followed by legislation to curb product availability (Room, in press). In the current climate of free markets and unfettered access, rising consumption of psychoactive substances and behavioural addictions may soon reach the point where societies push back against market forces through popular movements, ultimately leading to governmental controls.

The early twentieth-century push-back against alcohol marketing was a global effort at prohibition (Schrad, 2010). In the end this failed for alcohol (as well as for tobacco, prohibited for a few years in some US states); but on a second front—the fight against 'narcotics'—the social movement succeeded in building an international prohibition and control structure, the drug control treaties and institutions that are still with us today. As Courtwright (2005) has argued, the compromise conceptualization for much of the twentieth century was to firmly split discussion of addictive 'drugs' from discussion of tobacco and alcohol, which were just 'habits' not requiring strong market controls.

Conceptually, and in terms of scientific research, as Courtwright notes, this distinction began to break down in the 1970s. But the division remains, as a Manichean split, in the treatment of different substances under international law, including notably trade law and disputes. Though substances controlled by the drug treaties could be subject to trade disputes concerning the trade in them as medications, it is notable that none of them have been; we may guess that the treaties have informally rendered this a 'no-go' area. On the other hand, attempts by governments to move towards measures to control or discourage the use of alcohol or tobacco have been fought every inch of the way by the commercial interests concerned, both in the national political sphere and through trade disputes and other means internationally. Within the United States in particular, the Supreme Court's rulings that 'commercial speech' is constitutionally protected point toward a division where restrictions on promotion may only be constitutionally permissible if the substance or behaviour is prohibited.

Meanwhile, a substantial global public health movement continues to build steam around restricting the marketing and promotion of cigarettes. For alcohol, in countries which had strong temperance movements and a subsequent strong reaction against them, the reactive impulse seems largely spent, and it is primarily commercial forces which drive a politics of wide and deregulated availability (e.g. Room, 2010). As discussed in Chapter 3, a new dimension in the concept of addictive substances has opened up around the place of sugar in the epidemics of obesity that afflict many countries, both HICs and LMICs. Sugar, alcohol, and tobacco are now increasingly being thought of together in public health planning and action in the context of a growing global effort to reduce the rates of non-communicable diseases (NCDs) such as cancer, heart disease, chest disorders, and diabetes (Lustig et al., 2012). Tobacco smoking, alcohol consumption, and dietary factors are the major risk factors for these diseases, and will increasingly be linked together in public health thinking and action.

One complexity that is emerging in this context is the issue of the relation between the psychoactive (and thus addictive) quality of the substance and the aspect that carries the main health risk. For alcohol these are one and the same—although some psychopharmacologists are pursuing the idea of an alcohol substitute that would provide the pleasure without carrying the harms (Nutt, 2006), others doubt these can be separated (Room, 2006a). With sugar, there is the prospect of substituting other sweeteners (Mesure, 2014). With tobacco, most of the harm to health comes from the smoking mode itself and as well as from nitrosamines in tobacco; the psychoactive ingredient, nicotine, has relatively few negative effects on physical health (Ferrence et al., 2000). Swedish *snus* and now e-cigarettes (Boseley, 2014) offer alternatives to cigarette smoking that carry a relatively low risk in terms of consequences for physical health. At least for nicotine and sweetness, it seems possible that the dialectic of market promotion and the counteractive measures of public health controls concerning addictive behaviours may be transcended.

Acknowledgements

Text extract reproduced with permission from Padilla, M.B., Guilamo-Ramos, V., and Godbole, R. (2012), A syndemic analysis of alcohol use and sexual risk behavior among tourism employees in Sosúa, Dominican Republic, *Qualitative Health Research*, Volume 22, pp. 89–102, Copyright © 2012 SAGE Publications.

Text extracts from Robin Room, Pia Mäkelä, Laura Schmidt, and Jürgen Rehm, Alcohol, Health Disparities, and Development, World Health Organization, Geneva, Switzerland, 2006, reproduced with permission from the World Health Organization.

References

Almeida-Filho, N., Lessa, I., Magahães, L., et al. (2005). Social inequality and alcohol consumption-abuse in Bahia, Brazil: interactions of gender, ethnicity and social class. *Social Psychiatry and Psychiatric Epidemiology*, 40, 214–222.

Babor, T., Caulkins, J., Edwards, G., et al. (2010). *Drug Policy and the Public Good*. Oxford: Oxford University Press.

Blaszczynski, A., Sharpe, L., & Walker, M. (2001). *The Assessment of the Impact of the Reconfiguration on Electronic Gaming Machines as Harm Minimisation Strategies for Problem Gambling*. Sydney: University of Sydney Gambling Research Unit. Available at: http://www.psych.usyd.edu.au/gambling/GIO_report.pdf

Bloomfield, K., Grittner, U., Kramer, S., & Gmel, G. (2006). Social inequalities in alcohol consumption and alcohol-related problems in the study countries of the EU concerted action 'Gender, culture and alcohol problems: a multi-national study'. *Alcohol and Alcoholism*, 41(Suppl.), i26–i36.

Borch, A. (2012). The Real of problem gambling households. *Journal of Gambling Issues*, issue 27. Available at: http://jgi.camh.net/doi/pdf/10.4309/jgi.2012.27.6

Boseley, S. (2014). Boom in e-cigarette sales divides smoking campaigners. *The Guardian* (London), 21 February. URL: <http://www.theguardian.com/society/2014/feb/21/boom-ecigarette-sales-divides-campaigners>

Brooks, J.E. (1952). *The Mighty Leaf: Tobacco through the Centuries*. Boston: Little, Brown.

Campaign for Tobacco-Free Kids (2013). *Tobacco and Socioeconomic Status*. URL: <http://www.tobaccofreekids.org/research/factsheets/pdf/0260.pdf>

Caputo, R. (2001). Swahili coast: East Africa's ancient crossroads, *National Geographic*, October, pp. 104–119.

Caulkins, J.P., Reuter, P., & Coulson, C. (2011). Basing scheduling decisions on scientific ranking of drugs' harmfulness: false promise from false premises. *Addiction*, 106, 1886–1890.

Centers for Disease Control and Prevention (2012). *Global Tobacco Surveillance System*. URL: <http://www.cdc.gov/tobacco/global/spotlight/>

Challier, B., Chau, N., Predine, R., Choquet, M., & Legras, B. (2000). Associations of family environment and individual factors with tobacco, alcohol and illicit drug use in adolescents. *European Journal of Epidemiology*, 16, 33–42.

Chambliss, W. (1973). The Saints and the Roughnecks. *Society*, 11, 24–31.

Cisneros Örnberg, J. &Room, R. (2014). Impacts of tourism on drinking and alcohol policy in low- and middle-income countries: a selective thematic review. *Contemporary Drug Problems*, 41, 145–169.

Coffey, T.G. (1966).Beer Street, Gin Lane—some views of 18th century drinking. *Quarterly Journal of Studies on Alcohol*, 27, 669–692.

Courtwright, D. (2001). *Forces of Habit: Drugs and the Making of the Modern World*. Cambridge, MA: Harvard University Press.

Courtwright, D.T. (2005). Mr. ATOD's wild ride: what do alcohol, tobacco, and other drugs have in common? *Social History of Alcohol and Drugs*, 20, 105–140.

Degenhardt, L. & Hall, W. (2012).Extent of illicit drug use and dependence, and their contribution to the global burden of disease. *Lancet*, 379, 55–70.

Ferrence, R.G. (1989). *Deadly Fashion: The Rise and Fall of Cigarette Smoking in North America*. New York: Garland Publishing.

Ferrence, R., Slade, J., Room, R., & Pope, M. (ed.) (2000). *Nicotine and Public Health*. Washington, DC: American Public Health Association.

Gable, R.S. (2004). Comparison of acute lethal toxicity of commonly abused psychoactive substances. *Addiction*, 99, 686–696.

Galea, S. & Vlahov, D. (2002).Social determinants and the health of drug users: socioeconomic status, homelessness, and incarceration. *Public Health Reports*, 117(Suppl. 1), S135–S145.

Galea, S., Ahern, J., Vlahov, D., et al. (2003). Income distribution and risk of fatal drug overdose in New York City neighborhoods. *Drug and Alcohol Dependence*, 70, 139–148.

Goffman, E. (1967). Mental symptoms and public order. In: *Interaction Ritual; Essays in Face-to-Face Behavior*, pp. 137–148. Chicago: Aldine.

Hall, W., Room, R., & Bondy, S. (1999). Comparing the health and psychological effects of alcohol, cannabis, nicotine and opiate use. In: *The Health Effects of Cannabis* (ed. H. Kalant, W. Corrigall, W. Hall, & R. Smart), pp. 475–506. Toronto, ON: Centre for Addiction and Mental Health.

Harrison, L. & Gardiner, E. (1999). Do the rich really die young? Alcohol-related mortality and social class in Great Britain, 1988–1994. *Addiction*, 94, 1871–1880.

Hemström, Ö. (2002).Alcohol-related deaths contribute to socioeconomic differentials in mortality in Sweden. *European Journal of Public Health*, 12, 254–262.

Hilts, P.J. (1994). Is nicotine addictive? It depends on whose criteria you use: experts say the definition of addiction is evolving. *New York Times*, 2 August, p. C3. URL: <http://www.marijuanalibrary.org/NYT_addictive_080294.html>

Hradilova Selin, K. (2004). Dryckesvanor i den svenska befolkningen [Drinking habits among Swedes]. In: *Svenska Dryckesvanor och Deras Konsekvenser i Början av det Nya Millenniet* (ed. K. Hradilova Selin), pp. 75–94. Stockholm: SoRAD, Stockholms Universitet.

Hughes, E.C. (1945). Dilemmas and contradictions of status. *American Journal of Sociology*, 50, 353–359.

Humensky, J. (2010). Are adolescents with high socioeconomic status more likely to engage in alcohol and illicit drug use in early adulthood? *Substance Use Treatment, Prevention and Policy*, 5, 19.

INCB (2014). *Narcotic Drugs: Estimated World Requirements for 2014; Statistics for 2012.* New York: International Narcotics Control Board.

Jernigan, D. (1997). *Thirsting for Markets: The Global Impact of Corporate Alcohol.* San Rafael, CA: Marin Institute for the Prevention of Alcohol and Other Drug Problems.

Jernigan, D.H. (2010). The extent of global alcohol marketing and its impact on youth. *Contemporary Drug Problems*, 37, 57–89.

Jhingan, H.P., Shyangwa, P., Sharma, A., Prasad, K.M.R., & Khandelwal, S.K. (2003). Prevalence of alcohol dependence in a town in Nepal as assessed by the CAGE questionnaire. *Addiction*, 98, 339–343.

Johnson, W.T., Peterson, R.E., & Wells, L.E. (1977). Arrest probabilities for marijuana users as indicators of selective law enforcement. *American Journal of Sociology*, 83, 681–699.

Karriker-Jaffe, K.J. (2011). Areas of disadvantage: a systematic review of effects of area-level socioeconomic status on substance use outcomes. *Drug and Alcohol Review*, 30, 84–95.

Knupfer, G. (1989).The prevalence in various social groups of 8 different drinking patterns, from abstaining to frequent drunkenness: analysis of 10 U.S. surveys combined. *British Journal of Addiction*, 84, 1305–1318.

Kunst, A. (1997). *Cross-National Comparisons of Socioeconomic Differences in Mortality.* The Hague: CIP-Gegevens Koninklijke Bibltiotheek.

Lachenmeier, D.W., Rehm, J., & Gmel, G. (2007). Surrogate alcohol: what do we know and where do we go? *Alcoholism: Clinical and Experimental Research*, 31,1613–1624.

Leon, D.A., Saburova, L., Tomkins, S., et al. (2007). Hazardous alcohol drinking and premature mortality in Russia: a population based case-control study. *Lancet*, 369, 2001–2009.

Levine, H.G., Gettman, J.B., & Siegel, L. (2010). *Arresting Latinos for Marijuana in California: Possession Arrests in 33 Cities, 2006–2008.* Los Angeles: Drug Policy Alliance. URL: http://marijuana-arrests.com/docs/Arresting-Latinos-For-Marijuana-California.pdf

Lustig, R.H., Schmidt, L.A., & Brindis, C.D. (2012). The toxic truth about sugar. *Nature*, 487, 27–29.

McKee, M., Pomerlau, J., Robertson, A., et al. (2000). Alcohol consumption in the Baltic Republics. *Journal of Epidemiology and Community Health*, 54, 361–366.

Manchikanti, L., Heim, S. II, Fellows, B., et al. (2012). Opioid epidemic in the United States. *Pain Physician*, 15, ES9–ES38.

Melberg, H.O., Hakkarainen, P., Houborg, E., et al. (2011). Measuring the harm of illicit drug use on friends and family. *Nordic Studies on Alcohol and Drugs*, 28, 105–121.

Mendoza-Sassi, R.A. & Béria, J.U. (2003).Prevalence of alcohol use disorders and associated factors: a population-based study using AUDIT in southern Brazil. *Addiction*, 98, 799–804.

Mesure, S. (2014). Stevia wonder: the plant that's a super sugar alternative—and free from calories and carbs. *The Independent* (UK), 9 March. URL: <http://www.independent.co.uk/life-style/food-and-drink/news/stevia-wonder-the-plant-thats-a-super-sugar-alternative--and-free-from-calories-and-carbs-9179079.html#>

Mintz, S.W. (1985). *Sweetness and Power: The Place of Sugar in Modern History.* New York: Penguin Books.

Mäkelä, K. (1983). The uses of alcohol and their cultural regulation. *Acta Sociologica*, 26, 21–31.

Mäkelä, K., Room, R., Single, E., et al. (1981). *Alcohol, Society and the State: I. A Comparative Study of Alcohol Control.* Toronto, ON: Addiction Research Foundation.

Mäkelä, P. (1999). Alcohol-related mortality as a function of socioeconomic status. *Addiction*, 94, 867–886.

Mäkelä, P., Jansson, M., Keskimäki, I., & Koskinen, S. (2003).What underlies the high alcohol-related mortality of the disadvantaged: high morbidity or poor survival? *Journal of Epidemiology and Community Health*, 57, 981–986.

Najman, J.M., Williams, G.M., & Room, R. (2007). Increasing socioeconomic inequalities in male cirrhosis of the liver mortality: Australia 1981–2002. *Drug and Alcohol Review*, 26, 273–278.

Nutt, D.J. (2006). Alcohol alternatives—a goal for psychopharmacology? *Journal of Psychopharmacology*, 20, 318–320.

Nutt, D., King, L.A., Saulsbury, W., & Blakemore, C. (2007). Development of a rational scale to assess the harm of drugs of potential misuse. *Lancet*, 369, 1047–1053.

Nutt, D.J., King, L.A., & Phillips, L.D., for the Independent Scientific Committee on Drugs (2010). Drug harms in the UK: a multicriteria decision analysis. *Lancet*, 376,1558–1565.

O'Brien, P. (2013). Australia's double standard on Thailand's alcohol warning labels. *Drug and Alcohol Review*, 32, 5–10.

Padilla, M.B., Guilamo-Ramos, V., & Godbole, R. (2012). A syndemic analysis of alcohol use and sexual risk behavior among tourism employees in Sosúa, Dominican Republic. *Qualitative Health Research*, 22, 89–102.

Rehm, J., Patra, J., Baliunas, D., Popova, S., Roerecke, M., & Taylor, B. (2006). *Alcohol Consumption and Global Burden of Disease 2002.* Working paper prepared for the World Health Organization. Toronto, ON: Centre for Addiction and Mental Health.

Robicsek, F. (1978). *The Smoking Gods: Tobacco in Maya Art, History and Religion.* Norman, OK: University of Oklahoma Press.

Romero, S. (2006). Venezuela's cup runs over, and the Scotch whiskey flows. *New York Times,* 20 August. URL: <http://www.nytimes.com/2006/08/20/weekinreview/20romero. html?_r=0>

Room, R. (2005). Stigma, social inequality and alcohol and drug use. *Drug and Alcohol Review,* 24,143–155.

Room, R. (2006a). For alcohol alternatives, the science is not the hardest part. *Journal of Psychopharmacology,* 20, 323–324.

Room, R. (2006b). The dangerousness of drugs. *Addiction,* 101, 166–168.

Room, R. (2010). The long reaction against the wowser: the prehistory of alcohol deregulation in Australia. *Health Sociology Review,* 19, 151–163.

Room, R. (2011). Scales and blinkers, motes and beams: whose view is obstructed on drug scheduling? *Addiction,* 106, 1895–1896.

Room, R. (in press).The history of psychoactive substance use and problems and of social responses to them. In: Haber, P., Day, C. & Farrell, M., eds., *A Short Textbook of Addiction Medicine.* Melbourne: Palgrave, forthcoming.

Room, R. & Jernigan, D. (2000).The ambiguous role of alcohol in economic and social development. *Addiction,* 95(Suppl. 4), 523–535.

Room, R., Rehm, J., Trotter, R.T. II, Paglia, A., & Üstün, T.B. (2001).Cross-cultural views on stigma, valuation, parity and societal attitudes towards disability. In: *Disability and Culture: Universalism and Diversity* (ed. T.B. Üstün, S.Chatterji, J.E. Bickenbach, et al.), pp. 247–291. Seattle, WA: Hofgrebe & Huber.

Room, R., Jernigan, D., Carlini-Marlatt, B., et al. (2002). *Alcohol and Developing Societies: A Public Health Approach.* Helsinki: Finnish Foundation for Alcohol Studies.

Room, R., Ferris, J., Laslett, A.-M., Livingston, M., Mugavin, J., & Wilkinson, C. (2010).The drinker's effect on the social environment: a conceptual framework for studying alcohol's harm to others. *International Journal of Environmental Research and Public Health,* 7, 1855–1871.

Roques, B. (1999). *La Dangerosité de Drogues: Rapport au Secrétariat d'État à la Santé* [The Dangerousness of Drugs: Report to the State Secretariat for Health]. Paris: La Documentation Française–Odile Jacob.

Rose, N. (2007). Psychopharmaceuticals in Europe. In: *Mental Health Policy and Practices across Europe: The Future Direction of Mental Health Care* (ed. M. Knapp, D. McDaid, E. Mossialos, & G. Thornicroft), pp. 146–187. Maidenhead: Open University Press.

Saxena, S., Sharma, R., & Maulik, P.K. (2003). Impact of alcohol use on poor families: a study from North India. *Journal of Substance Use and Misuse,* 8, 78–84.

Schivelbusch, W. (1992). *Tastes of Paradise: A Social History of Spices, Stimulants and Intoxicants.* New York: Vintage Books.

Schmidt, L.A. & Room, R. (2012). Alcohol and the process of economic development: contributions from ethnographic research. *International Journal of Alcohol and Drug Research,* 1, 41–55.

Schmidt, L., Mäkelä, P., Rehm, J., & Room, R. (2010).Alcohol: equity and social determinants. In: *Equity, Social Determinants and Public Health Programmes* (ed. E. Blas & A. Sivasankara Kurup), pp. 11–29. Geneva: World Health Organization.

Scholten, W., Nygren-Krug, H., &Zucker, H.A. (2007). The World Health Organization paves the way for action to free people from the shackles of pain. *Anesthesia and Analgesia*, 105, 1–4.

Schrad, M.L. (2010). *The Political Power of Bad Ideas: Networks, Institutions, and the Global Prohibition Wave*. Oxford: Oxford University Press.

Shaffer, E.R., Brenner, J.E., & Houston, T.P. (2005). International trade agreements: a threat to tobacco control policy. *Tobacco Control*, 14(Suppl. II), ii19–ii25.

Shkolnikov, V.M., Leon, D.A., Adamets, S., Andreev, E., & Deev, A. (1998). Educational level and adult mortality in Russia: an analysis of routine data 1979 to 1994. *Social Science and Medicine*, 47, 357–369.

Singh, G.K. & Hoyert, D.L. (2000). Social epidemiology of chronic liver disease and cirrhosis mortality in the United States, 1935–1997: trends and differential by ethnicity, socioeconomic status, and alcohol consumption. *Human Biology*, 72, 801–820.

Storbjörk, J. &Room, R. (2008). The two worlds of alcohol problems: who is in treatment and who is not? *Addiction Research and Theory*, 16, 67–84.

Strategy Unit (2005). *Strategy Unit Drugs Report, May 2003*. London: Prime Minister's Strategy Unit. URL: <http://image.guardian.co.uk/sys-files/Guardian/documents/2005/07/05/Report.pdf>

Subramanian, S.V., Nandy, S., Irving, M., Gordon, D., & Davey Smith, G. (2005). Role of socioeconomic markers and state prohibition policy in predicting alcohol consumption among men and women in India: a multilevel statistical analysis. *Bulletin of the World Health Organization*, 83, 829–836.

Towns, C.B. (1915). *Habits That Handicap: The Menaces of Alcohol, Opium and Tobacco, and the Remedy*.New York:Century Co.

Wilkinson, R.G. (1996). *Unhealthy Societies: The Afflictions of Inequality*. New York: Routledge.

Wilkinson, R.G. & Marmot, M. (ed.) (2003). *Social Determinants of Health: The Solid Facts*, 2nd edn. Copenhagen: World Health Organization, European Office.

Wood, E., Montaner, J.S.G., Chan, K., et al. (2002). Socioeconomic status, access to triple therapy, and survival from HIV-disease since 1996. *AIDS*, 16, 2065–2072.

World Bank (2012). *The World Bank 'World Development Indicators'*. URL: <http://data.worldbank.org/data-catalog/world-development-indicators%3E>

World Health Organization (2007). *WHO Global Adult Tobacco Survey*. URL: <http://www.who.int/tobacco/surveillance/gats/en/>

World Health Organization (2013). *WHO Framework Convention on Tobacco Control*. URL: <http://www.who.int/fctc/guidelines/adopted/guidel_2011/en/>

Chapter 11

Addictive substances and behaviours and corruption, transparency, and governance

David Miller and Claire Harkins

11.1 Introduction to addictive substances and behaviours and corruption, transparency, and governance

In the case of addictive substances and behaviours, well-being is predominantly associated with either the effect on individuals of the substances or behaviours or their impacts on society more broadly. However, this chapter is concerned with the ways in which corporate and policy actions, or inactions, have impacts on well-being which are both significant and under-appreciated. These are effects on policy-makers, policy decisions, the way in which they are implemented, and the ultimate consequences of these policies in terms of well-being.

11.2 Well-being

The idea of well-being has become increasingly more prominent in policy circles. Both the Organisation for Economic Co-operation and Development (OECD) and the European Union (EU) have been working toward the inclusion and measurement of well-being in policy-making (OECD, 2006; European Commission, 2014a). The concept of well-being in public policy is relatively straightforward; it involves taking account of how societal factors can be detrimental to individual well-being. Poverty, physical and mental health, social exclusion, limited employment and educational prospects, and other forms of social disengagement can all exacerbate the likelihood of dependence on substances or behaviours that can be harmful. Well-being is recognized as an important concept because it acknowledges the social as well as the individual factors underlying both harm and positive health. The OECD framework regards societal well-being as comprising three dimensions: quality of life, material conditions, and sustainability of well-being over time.

Governance attuned to well-being is thus an important component of well-being programmes. In our view it is important to ensure that this includes not just measures intended to directly improve well-being, such as conventional public health policies on tobacco, alcohol, or food, but also to focus on up-stream, indirect actions which affect well-being by making public health policies easier to implement and enforce. We focus here on increasing transparency and decreasing corruption, which can help to make sectional interests both more visible and less powerful. 'Addictive' industries, such as tobacco, alcohol, food, or gambling have enormous economic resources and use them to create and foster conditions to maintain and protect their business interests. The same industries are also increasingly involved in policy development and implementation—in a word, governance.

11.3 **Governance in theory**

Theoretical perspectives on governance increasingly recognize that the nature of governance relies on multiple actors, including corporate and economic actors (Rhodes, 2000; Kooiman, 2003). Kooiman (2003) argues that changes to the way states govern lead to an increasing reliance on external expertise in policy, while Vibert (2006) argues that the rise of what he calls the 'unelected' in systems of governance should be encouraged as the private sector will deliver services and have a positive impact on governance. Others fear that the rise of unelected economic and corporate actors, particularly in relation to public health, works to the advantage of corporations and to the detriment of public health and has the effect of exacerbating inequalities (Anderson and Baumberg, 2007; Miller and Harkins, 2010). Theoretical accounts accept that there are multiple actors involved in policy development; however, few have attempted to assess how these actors impact upon governance, policy, and ultimately well-being.

11.4 **Crime, corruption, and institutional corruption**

Not all crimes involve corruption and not all corruption is crime. Indeed the terms used to denote the phenomena are socially and politically constructed and historically variable. In other words, what is defined as illegal in a society creates crime in a straightforward way. This is important, because what is and what 'should' count as corruption in relation to addictive industries is subject to a continual struggle. We outline this, put it into historical context, and describe the main areas of corruption to which addictive industries might be said to be connected.

Crime, corruption, and indeed addiction are all subject to both scientific and policy debate and dispute. The history of the changing conceptualization of addiction as a notion and the particular attachment of the notion to specific substances—cocaine, heroin, alcohol, tobacco, so-called 'legal highs'—illustrates this very well (Anderson et al., 2010). Debates over whether sugar is addictive or whether obesity is a consequence of addiction illustrate the difficulties of defining addiction. Indeed, some argue that sugar and added sweeteners are addictive and should be subject to control in the same way as alcohol (Lustig et al., 2012). Alternatively, it has been argued that 'since the human body does not become physically dependent on sugar the way it does on opiates like morphine and heroin, sugar is not addictive' (Duchene, 2006). Ziauddeen et al. (2012) challenge the view that obesity and overeating can be described as addiction, suggesting that the application of a single model, in this case the model of addiction, is unhelpful at best.

If sugar was agreed to be addictive there would be serious implications for policy, research, and public health. Which is why we have seen the sugar industry, and other commercial sectors become involved in debates and discourses around health, policy research and addiction. (Miller and Harkins 2013 a). These examples illustrate the contest over definitions of addiction across disciplines, substances, and behaviours. The concept of addiction is fluid and contestable and changes over time and as a result of increased knowledge and the level of political or policy debate.

We can think of the impact of the outcomes of these debates in two ways—definitional and material. Defining a particular substance as having particularly addictive or harmful effects to individuals or society is part of the process of delineating whether a 'crime' is committed in possessing, using, or trading in a particular substance. To put it most simply, policy and legal processes create criminality merely by creating laws that define existing conduct as criminal. Thus—in a recent example—users of mephedrone one day were indulging in a behaviour that was entirely legal, while the next day they were vulnerable to being defined as criminals by virtue of a change in the law (BBC News, 2010; Nutt, 2010). This is to say nothing of the effects that such a declaration has on existing conduct. This is a second and important way in which definitions produce changes in material behaviours. Thus prohibition of alcohol in the United States in 1920 created a whole new class of criminals, but the bootlegging industry that grew up in response transformed the way in which alcohol was produced, traded, and consumed. The involvement of organized crime is well known in that case. Similar issues are found in all other examples of substance use, and indeed in relation to other behaviours that might be subject to discussion as 'addictions' or 'crimes', such as gambling. Our approach, therefore, can be said to be relativist or constructivist at the level of epistemology in the sense that knowledge of the world is inevitably constructed by humans and is thus provisional. However, in the wider sense our position is ontologically anti-constructivist since we see both the material world (nature, economics, and social and cultural organization) as existing independently of our understanding of it, as providing the circumstances in which we pursue knowledge, and as disciplining knowledge if we let it—and sometimes even if we do not (Miller and Reilly, 1995; Miller, 1998, 1999; Maxwell, 2008). Any attempt to understand the world, we contend, must be able to distinguish—at least analytically—between truth and fiction, between propaganda and communicative good faith. As Nick Crossley (2004, p. 89) notes:

> A position which refused to acknowledge, in principle, a distinction between the force of good reasons and the effect of power, bribery or trickery would have no basis for critique . . . Furthermore, it would have no basis from which to speak of communicative distortion.

The question of communicative distortion is at the centre of many of the issues that come under the rubric of institutional corruption. The question of bias in science and the role of, for example, industry funding in this, the area of evidence-based policy, and the role of think tanks and lobby groups in policy-making all depend on notions of communicative distortion or bias.

11.4.1 Corruption and corporate capture

In line with the main focus of this chapter, the main forms of corruption that we will discuss in relation to addiction are those related to the political system. It is of course the case that corruption can affect the economy, but the extent to which this becomes a public issue is determined by how it is dealt with (or not) by the political system. Forms of corruption like bribery, fraud, and theft remain commonplace in some jurisdictions but the question of what constitutes corruption is itself subject to debate and dispute in society. Activities that tend to undermine the rule of law or of democratic processes may not be illegal, but they may have far-reaching consequences for the ability of addictive industries to pursue a market share in ways that harm public health. It is perhaps useful to describe this as 'institutional corruption', which has been defined by Lessig (2013) as:

> a systemic and strategic influence which is legal, or even currently ethical, that undermines the institution's effectiveness by diverting it from its purpose or weakening its ability to achieve its purpose, including, to the extent relevant to its purpose, weakening either the public's trust in that institution or the institution's inherent trustworthiness.

This is a reasonable starting point, but it does assume that institutions become corrupt as opposed to being corrupt at their creation, perhaps in a deliberate deception or ideological process. This can be argued to occur, especially when a large number of the institutions in a society have become institutionally corrupt (Robinson, 1998; Brown and Cloke, 2004; Miller, 2004).

The UK today is arguably affected by widespread institutional corruption, as one of the leading neoliberal societies on the planet along with the United States. Briefly, the process of neoliberalization is widely recognized to have been inaugurated by reforming market-friendly governments in the UK and United States from 1979 and 1980, respectively. Since then, most countries in the world have been progressively, if unevenly, affected. Neoliberalism has been defined by David Harvey (2005) as the 'doctrine that market exchange is an ethic in itself, capable of acting as a guide for all human action'. This definition is useful because it draws attention to the fact that neoliberalism is a doctrine as opposed to a description of how any given society functions. This is important because, first, societies adopt or adapt to neoliberalism in their own, uneven and sometimes unpredictable ways and, more importantly, because it signals that the doctrine is a way of explaining what is wrong with a society or a relationship in order to reform it, but it does not necessarily result or indeed intend to result in a set of social relations as envisaged or claimed by its advocates. Thus, the oft remarked gap between the advocates of the 'shrinking state' and the empirical reality of the need for a 'strong state' to sustain the 'free market' and defend neoliberal-inspired reform from the population (Gamble, 1994). The gap is produced in part because reality did not measure up to the theorist's ideas and because the doctrine is a means of pursuing certain interests—it is in other words ideological.

Practically speaking, in relation to corruption, neoliberalism transferred very significant property and resources from public hands to private, thus reducing at a stroke the potential for democratic control over the economy. The corollary was an increase in the power of private capital to make its own investment decisions. This power was increased by an attack across the Western world on the rights of workers to organize and defend their interests against those of capital (Leys, 2001). The subsequent waves of neoliberal reform including the contracting out of services, the marketization of government itself, the introduction of private finance into the public sector, and a myriad of other measures that also increased both the direct role of capital in (what had become) market decisions but also directly in political decisions (Crouch, 2004). Alongside this, both in the process of privatizing public assets and in dividing the spoils afterwards, there was a massive expansion of intermediary professions (lobbyists, accountants, consultants) that were used to pursue direct corporate interests in areas vacated or opened to competition by the public sector. We can highlight in particular the rise of public relations and lobbying consultancies. The UK was the most significant laboratory for this process because the United States had been a more market-friendly society for some decades, because the UK took a lead in neoliberal reform, and because of the importance to emerging transnational business of London as a financial centre. In the period between 1979 and 1998 the public relations industry expanded 4.3 times in real terms (Miller and Dinan, 2000). The lobbying industry did exist before 1979, but it has expanded out of all recognition in the intervening decades (Miller and Dinan, 2008).

With PR comes the chronic inability of private and public institutions to communicate honestly (Dinan and Miller, 2007), and with the lobbying industry has come the hugely enhanced role of money in politics. Both have been at the cutting edge of undermining ethics and standards in public life and—consequently—in the perilous decline of public faith in formal politics as expressed in countless opinion polls and indeed in the UK in the precipitous decline after the turn of the century in the proportion of the electorate voting in elections (Miller, 2004). The widespread nature of the malaise has affected almost every single political institution in the UK in the past 5 years. We can list, for example, the banking crisis and the inability of the political system to deal with the endemic corruption of the financial institutions and their supposed regulators, the House of Lords, MPs' expenses, lobbying scandals, and police violence and corruption and collaboration with an out of control media system. This is not to mention the apparent endemic corruption and bloodshed that has accompanied the Western interventions in Iraq and Afghanistan—a bloody mess by any account. Social science struggles to keep up with the sheer scope of the issues. Scholars from a variety of perspectives have discussed the 'rise of the unelected' or 'post-democracy'. But, as if to illustrate our core thesis of the intrusion of corporate interests into every sphere of society, the first of these quotes is from the title of an academic (Vibert, 2006) who applauded the declining role of the elected in governance. Vibert is a co-founder and director of the free-market think-tank the European Policy Forum, which has received donations from the same conservative foundations that bankroll better-known think-tanks such as the Centre for Policy Studies—one of the original triumvirate of Thatcherite think-tanks (Powerbase, 2014a).

A key reason for using the term 'institutional corruption' as opposed to just a lot of corruption is that it is not just a question of specific individuals or firms bending the rules but that the whole political and economic system has been skewed by corporate interests in general. We describe this as 'corporate capture'.

How does this happen? We think that it is useful to discuss the impact of addictive industries on well-being through an understanding of corporate strategy. It is necessary to examine the breadth of corporate political activity in order to understand one element such as social responsibility or the question of bias in science. Rather than look at the influence on a particular policy or department, we start with the corporations and try and follow what they do (Miller & Harkins 2014).

We find that corporations are active in a wide variety of policy-relevant areas as well as in a number of arenas that, at first sight, might appear not to be centrally relevant to corporate political activity, such as social responsibility and relations with science or civil society and apparently arcane policy issues.

Policy and political decision making has always taken place at a variety of levels, but recent trends up to supranational governance and down to subsidiarity/devolution have created a range of new venues for decision making. Most obvious in Europe is the EU itself with its range of institutional forums and decision-making bodies. Large corporations differentiate their policy activities to target decision making wherever it takes place. As a result corporations attempt to act through a complex web of influence. They act directly, through trade associations (organized at national and transnational levels), and they engage with or fund a complex network of lobbying, public relations, legal, financial, and other consultancies as well as other ventures in civil society.

Here we will examine attempts to capture science, civil society, and policy, which are among the most important areas for addictions.

11.4.2 **Science**

Scientific expertise is a key resource for corporations. The tobacco industry successfully muddied the waters about the health effects of tobacco for 30 years (Holden and Lee, 2009). Similar tactics are currently being used by the food (Brownell and Warner, 2009) and alcohol industries (Miller and Harkins 2014).

Such strategies involve more than 'spinning' science and encompass very wide-ranging attempts to skew the scientific evidence base and to manage the whole scientific enterprise. McGarrity and Wagner (2008, p. 10) describe the 'tools for bending science' as 'shaping, hiding, attacking, harassing, packaging and spinning'—tools that encompass the entire range of the scientific process from funding science to attempting to undermine science that is not useful and from managing how science is reported and used in policy processes to attempting to influence scientific experts to influence both the evidence base and the regulatory and policy process (Krimsky, 1995; Kassirer, 2005; Mooney, 2006; McGarrity and Wagner, 2008; Michaels, 2008; Wiist, 2010).

These techniques of 'corrupting' science are said to have increased in recent years as a result of the increased importance of private finance in scientific research. Public funding for higher education in general and research specifically has been cut (Soley, 1995). In addition we have seen significant investment by the private sector in science-related areas, including especially those connected to biotechnology and genomics (Rose and Rose, 2012).

As a result, the effects of corporate funding and conflicts of interest in science have become a live issue in scientific debate. Some have maintained that the sources of funding make little difference to science, or that declarations of interest escalate cynicism about the motives of scientists. Such views come from a variety of sources such as the UK's Science Media Centre. It says it is 'an independent press office helping to ensure that the public have access to the best scientific evidence and expertise through the news media' (Science Media Centre, 2014a). Its CEO Fiona Fox (2013) has argued:

> while 'industry funded' is technically accurate it is also misleading and perhaps reveals as much about the bias of the critics . . . It is deeply insulting to an eminent scientist to suggest that an outside influence, financial or otherwise, would distort their scientific findings.

Similar views are to be found in the publications of the US-based American Council on Science and Health. It has argued that 'most conflicts of interest activists clearly have prior strong ideological commitments against markets and corporations' (Bailey, 2008). Colin Blakemore, former Chief Executive of the UK Medical Research Council, is reported as saying: 'the idea that because a scientist has some links with industry they are automatically tainted and evil is just ridiculous' (cited in Fox, 2006). In the addiction field some argue that conflict of interest declarations can stigmatize honest scientists. Even if bias exists it can be handled via peer review and replication of studies, they say (Gmel, 2010; Peele, 2010).

Whether it is ridiculous or insulting, or not, the question cannot be settled by rhetorical flourishes. Nor can it be resolved by pointing to the significant corporate funding received by the Science Media Centre or the American Council on Science and Health (Science Media Centre, 2014b; Powerbase, 2014b). It is, though, capable of being answered by science. An emerging literature on the effects of corporate funding on the findings of scientific studies suggests that there is a relationship between corporate funding and research findings. Babor and Miller (2014) cite more than twenty such studies. We can also note other studies on nutrition research (Lesser et al., 2007) as well as in drug trials (Jørgensen et al., 2006), all of which point in the same direction.

It is important to note that the significant role of corporate funding and potential conflicts of interest also have very significant consequences for the policy process, since the extent to which experts involved in policy processes have conflicts of interest and the extent to which they are disclosed, tolerated, or managed is a significant issue in policy, as we will see shortly.

11.4.3 Civil society

Civil society is also targeted by corporate strategy, which we define to exclude those organizations that are under the direct and open control of business (such as trade associations and lobbying and PR firms). We therefore include only those that are not, or claim not to be, under direct control. This is obviously not a matter of a clear dividing line and we acknowledge the debate on the meaning of the term (Edwards, 2005). It is important to take this approach since one of the oldest corporate techniques is the creation of front groups—organizations claiming to be independent but actually controlled by corporations (Miller and Dinan, 2008). Such fake grassroots groups have been called 'astroturf' organizations (Anderson, 1996; Silverstein, 1996). In addition to astroturf groups there are a myriad of policy-active civil society groups that act indirectly or are partly influenced by the corporations. Again we can refer to this as the institutional corruption of civil society: in particular we can point to think-tanks, policy-planning groups, social responsibility ventures, and organizations set up to inform or manage the news media.

In the addiction field many of these groups have a science-related orientation. Some suggest that they are science-based organizations and they do not always disguise or fail to disclose their sources of funding. But some do. For example the British Nutrition Foundation, the European Food Information Council (EUFIC), and the International Life Sciences Institute (ILSI) all claim to be 'independent' or 'science-based' but all are corporate funded—a fact not always made clear (Chamberlain, 2010). It should be noted that the EUFIC is co-financed by the European Commission. All are also deeply involved in policy-making—in supplying experts for official committees and in revolving-door connections with regulatory bodies (Corporate Europe Observatory, 2011). The Center for Science in the Public Interest (2003) compiled a list of scores of similar organizations.

The rise of the think-tank has again been a widely remarked feature of the neoliberal period. While the earliest think-tanks go back to the beginning of the twentieth century there has been a very significant expansion of think-tanks in the past three decades, especially those devoted to 'free market' policies (Mirowski and Plehwe, 2009). Think-tanks are usually not so obviously funded by corporations and tend to describe themselves as independent research institutions, yet very few are open about their funding sources. Nevertheless some details about the links between the tobacco, food, retailing, and alcohol industries and two long-established UK-based market think-tanks are available.

The Institute of Economic Affairs (IEA) is the oldest market-liberal think-tank in the UK, coming into existence in the 1950s. The Adam Smith Institute was created some two decades later. Both refuse to disclose the sources of their funding, but both have recently been revealed to be multiyear recipients of funding from the tobacco industry (Doward, 2013; Tobacco Tactics, 2014a,b).

Subsequently it was revealed that the IEA is in receipt of funding from the alcohol and retail industries as well (Snowdon, 2014).

Corporate influence on the organizations of civil society is plainly quite significant, but a recurring problem in assessing both the extent and the importance of corporate influence is the endemic secrecy and lack of transparency about sources of funding.

11.5 **Capturing policy**

We have suggested that the attempt to capture varying arenas of debate and decision can be analysed separately, as we have tried to do here. But, of course, as we noted at the beginning, separating them, while analytically useful, is by no means a tidy process. The very extensive engagement of the corporations with science is intended to enable them to use science as a resource in policy capture. Civil society is a means for the corporations to see off the opposition of activist groups and the trades unions.

Policy capture of one sort or another is the ultimate aim of all the strategies outlined here and many others. As we have noted, this can be done directly or indirectly. The most obvious way in which corporations directly pursue their interests is via interaction with policy-makers either on their own account, via trade associations, or through lobbying consultancies. It is central to our argument, however, that this is buttressed and supported by the use they make of other domains—such as science and civil society.

Taking the example of the UK government's U-turn on the minimum unit pricing of alcohol we can see the way in which the alcohol industry variously attempted to mobilize science, civil society, and direct lobbying of government to undermine the policy. The industry funded a number of critiques of the Sheffield University modelling that underpinned the policy, mobilized think tanks, and met and communicated directly with government (Miller and Harkins, 2012; Gornall, 2014).

Policy capture is most obvious in institutions of partnership governance where government decision making or policy implementation is partially given over to private interests or to a mixture of private and civil society interests. Partnership governance has become popular in recent years—particularly in the addictions field with the creation of Change4Life and the Responsibility Deal in the UK and the European Alcohol and Health Forum and the EU Platform on Diet Physical Activity and Health at the EU level. Partnership governance erodes barriers between government and the private sectors and hinders the pursuit of social objectives that might challenge the perceived interests of business (Miller and Harkins, 2010).

11.5.1 **Capturing policy and the revolving door**

The revolving door is a significant problem across the Western world, as recognized by intergovernmental bodies like the OECD. It recognizes that these issues have become more acute in the neoliberal age:

> New forms of relationship have developed between the public sector and the business and non-profit sectors . . . In consequence, there is clearly an emerging potential for new forms of conflict of interest involving an individual official's private interests and public duties. (Bertók, 2003, p. 3)

The financial crisis certainly helped to put on the agenda the extent of revolving-door connections between the financial services industry, government, and regulatory agencies. An OECD study found that the banks with the densest revolving-door connections had their headquarters in the United States, Switzerland, and UK. In the EU and the UK the means of regulating the revolving door is widely regarded in policy circles as inadequate (Miller and Dinan, 2009b).

The phenomenon of the revolving door refers to the movement of staff into and out of key policy-making posts in the executive and legislative branches and regulatory agencies. This can carry the risk of increasing the likelihood that those making policies are overly sympathetic to the needs (particularly) of business, either because they come from that world or they plan to move or return to the private sector after working in government. Four main routes through the 'revolving door' can be identified (Revolving Door Working Group, 2005).

The tobacco, alcohol, food, and gambling industries attempt to make sure that the people they retain to engage in lobbying and policy work have as much insider or specialist knowledge of the policy-making world as possible. That is why corporations themselves, as well as lobby firms and think-tanks, have helped to spin the so-called revolving door both ways, by sending their employees into government at the national or EU level on secondment or on a career path that may not gain them immediate advantage but on which they can later capitalize, perhaps when the former staffer returns to their employ or when a career civil servant leave the 'public service' to pursue the private interests of the industry (Miller and Harkins, 2013b).

We can conclude this section by noting that the problems of crime and corruption related to the illicit status of certain substances or the illegal status of certain behaviours can be most effectively targeted by redefining them as licit and legal. This will—at a stroke—abolish the criminality associated with possession and consumption. When allied with measures to ensure the quality of newly legal products, it will also in many cases reduce harm significantly. We will return to the question of the governance measures needed to reduce harm most effectively in Section 11.7.

In relation to licit products, the means of targeting the problems of corruption, and especially institutional corruption, are mostly different. With the exception of industry involvement in criminal practices such as smuggling, counterfeit goods, organized crime, and the like, the main way to target corruption is in reforms of the political system, either in general or specifically targeted at a particular sector of industry (Rowell and Cookson, 2000; Rowell and Bates, 2000).

11.6 Transparency

Transparency is often suggested as a solution to problems of corruption. It can be. But matters are more complicated since political and economic transparency can pull in different directions. In addition, enforcement is not always effective and transparency is not a panacea for appropriate governance of addictive industries with the aim of directly improving public health and well-being.

We can start by noting that addictive industries are not in general fully transparent about the science that they undertake or sponsor or the donations and contributions they make to political parties, civil society groups, or lobbying, PR, marketing, and advertising agencies.

11.6.1 Transparency in science

The 'corruption' of science is a significant issue in parts of the scientific community and has sparked a lively debate and evolving transparency guidance and rules in the medical and addiction journals. Journal editors have collaborated to deal with the challenges of potential conflicts of interest, including the Committee on Publication Ethics (COPE), the International Committee of Medical Journal Editors (ICMJE), and the International Society of Addiction Journal Editors (ISAJE). COPE was started in 1997 by a small group of medical editors but now has over 9000 journal editor members worldwide. The COPE code lists minimum standards which are focused mostly on transparency, ethical conduct, and conflict of interest (COPE, 2011). The ICMJE adds further detail specifically on conflict of interest noting that (ICMJE, 2013):

> A conflict of interest exists when professional judgment concerning a primary interest (such as patients' welfare or the validity of research) may be influenced by a secondary interest (such as financial gain). Perceptions of conflict of interest are as important as actual conflicts of interest.
> [...]
> Financial relationships (such as employment, consultancies, stock ownership or options, honoraria, patents, and paid expert testimony) are the most easily identifiable conflicts of interest and the most likely to undermine the credibility of the journal, the authors, and of science itself. However, conflicts can occur for other reasons, such as personal relationships or rivalries, academic competition, and intellectual beliefs.

The ISAJE adds the following kinds of financial interests: research funding, payment for lectures or travel, and company support for staff (ISAJE, 2013). Babor and Miller (2014, p. 342) note that academic work on the relation between declared interests and findings has 'ironically [been] made possible in part by COI [conflict of interest] declaration policies instituted by the major biomedical journals'.

11.6.2 **Transparency in civil society**

Medical journals have led the way on conflict of interest guidelines, but the extent of compliance is uncertain. The presumption may be that the potential reputational damage faced by academic authors who fail to disclose relevant funding or who submit false statements is an adequate incentive to keep the system functioning. It is less clear, however, that such incentives worry authors from outside the universities—such as those in think-tanks and similar civil society groups. Two examples indicate the difficulties. First the case of the IEA which 'has a policy of donor confidentiality' (Snowdon, 2014). In a contribution to the *British Medical Journal* (BMJ) admonishing the journal for publishing an account of the influence of the alcohol industry on government policy, the IEA head of 'lifestyle economics', Christopher Snowdon declared only minor personal conflicts of interest. The BMJ requires authors to declare competing interests both 'personal or organisational'. Snowdon's statement could be queried on the grounds that his article itself admitted funding from the alcohol and retail industries and on the basis that the IEA has received multiyear funding from a variety of tobacco companies and has played a role in the tobacco industry's well-documented attempts to create doubt about the health impacts of second-hand smoke and to influence the general way that risk is dealt with (Tobacco Tactics, 2014b). The opaque nature of IEA funding arrangements, and the apparent lengths that some think-tanks go to to disguise their funding sources, makes it difficult to accurately assess the extent of any conflict of interest (Miller et al. 2014).

A second example is that of the Democracy Institute which has collaborated with the IEA and other think-tanks to advocate industry-friendly messages on public health. The Institute which claims to have offices in London and Washington, DC appears to have no institutional existence as a company or a charity in the UK, in Washington, DC, or in surrounding states. It does not disclose donors and so it is unclear how—when its director Patrick Basham writes in the BMJ—his null claim of competing interests statement should be interpreted (Basham and Luik, 2008). His claim that he had been awarded a PhD turned out, when checked by the present authors, to be untrue. Journals like the BMJ do not have the resources to check the disclosure statements of all contributors, which suggests that one of the weaknesses of current policy is that it depends on the honesty and openness of contributors. On the other hand it may be that journal transparency rules will need to move towards total disclosures from think-tanks and other similar bodies if proper assessments of conflict of interest are to be made. Even then transparency policies appear necessary but not sufficient to defend the integrity of science.

What would help would be enhanced transparency rules in civil society. These would make it easier for other domains—science, the media, policy-makers—to more effectively evaluate the role and conduct of think-tanks and other civil society bodies. The extent of the regulation of non-profits (known as 'charities' or non-profit companies in the UK, 'association sans but lucratif' in Brussels, and as tax exempt '501(c)3' organizations in the United States) is variable. In no country is it an uncomplicated window on how funds flow from corporations and corporate-linked foundations to campaign groups, think-tanks, and a wide variety of other lobby groups. In the UK, for example, there is no requirement to disclose the names of large institutional donors to charities and the practice of disclosing where charities donate is uneven. The same is true in the United States. In the UK such records as are kept are held for only 7 years and then destroyed for legal reasons, making it impossible to track historical data. In other countries, Germany or Belgium, for example, the rules are looser and less information is available.

Think-tanks and other similar policy-related bodies in civil society are often reluctant to disclose their sources of funding and are unlikely to campaign for transparency in politics. Take the example of the IEA, the oldest market-liberal think-tank in the UK, which 'has a policy of donor confidentiality'. It appears that some donors deliberately seek anonymity, indeed some go to considerable lengths to disguise their donations. In 1999 conservative funders created secretive US-based foundations—the Donors Trust and associated Donors Capital Fund (Mashey, 2012). These are described as 'donor advised', meaning that donors can, as the Donors Trust states, 'keep your charitable giving private, especially gifts funding sensitive or controversial issues' (Donors Trust, 2014). Since their creation the two bodies have given nearly $400 million to support climate contrarianism and a range of other conservative causes. The 'American Friends of the IEA' received some $215,000 between 2004 and 2010 from this source (Mashey, 2012).

In the UK a charity called the Institute for Policy Research (IPR) distributes resources to conservative think-tanks and similar groups. These include the IEA as well as other well-known neoliberal think tanks such as the Centre for Policy Studies, Open Europe, and Politeia (Powerbase, 2014a). However, in its annual report and accounts it does not reveal where the money comes from. It is possible to trace the source of some of the money via other conservative foundations, which list donations to the IPR. But there is no way to link the donations from the foundations through to the ultimate destination with particular think-tanks, so which interests are funding which think-tanks remains obscure. We can note that one of the donors to the IPR is the Garfield Weston Foundation, which is controlled by the Weston family, owners of Associated British Foods a diversified international food, agri-business, and retail group including British Sugar plc, with global sales of £6 billion. Documents lodged with the UK Charity Commission reveal further donations to the IEA from the Garfield Weston Foundation of £100,000 between 2005 and 2011. In addition the MJC Stone Charitable Trust gave the IEA over £50,000 between 2004 and 2011. It is associated with the former sugar and commodities trader Michael Smith.

These brief examples of the complexity of the funding of one think-tank suggest the difficulties in establishing, within current rules, how civil society organizations like think-tanks are funded and the possible need for further measures to open up the policy process.

11.6.3 Lobbying transparency

Lobbying transparency is one key mechanism adopted in a variety of countries to open up the political process. It has its longest history in the United States where the Foreign Agents Registration Act was first enacted in 1938 as a result of attempts by lobbyists acting for Nazi Germany to influence US policy. In 1946 the Federal Regulation of Lobbying Act was passed. Since then regulation of lobbying has spread to many other countries and has been progressively tightened in the United States as well as being extended to all 50 states in some form (Schuman, 2011). In the EU, lobbying transparency is a much newer phenomenon. No EU country has lobbying regulation comparable to that in the United States. Some European states such as Lithuania (2001), Poland (2005), Hungary (2006), Slovenia (2010), the Netherlands (2012), and Austria (2012) have introduced legislation. In early 2014 the UK passed a lobbying regulation bill of sorts for the first time. In the past 5 years the European Commission and the European Parliament have made tentative steps towards a lobby register, but so far this remains at the level of a voluntary register with no compulsion for lobbyists to join (European Commission, 2014b). Critics have charged that 'all the signs emerging from the Commission are that they would prefer to retain their voluntary and "light touch" approach to lobbying regulation . . . the evidence presented in this report, clearly shows that the effectiveness of the voluntary register is unconvincing at best, and dismal at worst'. (Arauzo et al., 2013, p. 3).

It is clear that moves towards transparency are being made across Europe, though in many cases these are gradual, voluntary, or limited. The experience in the United States is that a relatively advanced system of lobbying disclosure can be a useful means for citizen interests to track the role of private interests and monitor conflicts of interest and corruption. However, it is also clear from the United States that transparency is no panacea for effective action to target social problems such as in the area of public health and addictions.

11.6.4 Transparency and the revolving door

Associated with lobbying transparency, though often dealt with separately, is the question of the revolving door. In the UK and EU the regulation of the revolving door is in its infancy, compared with, for example, the United States where there is a much longer institutional history of regulatory measures. In the United States, where more information is available, we can tell that 10 of the 21 lobbyists working for Diageo in 2013 previously held government jobs (Open Secrets, 2014). No such information is available in the UK or EU.

In the UK issues related to the revolving door are not regulated in any meaningful way. Instead there is the Advisory Committee on Business Appointments (ACOBA), which as its name suggests simply advises public servants on cooling-off periods or whether to take particular posts or contacts. It has no mechanism for monitoring compliance and no powers to sanction any breach of its advice. It is widely regarded as not fit for purpose (Miller et al., 2012). The most recent official enquiry on the revolving door, carried out by the Public Administration Select Committee, recommended in 2012 that ACOBA should be 'abolished' and ethics regulation placed on a 'statutory' footing (Public Administration Select Committee, 2012).

Moreover, critics charge that although the EU institutions have rules to govern the revolving door, they are 'weak and are not effectively implemented' (Clausen and Cann, 2011). On conflict of interest a similar pattern prevails. Take the case of the European Food Safety Authority (EFSA), which after heavy criticism, adopted in spring 2012 a new conflict of interest policy. Although having the effect of screening out 85 experts for conflicts of interest, one study (utilizing only data declared by the experts themselves) found that of those who had been passed by the new policy some 58.37% had at least one conflict of interest (Horel and Corporate Europe Observatory, 2013). In addition there are many cases of the revolving door between corporate funded groups such as EUFIC and ILSI and the EFSA (Corporate Europe Observatory and Earth Open Source, 2012). Reforms are under way; however, there remain inadequate mechanisms for gathering, monitoring, and managing conflicts.

One key implication is that much clearer advice and regulation of post-employment opportunities is needed. Much more transparency is also required about which offers are taken up and which rules govern them. In addition, while the issue of conflict of interest is partly about recognizing the issue and making it public, a more significant question that many countries and the European institutions have not yet fully come to terms with is that of managing conflicts of interest to minimize them. That might mean prohibiting certain sorts of post-employment, increasing cooling-off periods, or being much more specific about what is allowed and what is not. Along with this there must be an effective and transparent way to monitor and evaluate compliance and sanctions for non-compliance.

A final point is that the EU has no locus in managing revolving-door processes in member states, just as member states have no locus in overseeing cases of EU officials moving to 'national' organizations.

In a world where the national/EU boundary is porous and 'national' organizations blur with transnational corporations and where some trade associations, such as the Scotch Whisky Association, operate at both national and EU-level, monitoring and management of conflict of interest have become more complex and the interaction between levels has barely been considered. Until it is effectively dealt with, the potentially negative impact of the addictive industries on the development of public health policies will be heightened.

11.7 **Governance**

The means of reducing harm is different in relation to licit products. It may mean additional or varied regulation of the product itself or its promotion or availability, as seen in differing strategies with tobacco, alcohol, gambling, and food.

Governance for well-being, though, is of crucial importance. It can help to make transparency effective by making it meaningful and enforcing the rules that do exist. However, governance for well-being would also need to take several steps beyond transparency for well-being to be enhanced significantly. This means taking direct and effective action against industries the activities of which cause significant harm to public health and well-being.

Such measures might include: regulating the availability of the product; who can buy it; how it is promoted; its price. Associated measures might include transparency measures as well as regulating access of industry representatives to policy or scientific information, meetings, decision making, etc.

11.8 **Conclusion**

In conclusion, a key consequence of our argument is that policy responses to enhance well-being should, in addition to comforting those afflicted by addictions or their effects, also focus on those economic and policy levers that can have very significant effects downstream in terms of both individual behaviours and the wider societal impact.

To encourage well-being, it is necessary to take a determined public health approach to the regulation of products that are implicated in harms to health and well-being. However, if these policies are to be effective they must be supplemented with approaches that also focus on significant reforms to transparency. These must aim to protect the evidence base from corruption by vested interests, and open up of the work of lobbyists to public and policy scrutiny. But transparency will not be enough. Measures will also need to be taken to create a level playing field, to stop corporate actors engaged in the production of potentially harmful products from gaining privileged access to policy-making and to determinedly resist the phenomenon of corporate capture.

Acknowledgements

Text extract from Lessig, L., Foreword: 'Institutional Corruption' Defined, Journal of Law, Medicine and Ethics, Volume 41, Number 3, pp. 553–5, Copyright © 2013 American Society of Law, Medicine and Ethics, Inc. reproduced by permission of Wiley and Sons Ltd.

Text extracts from International Committee of Medical Journal Editors, Recommendations for the Conduct, Reporting, Editing, and Publication of Scholarly Work in Medical Journals, Updated December 2013, Copyright © ICMJE 2013, reproduced with permission from International Committee of Medical Journal Editors, available from http://www.icmje.org/icmje-recommendations. pdf. Please note that the recommendations are subject to change, to see updates visit www.icmje.org.

References

Anderson, W.T. (1996). Astroturf—the big business of fake grassroots politics. *Jinn Magazine*, 5 January. URL: <https://web.archive.org/web/20110129034915/http://www.pacificnews.org/jinn/stories/2.01/960105-astroturf.html

Anderson, P. & Baumberg, B. (2007). Alcohol policy: who should sit at the table? *Addiction*, **102**, 335–336.

Anderson, T., Swan, H., & Lane, D. (2010). Institutional fads and the medicalization of drug addiction. *Sociology Compass*, **4**, 476–494.

Arauzo, E., Hoedeman, O., & Tansey, R. (2013). *Rescue the Register! How to Make EU Lobby Transparency Credible and Reliable*. Brussels: Alliance for Lobbying Transparency and Ethics Regulation.

Babor, T. & Miller, P. (2014). McCarthyism, conflict of interest and Addiction's new transparency declaration procedures. *Addiction*, **109**, 341–344.

Bailey, R. (2008). *Scrutinizing Industry-Funded Science: The Crusade Against Conflicts of Interest*. New York: American Council on Science and Health.

Basham, P. & Luik, J. (2008) Is the obesity epidemic exaggerated? Yes. *British Medical Journal*, **336**, 244.

BBC News (2010). Mephedrone to be made Class B drug within days. *BBC News website*, 12 April. URL: <http://news.bbc.co.uk/1/hi/uk/8616758.stm>

Bertók, J. (2003). *Managing Conflict of Interest in the Public Service OECD Guidelines and Overview*. Paris: OECD.

Brown, E. & Cloke, J. (2004). Neoliberal reform, governance and corruption in the South: assessing the international anti-corruption crusade. *Antipode*, **36**, 272–294.

Brownell, K. & Warner, K. (2009). The perils of ignoring history: big tobacco played dirty and millions died. How similar is big food? *The Milbank Quarterly*, **87**, 259–294.

Center for Science in the Public Interest (2003). *Lifting the Veil of Secrecy: Corporate Support for Health and Environmental Professional Associations, Charities, and Industry Front Groups*. Washington, DC: Integrity in Science Project, Center for Science in the Public Interest.

Chamberlain, P. (2010). Competing interests: independence of nutritional information? *British Medical Journal*, **340**, c1438.

Clausen, J. & Cann, V. (2011). *Block the Revolving Door: Why We Need to Stop EU Officials Becoming Lobbyists*. Brussels: ALTER-EU.

Committee on Publication Ethics (2011). *Code of Conduct and Best Practice Guidelines for Journal Editors*. URL: <http://publicationethics.org/files/Code_of_conduct_for_journal_editors_Mar11.pdf>

Corporate Europe Observatory (2011). *Serial Conflicts of Interest on EFSA's Management Board*. URL: <http://corporateeurope.org/sites/default/files/2011-02-23_mb_report.pdf>

Corporate Europe Observatory and Earth Open Source (2012). *Conflicts on the Menu. A Decade of Industry Influence at the European Food Safety Authority (EFSA)*. URL: <http://corporateeurope.org/sites/default/files/publications/conflicts_on_the_menu_final_0.pdf>

Crossley, N. (2004). On systematically distorted communication: Bourdieu and the socio-analysis of publics. *Sociological Review*, **52**(Suppl. s1), 88–112.

Crouch, C. (2004). *Post-Democracy*. Cambridge: Polity Press.

Dinan, W. & Miller, D. (ed.) (2007). *Thinker, Faker, Spinner, Spy: Corporate PR and the Assault on Democracy*. London: Pluto Press.

Donors Trust (2014). *Donors Trust website FAQs*. URL: <http://www.donorstrust.org/AboutUs/FAQs.aspx>

Doward, J. (2013). Health groups dismayed by news 'big tobacco' funded rightwing think tanks. *The Observer*, 1 June. URL: <http://www.theguardian.com/society/2013/jun/01/thinktanks-big-tobacco-funds-smoking>

Duchene, L. (2006). Probing question: is sugar addictive? *Penn State University News*, 16 January. URL: <http://news.psu.edu/story/141336/2006/01/16/research/probing-question-sugar-addictive>

Edwards, M. (2005). *The Oxford Handbook of Civil Society*. New York: Open University Press.

European Commission (2014a). What is the 'Beyond GDP' initiative? URL: <http://ec.europa.eu/environment/beyond_gdp/index_en.html>

European Commission (2014b). *Transparency Register*. URL: <http://ec.europa.eu/transparencyregister/info/homePage.do>

Fox, F. (2006). Richard Doll: supping with the Devil? *On Science and the Media*, 11 December. URL: <http://fionafox.blogspot.co.uk/2006/12/richard-doll-supping-with-devil.html>

Fox, F. (2013). Following the money misses the point. *Science Media Centre Blog*, 25 June. URL: <http://www.sciencemediacentre.org/following-the-money-misses-the-point/>

Gamble, A. (1994). *The Free Economy and the Strong State: The Politics of Thatcherism*, 2nd edn. Basingstoke: Palgrave Macmillan.

Gmel, G. (2010). The good, the bad and the ugly. *Addiction*, **105**, 203–205.

Gornall, J. (2014). Under the influence. *British Medical Journal*, **348**, f7646.

Harvey, D. (2005). *A Brief History of Neoliberalism*. Oxford: Oxford University Press.

Holden, C. & Lee, K. (2009). Corporate power and social policy: the political economy of the transnational tobacco companies. *Global Social Policy*, **9**, 328–325.

Horel, S. & Corporate Europe Observatory (2013). *Unhappy Meal: The European Food Safety Authority's Independence Problem*. URL: <http://corporateeurope.org/sites/default/files/attachments/unhappy_meal_report_23_10_2013.pdf>

ICMJE (International Committee of Medical Journal Editors) (2013). *Recommendations for the Conduct, Reporting, Editing, and Publication of Scholarly Work in Medical Journals*, updated December 2013. URL: <http://www.icmje.org/icmje-recommendations.pdf>

ISAJE (International Society of Addiction Journal Editors) (2013). *Ethical Practice Guidelines in Addiction Publishing: A Model for Authors, Journal Editors and Other Partners*. URL: <http://www.parint.org/isajewebsite/ethics.htm>

Jørgensen, A.W, Hilden, J., & Gotzsche, P.C. (2006). Cochrane reviews compared with industry supported meta-analyses and other meta-analyses of the same drugs: systematic review. *British Medical Journal*, **333**, 782–785.

Kassirer, J.P. (2005). *On the Take: How Medicine's Complicity with Big Business Can Endanger Your Health*. Oxford: Oxford University Press.

Kooiman, J. (2003). *Governing as Governance*. New York: Sage.

Krimsky, S. (1995). *Science in the Private Interest*. New York: Rowman and Littlefield.

Lesser, L., Ebbeling, C.B., Goozner, M., Wypij, D., & Ludwig, D.S. (2007). Relationship between funding source and conclusion among nutrition-related scientific articles. *PLoS Medicine*, **4**(1), e5. doi: 10.1371/journal.pmed.0040005

Lessig, L. (2013). Foreword: 'institutional corruption' defined. *Journal of Law, Medicine and Ethics*, **41**, 553–555.

Leys, C. (2001). *Market-Driven Politics: Neoliberal Democracy and the Public Interest*. London: Verso.

Lustig, R., Schmidt, L., & Brindis, C. (2012). Public health: the toxic truth about sugar. *Nature*, **482**, 27–29.

McGarrity, T. & Warner, W. (2008). *Bending Science*. Cambridge, MA: Harvard University Press.

Mashey, J. (2012). Fakery 2: more funny finances, free of tax. *Desmogblog*, 25 October. URL: <http://desmogblog.com/2012/10/23/fakery-2-more-funny-finances-free-tax>

Maxwell, J.A. (2008). The value of a realist understanding of causality for qualitative research. In: *Qualitative Inquiry and the Politics of Evidence* (ed. N.K. Denzin & G.D. Giardina), pp. 163–181. Walnut Creek, CA: Left Coast Press.

Michaels, D. (2008). *Doubt is Their Product: How Industry's Assault on Science Threatens Your Health*. Oxford: Oxford University Press.

Miller, D. (1998). Mediating science: promotional strategies, media coverage, public belief and decision making. In: *Communicating Science: Contexts and Channels* (ed. E. Scanlon, E. Whitelegg, & S. Yates), pp. 206–226. London: Routledge.

Miller, D. (1999). Risk, science and policy: definitional struggles, information management, the media and BSE. *Social Science and Medicine*, **49**, 1239–1255.

Miller, D. (2004). System failure: it's not just the media—the whole political system has failed. *Journal of Public Affairs*, **4**, 374–383.

Miller, D. & Dinan, W. (2000). The rise of the PR industry in Britain 1979–98. *European Journal of Communication*, **15**, 5–35.

Miller, D. & Dinan, W. (2008). *A Century of Spin*. London: Pluto.

Miller, D. & Dinan, W. (2009a). Journalism, public relations and spin. In: *Handbook of Journalism Studies* (ed. K. Wahl-Jorgensen & T. Hanitzsch), pp. 250–264. New York: Routledge.

Miller, D. & Dinan, W. (2009b). *Revolving Doors, Accountability and Transparency— Emerging Regulatory Concerns and Policy Solutions in the Financial Crisis*. URL: <http://www.oecd.org/officialdocuments/publicdisplaydocumentpdf/?cote=GOV/PGC/ETH%282009%292&docLanguage=En>

Miller, D. & Harkins, C. (2010). Corporate strategy and corporate capture: food and alcohol industry and lobbying and public health. *Critical Social Policy*, **30**, 564–589.

Miller, D. & Harkins, C. (2012). The struggle over minimum unit pricing for alcohol has only just begun. *ALICE RAP Blog*, 21 May 2012. URL: <http://www.alicerap.eu/blog/71-the-struggle-over-minimum-pricing-for-alcohol-has-only-just-begun-2.html>

Miller, D. & Harkins, C. (2013a). Sugar , industry documents and research on corporate influences on addiction. *ALICE RAP Blog*, 28 April 2013. URL: <http://www.alicerap.eu/blog/102-sugar,-industry-documents-and-research-on-corporate-influences-on-addiction.html>

Miller, D. & Harkins, C. (2013b). Revolving doors and alcohol policy: a cautionary tale. *ALICE RAP Blog*, 23 October 2013. URL: <http://www.alicerap.eu/blog/120-revolving-doors-and-alcohol-policy-a-cautionary-tale.html>

Miller, D. & Harkins, C. (2014). Can the influence of the alcohol industry be curtailed? *BMJ Blog*, 7 January 2014. URL: <http://blogs.bmj.com/bmj/2014/01/08/david-miller-and-claire-harkins-can-the-influence-of-the-alcohol-industry-be-curtailed/>

Miller, D. & Reilly, J. (1995). Making an issue of food safety: the media, pressure groups and the public sphere. In: *Eating Agendas: Food, Eating and Nutrition as Social Problems* (ed. D. Maurer & J. Sobal), pp. 305–336. New York: Aldine De Gruyter.

Miller, D., Dinan, W., Cave, T., & Jones, M. (2012). *Public Administration Committee. Written Evidence Submitted by Spinwatch (BA 04)*. URL: <http://www.publications.parliament.uk/pa/cm201213/cmselect/cmpubadm/404/404we05.htm>

Miller, D., Gilmore, A.B., Sheron, N., Britton, J., & Babor, T.F. (2014). Re: Costs of minimum alcohol pricing would outweigh benefits. *British Medical Journal*, **348**, g1572.

Mirowski, P. & Plehwe, D. (ed.) (2009). *The Road from Mont Pelerin: The Making of the Neoliberal Thought Collective*. Cambridge, MA: Harvard University Press.

Mooney, C. (2006). *The Republican War on Science*. New York: Basic Books.

Nutt, D. (2010). Lessons from the mephedrone ban. *theguardian.com*, 28 May 2010. URL: <http://www.theguardian.com/commentisfree/2010/may/28/mephedrone-ban-drug-classification>

OECD (2006). *Compendium of OECD Well-Being Indicators*. URL: <http://www.oecd.org/std/47917288.pdf>

Open Secrets (2014). *Diageo PLC*. URL: <http://www.opensecrets.org/orgs/summary.php?id=D000025490>

Peele, S. (2010). Civil war in alcohol policy: northern versus southern Europe. *Addiction Research and Theory*, **18**, 389–391.

Powerbase (2014a). *Institute for Policy Research*. URL: <http://www.powerbase.info/index.php/Institute_for_Policy_Research>

Powerbase (2014b). *American Council on Science and Health*. URL: <http://www.powerbase.info/index.php/American_Council_on_Science_and_Health>

Public Administration Select Committee (2012). *Business Appointment Rules Third Report of Session 2012–13 Report, Together With Formal Minutes, Oral and Written Evidence*. URL: <http://www.publications.parliament.uk/pa/cm201213/cmselect/cmpubadm/404/404.pdf>

Revolving Door Working Group (2005). *A Matter of Trust: How the Revolving Door Undermines Public Confidence in government—And What To do About it*. URL: <http://pogoarchives.org/m/gc/a-matter-of-trust-20051001.pdf>

Rhodes, R.A.W. (2000). Governance and public administration. In: *Debating Governance: Authority, Steering, and Democracy* (ed. J. Pierre), pp. 54–90. Oxford: Oxford University Press.

Robinson, M. (1998). Corruption and development: an introduction. In: *Corruption and Development* (ed. M. Robinson), pp. 1–14. London: Frank Cass.

Rose, H. & Rose, S. (2012). *Genes, Cells and Brains: The Promethean Promises of the New Biology*. London: Verso.

Rowell, A. & Bates, C. (2000). *Tobacco smuggling in the UK*. London: Action on Smoking and Health. URL: <http://www.ash.org.uk/files/documents/ASH_257.pdf>

Rowell, A. & Cookson, R. (2000). No smoke without fire. *Spinwatch*. URL: <http://www.spinwatch.org/index.php/issues/health/itemlist/category/29-tobacco-industry>

Schuman, D. (2011). A state by state look at lobbyist disclosure. *Sunlight Foundation*, 19 July. URL: < http://sunlightfoundation.com/blog/2011/07/19/a-state-by-state-look-at-lobbyist-disclosure/>

Science Media Centre (2014a). *Welcome to the Science Media Centre*. URL: <http://www.sciencemediacentre.org/>

Science Media Centre (2014b). *Funding*. URL: <http://www.sciencemediacentre.org/about-us/funding/>

Silverstein, K. (1996). APCO: astroturf makers. *Multinational Monitor*, 17(3). URL: <http://www.multinationalmonitor.org/hyper/mm0396.09.html>

Snowdon, C. (2014). Costs of minimum alcohol pricing would outweigh benefits. *British Medical Journal*, **348**, f7531.

Soley, L. (1995). *Leasing the Ivory tower: The Corporate Takeover of Academia*. Boston MA: South End Press.

Tobacco Tactics (2014a). *IEA: History of Close Ties with the Tobacco Industry*. URL: <http://www.tobaccotactics.org/index.php/IEA:_History_of_Close_Ties_with_the_Tobacco_Industry

Tobacco Tactics (2014b). *IEA: Working with RJ Reynolds, BAT and Philip Morris on Environmental Risk*. URL: <http://www.tobaccotactics.org/index.php/IEA:_Working_with_RJ_Reynolds,_BAT_and_Philip_Morris_on_Environmental_Risk>

Vibert, F. (2006). *The Rise of the Unelected: Democracy and the New Separation of Powers*. Cambridge: Cambridge University Press.

Wiist, W. (2010). *The Bottom Line or Public Health: Tactics Corporations Use to Influence Health and Health Policy, and What We Can Do to Counter Them*. New York: Oxford University Press.

Ziauddeen, H., Farooqi, I., & Fletcher, P. (2012). Obesity and the brain: how convincing is the addiction model? *Nature Reviews Neuroscience*, **13**, 279–286.

Chapter 12

Conclusion

Jürgen Rehm, Robin Room,
and Peter Anderson

12.1 **Our conclusion: an introduction**

This book has proposed individual and societal well-being and its domains as a framework for a better understanding of addictive substances and behaviours. We have tried to show that the use of addictive substances and addictive behaviours permeate many aspects of modern society and that they contribute to everyday life. This means that modern societies also have to understand addictions in order to minimize the harm and increase the well-being associated with them, for example for tobacco (Shibuya et al., 2003; WHO Framework Convention on Tobacco Control, 2014), alcohol (Anderson et al., 2009; Babor et al., 2010a; World Health Organization, 2010); illegal drugs and misuse of pharmaceutical drugs (Babor et al., 2010b), and gambling (Williams et al., 2011). These cited references already point to one problem in our understanding: we lack a common framework for use with all addictive substances and behaviours (and there may be good reasons to include more than the substance and behavioural addictions mentioned; see Chapter 3 or Lustig et al. (2012)), and most prevention and other interventions are discussed specifically for one type of behaviour only. One problem with this approach becomes immediately obvious: in the current monitoring structure we lack knowledge about substitution effects, such as use of cannabis potentially increasing if alcohol controls are increased, or vice versa.

In this concluding chapter we will try to point out some commonalities and conclusions for the wider field from the work presented in the different chapters of this book.

12.2 **Use of addictive substances and addictive behaviour can be described on a continuum, and addiction can be seen as one way of framing heavy use, i.e. one end of the continuum**

Many people who use addictive substances or who show potentially addictive behaviours are not heavy users. Many people try out such behaviours: some stop after first use, others go on to use occasionally, and others will use moderately or heavily over time. But patterns of use do not just go in one direction: people cease or reduce their behaviours, and they may change in different directions several times during their lives. People who have been at the high end of consumption or behaviour are no exception here. To give an example for one substance, alcohol: longitudinal studies on people who experience alcohol dependence at some time in their lives paint a picture of changing behaviours over time, and even if there is a general trend for reduction of drinking among survivors after decades, the time in between can often be best described as an ebb and flow of drinking (see work on the Barcelona cohort (Gual et al., 1989, 1999, 2004, 2009) or the famous Vaillant cohorts (Vaillant, 1983, 2003)). Similar effects can be found in the population of drinkers as a whole (Skog and Rossow, 2006).

If lifetime use of addictive substances or addictive behaviour fluctuates in both directions, it is best conceptualized as a continuum, with individuals undertaking such behaviours being active agent users, as Sullivan and Hagen show in Chapter 2. This does not mean that mechanisms do not differ at various points on the continuum, i.e. the reasons for first use may often be different from the reasons for continued use, or for continued heavy use over time (Sullivan and Hagen, 2002; Sullivan et al., 2008). For example, it has been found that initiation of use or behaviour is much more socially determined than continued heavy use over time, when individual traits and characteristics play a larger role (Hradilova Selin, 2005; Rehm et al., in press b).

One consequence of this concept of a continuum of behaviour is that there is no mystical significance about addiction: rather it is one point or region on that continuum. All the points subsumed by this term can be better captured by the term 'heavy use over time'. In other words, from a public health perspective everything that is needed to define addiction and its impact on individuals and societies is captured by 'heavy use over time' (Rehm et al., 2013, 2014); see also the comments of Bradley and Rubinsky (2013), Heather (2013), Saunders (2013), and Rice (2013). Thus, heavy use over time is responsible for the changes in the brain and other physiological characteristics of substance use disorders; it is responsible for intoxication, and for the withdrawal and tolerance phenomena regarded as central to current definitions of addiction or dependence; it is responsible for the main social consequences of substance use disorders such as problems in fulfilling social roles; and it is responsible for the majority of the substance-attributable burden of disease and mortality. The addiction concept may provide an explanation for heavy drinking over time in terms of a postulated psychic or brain disorder, and the concept may sometimes be therapeutically useful for a heavy user who wishes to change, but the concept is superfluous for public health and policy (MacCoun, 2003). In terms of public health thinking and policy, heavy use over time as a definition better fits the empirical data and will also eliminate some of the current problems with definitions and operationalization (Rehm et al., 2013, in press a).

12.3 **Impacts on consumption and consumption-related harm**

Why is the study of addictive substances and behaviour so important? The simplest answer would be the amount of harm which is associated with such substances. One measure of harm to society, albeit associated with a number of conceptual problems, would be the economic and social costs which are caused by the use of addictive substances and addictive behaviour, as summarized by Shield et al. in Chapter 9. Even though details of particular costs may be contested and depend on specific operationalizations and the economic approach chosen, the overall costs of substance use and addictive behaviours are clearly enormous, in Europe as elsewhere. In Chapter 9, Shield et al. provide an overview of the European studies to date, and their shortcomings. But what is probably more important is that they sketch out a way forward to arrive at more informative, comparable, and useful studies for the future.

Other measures used to describe the harm from addictive substances and behaviour comprise a variety of public health measures, such as deaths, years of life lost, or burden of disease: most notable here are the Global Burden of Disease and Injury studies and their regional and country reports (Lim et al., 2012; Institute for Health Metrics and Evaluation, 2014), and the efforts of the World Health Organization in their Global Health Estimates, including the yearly World Health Reports and the various Global Status Reports such as the Global Status Report on Alcohol and Health (World Health Organization, 2014a,b). All of these reports point to the high health burden caused by alcohol use, smoking, and use of illegal drugs (gambling is not usually included). This is not surprising, given the numerous disease and injury categories which are causally related to the consumption of addictive substances and addictive behaviour (see the overview in Chapter 4). The health harm is not limited to the harm to users themselves, but extends to others around them. Examples include second-hand tobacco smoke and its effect on the non-smokers inhaling it (Office on Smoking and Health, 2006), the impact of a mother's drinking on the health of the newborn (National Institute of Alcohol Abuse and Alcoholism, 2011; Patra et al., 2011), or the effects of any psychoactive substances on traffic and other injuries (Vitale and van de Mheen, 2006; Taylor et al., 2010; Asbridge et al., 2012).

However, while the impact of substances on health is large, a detailed analysis of the results of studies of their social cost reveals that costs in welfare, law enforcement, and other sectors are high as well, and may even be higher under certain circumstances. For gambling, most research shows increases in overall crime rates following legalization or increases in gambling from changes such as opening casinos (Stitt, 2000; Evans and Topoleski, 2002; Grinols and Mustard, 2006), mainly driven by financial fraud and/or property crimes, and also increases in rates of reported problems from gambling (Room et al., 1999).

12.4 Implications for future policies concerning use of addictive substances and behaviours in modern society

This book has shown that the harms to society and health caused by addictive substances and behaviours are large in modern societies. How should these harms be best reduced? For all substance and behaviours, less harm will occur if use is shifted to lower levels on the continuum. For both the use of addictive substances and gambling there is a dose–response relationship between level of use and harm: in general, the lower the overall levels of use the less the harm. So we are looking to reduce levels of use. Simply banning certain substances categorically or banning gambling do not seem to be options which work well in modern multivalent societies, at least not with respect to known substances (for drugs, see Room and Reuter, 2012). While the health balance of bans may not necessarily be negative (e.g. the effects of alcohol prohibition on rates of liver cirrhosis; Dills and Miron (2004)), modern societies stress civil liberties and more voluntary ways to reduce risks. These trends include classes of drug currently categorized as illegal where recent policy shifts clearly point towards legalization or decriminalization (e.g. Global Commission on Drug Policy, 2011).

How can public health be preserved or increased in such circumstances? There are initiatives in public health which stress favourable environments and health-promoting societal contexts (Davies et al., 2014). Such contexts are characterized by cultures in which healthy behaviours are the norm, and in which the institutional, social, and physical environment supports such mind-sets. Achievement of this ambition will require a positive, holistic, eclectic, and collaborative effort, involving a broad range of stakeholders. To achieve this goal, the value of health and incentives for healthy behaviour should be emphasized, healthy choices in behaviour should become the default, and factors that create a culture and environment which promote unhealthy behaviour should be minimized.

Some of these principles point directly to policies which have long been propagated by the World Health Organization as 'best buys' but are rarely applied in the current policy climate, such as high taxation of addictive substances and gambling or a ban on advertising and marketing for such behaviours (World Health Organization, 2011). Quite often, attempts to implement such policies are hindered by the influence of industry and other stakeholders who profit from the unhealthy behaviours (such as the tobacco industry from smoking, or the alcohol industry and retail stores from heavy drinking). Modern public health professionals have to be aware of the impact of these stakeholders (as described by Miller and Harkin in Chapter 11). Policy changes can often be achieved, but require substantial popular organization and support in opposition to the vested interests, and the ability to take advantage of a 'policy window' when it opens (Kingdon, 1984; Keeler, 1993). Changes such as tax rises or restrictions on hours of sale have the advantage of not singling out and publicly identifying individual heavy consumers, and can be regarded as a form of 'nudging' (Thaler and Sunstein, 2008), impacting subtly on consumers' decisions. However, under pressure from interested stakeholders, governments often seem to retreat to redefining 'nudging' in terms of measures with minimal impact on the market and with limited or no evidence of effectiveness (Marteau et al., 2011; Loewenstein et al., 2012).

While some success has been shown for nudging in public health, there is a fear that we miss out the lower socioeconomic classes, where there is the highest impact of addictive substances and behaviours (see Chapter 7 by Moskalewicz and Klingemann) (Redonnet et al., 2012; Probst et al., 2014).

Overall, we should stress the need for change but realize that it cannot be achieved by simply repeating the call for more/higher taxes or reduction in availability all the time. As the changes in behaviour and rates of harm from tobacco smoking and from drink driving illustrate, changes in cultural norms as well as in legislation are required. For entrenched popular behaviours, pushing forward the public health interest requires persuading the public as well as regulatory change; the two factors support each other. It will have to happen in modern societies which stress capitalist principles and civil liberties, at least for the rich. Regulatory and structural measures are necessary but may have to be adopted in different formats; they should be complemented by softer techniques such as incentive-based nudging (Anderson et al., 2011) and better, more evidence-based prevention such as personalized prevention (see Chapter 6 by Conrod et al.; Conrod et al., 2013).

References

Anderson, P., Chisholm, D., & Fuhr, D. (2009). Effectiveness and cost-effectiveness of policies and programmes to reduce the harm caused by alcohol. *Lancet*, **373**, 2234–2246.

Anderson, P., Harrison, O., Cooper, C., & Jané-Llopis, E. (2011). Incentives for health. *Journal of Health Communication*, **16**(Suppl. 2), 107–133.

Asbridge, M., Hayden, J.A., & Cartwright, J.L. (2012). Acute cannabis consumption and motor vehicle collision risk: systematic review of observational studies and meta-analysis. *British Medical Journal*, **344**, e536.

Babor, T., Caetano, R., Casswell, S., et al. (2010a). *Alcohol: No Ordinary Commodity. Research and Public Policy*, 2nd edn. Oxford: Oxford University Press.

Babor, T.F., Caulkins, J.P., Edwards, G., et al. (2010b). *Drug Policy and the Public Good*. Oxford: Oxford University Press.

Bradley, K.A. & Rubinsky, A.D. (2013). Why not add consumption measures to current definitions of substance use disorders? Commentary on Rehm et al. 'Defining substance use disorders: Do we really need more than heavy use?'. *Alcohol and Alcoholism*, **48**, 642–643.

Conrod, P.J., O'Leary-Barrett, M., Newton, N., et al. (2013). Effectiveness of a selective, personality-targeted prevention program for adolescent alcohol use and misuse: a cluster randomized controlled trial. *Journal of the American Medical Association—Psychiatry*, **70**, 334–342.

Davies, S.C., Winpenny, E., Ball, S., Fowler, T., Rubin, J., & Nolte, E. (2014). For debate: a new wave in public health improvement. *Lancet*, doi: 10.1016/S0140-6736(13)62341-7

Dills, A.K. & Miron, J.A. (2004). Alcohol prohibition and Cirrhosis. *American Law and Economics Review*, **6**, 285–318.

Evans, W.N. & Topoleski, J.H. (2002). The social and economic impact of Native American casinos. NBER Working Paper No. 9198. URL: <http://www.nber.org/papers/w9198>

Global Commission on Drug Policy (2011). *War on drugs. Report of the Global Commission on Drug Policy*. URL: <http://www.globalcommissionondrugs.org/wp-content/themes/gcdp_v1/pdf/Global_Commission_Report_English.pdf>

Grinols, E.L. & Mustard, D.B. (2006). Casinos, crime and community costs. *Review of Economics and Statistics*, **88**, 28–45.

Gual, A., Bravo, F., Lligoña, A., & Colom, J. (2009). Treatment for alcohol dependence in Catalonia: health outcomes and stability of drinking patterns over 20 years in 850 patients. *Alcohol and Alcoholism*, **44**, 409–415.

Gual, A., Bruguera, E., Heras, S., & Lligoña, A. (1989). Caracteristicas de los alcoholicos que solicitan tratamiento en Catalunya. *Libro de Ponencias de las XVII Jornadas Nacionales de Socidrogalcohol*, 65–88.

Gual, A., Lligoña, A., & Colom, J. (1999). Five-year outcome in alcohol dependence. A naturalistic study of 850 patients in Catalonia. *Alcohol and Alcoholism*, **34**, 183–192.

Gual, A., Lligoña, A., Costa, S., Segura, L., & Colom, J. (2004). Long term impact of treatment in alcoholics. Results from a 10-year longitudinal follow-up study of 850 patients. *Medicina Clinica (Barcelona)*, **123**, 364–369.

Heather, N. (2013). A radical but flawed proposal: comments on Rehm et al. 'Defining substance use disorders: do we really need more than heavy use?'. *Alcohol and Alcoholism*, **48**, 646–647.

Hradilova Selin, K. (2005). Predicting alcohol-related harm by sociodemographic background: high prevalence versus high risk. *Contemporary Drug Problems*, **32**, 547–588.

Institute for Health Metrics and Evaluation (2014). *Global Burden of Disease (GBD)*. URL: <http://www.healthdata.org/gbd>

Keeler, J.T.S. (1993). Opening the window for reform: mandates, crises and extraordinary policy-making. *Comparative Political Studies*, **25**, 433–486.

Kingdon, J.W. (1984). *Agendas, Alternatives and Public Policies*. Boston: Little-Brown.

Lim, S.S., Vos, T., Flaxman, A.D., et al. (2012). A comparative risk assessment of burden of disease and injury attributable to 67 risk factors and risk factor clusters in 21 regions, 1990–2010: a systematic analysis for the Global Burden of Disease Study 2010. *Lancet*, **380**, 2224–2260.

Loewenstein, G., Asch, D.A., Friedman, J.Y., Melichar, L.A., & Volpp, K.G. (2012). Can behavioural economics make us healthier? *British Medical Journal*, **344**, e3482.

Lustig, R.H., Schmidt, L.A., & Brindis, C.D. (2012). The toxic truth about sugar. *Nature*, **487**, 27–29.

MacCoun, R. (2003). Is the addiction concept useful for drug policy? In: *Choice, Behavioral Economics and Addiction* (ed. N. Heather & R.E. Vuchinich), pp. 383–401. Oxford: Pergamon.

Marteau, T.M., Ogilvie, D., Roland, M., Suhrcke, M., & Kelly, M.P. (2011). Judging nudging: can nudging improve population health? *British Medical Journal*, **342**, d228.

National Institute of Alcohol Abuse and Alcoholism (2011). *Alcohol Research and Health*. Special issue on fetal alcohol spectrum disorders. URL: <http://pubs.niaaa.nih.gov/publications/arh341/toc34_1.htm>

Office on Smoking and Health (2006). *The Health Consequences of Involuntary Exposure to Tobacco Smoke. A Report of the Surgeon General*. Atlanta, GA: Centers for Disease Control and Prevention.

Patra, J., Bakker, R., Irving, H., Jaddoe, V.W.V., Malini, S., & Rehm, J. (2011). Dose–response relationship between alcohol consumption before and during pregnancy and the risks of low birthweight, preterm birth and small for gestational age (SGA)-a systematic review and meta-analyses. *BJOG: International Journal of Obstetrics and Gynaecology*, **118**, 1411–1421.

Probst, C., Roerecke, M., Behrendt, S., & Rehm, J. (2014). Socioeconomic differences in alcohol-attributable mortality compared to all-cause mortality: a systematic review and meta-analysis. *International Journal of Epidemiology*, **43**, 1314–1327.

Redonnet, B., Chollet, A., Fombonne, E., Bowes, L., & Melchior, M. (2012). Tobacco, alcohol, cannabis and other illegal drug use among young adults: the socioeconomic context. *Drug and Alcohol Dependence*, **121**, 231–239.

Rehm, J., Marmet, S., Anderson, P., et al. (2013). Defining substance use disorders: do we really need more than heavy use? *Alcohol and Alcoholism*, **48**, 633–640.

Rehm, J., Anderson, P., Gual, A., et al. (2014). The tangible common denominator of substance use disorders: a reply to commentaries to Rehm et al. (2013). *Alcohol and Alcoholism*, **49**, 118–122.

Rehm, J., Probst, C., Kraus, L., & Lev-Ran, S. (in press a). What is addiction? In: *Governance of Addictions in Europe: Policies, Processes and Pressures* (ed. P. Anderson, G. Bühringer, & J. Colom). Barcelona: ALICE RAP.

Rehm, J., Probst, C., & Shield, K.D. (in press b). Burden of disease: the epidemiological aspects of addiction. In: *Textbook of Addiction Treatment. An International Perspective* (ed. N. el Guebaly). Heidelberg: Springer. doi: 10.1007/978-88-470-5322-9

Rice, P. (2013). A commentary on defining substance use disorders: do we really need more than heavy use? *Alcohol and Alcoholism*, **48**, 641.

Room, R. & Reuter, P. (2012). How well do international drug conventions protect public health? *Lancet*, **379**, 84–91.

Room, R., Turner, N.E., & Ialomiteanu, A. (1999). Community effects of the opening of the Niagara casino. *Addiction*, **94**, 1449–1466.

Saunders, J.B. (2013). The concept of substance use disorders. A commentary on 'Defining substance use disorders: do we really need more than heavy use' by Rehm et al. *Alcohol and Alcoholism*, **48**, 644–645.

Shibuya, K., Ciecierski, C., Guindon, E., Bettcher, D., Evans, D., & Murray, C. (2003). WHO framework convention on tobacco control: development of an evidence based global public health treaty. *British Medical Journal*, **327**, 154–157.

Skog, O.-J. & Rossow, I. (2006). Flux and stability: individual fluctuations, regression towards the mean and collective changes in alcohol consumption. *Addiction*, **101**, 959–970.

Stitt, G. (2000). *Effects of Casino Gambling on Crime and Quality of Life in New Casino Jurisdictions, Final Report*. Rockville, MD. National Institute of Justice.

Sullivan, R.J. & Hagen, E.H. (2002). Psychotropic substance-seeking: evolutionary pathology or adaptation?. *Addiction*, **97**, 389–400.

Sullivan, R.J., Hagen, E.H., & Hammerstein, P. (2008). Revealing the paradox of drug reward in human evolution. *Proceedings of the Royal Society B: Biological Sciences*, **275**, 1231–1241.

Taylor, B., Irving, H.M., Kanteres, F., et al. (2010). The more you drink, the harder you fall: a systematic review and meta-analysis of how acute alcohol consumption and injury or collision risk increase together. *Drug and Alcohol Dependence*, **110**, 108–116.

Thaler, R.H. & Sunstein, C. (2008). *Nudge: Improving Decisions About Health, Wealth, and Happiness*. New Haven, CT: Yale University Press.

Vaillant, G.E. (1983). *The Natural History of Alcoholism: Paths to Recovery*. Cambridge, MA: Harvard University Press.

Vaillant, G.E. (2003). 60-year follow-up of alcoholic men. *Addiction*, **98**, 1043–1051.

Vitale, S. & Van De Mheen, H.D. (2006). Illicit drug use and injuries: a review of emergency room studies. *Drug and Alcohol Dependence*, **82**, 1–9.

Williams, R.J., Rehm, J., & Stevens, R.M.G. (2011). *The Social and Economic Impacts of Gambling. Final Report for the Canadian Consortium for Gambling Research*. URL: <https://www.uleth.ca/dspace/bitstream/handle/10133/1286/SEIG_FINAL_REPORT_2011.pdf?sequence=1>

WHO Framework Convention on Tobacco Control (2014). Head of the Convention Secretariat strongly supports 100% smoke-free Tokyo. URL: <http://www.who.int/fctc/implementation/cooperation/japan/en/>

World Health Organization (2010). *Global Strategy to Reduce the Harmful Use of Alcohol*. Geneva: World Health Organization.

World Health Organization (2011). *Global Status Report on Noncommunicable Diseases 2010. Description of the Global Burden of NCDs, Their Risk Factors and Determinants*. Geneva: World Health Organization.

World Health Organization (2014a). *Global Health Estimates*. URL: <http://www.who.int/healthinfo/global_burden_disease/en/>

World Health Organization (2014b). *Global Status Report on Alcohol and Health*. Geneva: World Health Organization.

Index

A
abstinence-oriented therapy 67
Adam Smith Institute 223
adaptive immunity 79
addiction
  changing conceptualization 216–17
  conceptual frame of addictive
    behaviours 1–2
  continuum of behaviour 239–42
  definition 38–9
  dosage and 43
  as heavy use over time 240–1
  medicalization 153–4
  net-widening 37–8, 41–5
  pan-addiction model 39–41
ADH1B 105
ADH1C 105
administration routes 18, 25
adolescent substance use
  consequences 120
  economic recession 168
  evidence-based psychosocial
    interventions 126–32
  harm 120–3
  policy issues 123–4, 133–4
  prevalence 119
  prevention and intervention
    approaches 123–6
  risk factors 120–3
Adventure Effectiveness Trial 128
Advisory Committee on Business
  Appointments 230
Africa
  amphetamine use 201
  ancient use of khat 17
  injecting drug use 202
  tobacco consumption 99, 205
  traditional beer brewing 44
African Americans 150, 151
African 'pygmy' men 30
age
  burden of addictive substances 99, 103
  onset of alcohol use 119
aggression 89–90
AIDS 84
alcohol
  automatic attitudes to 131
  as a habit-forming substance 37
  harm ranking 190–1
  human evolution 5–6
  minimum pricing 224

production methods 193–5
alcohol consumption
  adolescents 119, 120
  age of onset 119
  alcoholism 41
  anxiety and depression 122
  binge-drinking 88, 89, 119, 120, 175, 198
  burden of 96, 97–8, 100–2, 197–8
  continuum of behaviour 240
  drunkenness 131, 147, 193
  economic conditions 166–7, 169–70
  genetics of cancer risk 85, 105
  health effects 82–90, 102
  income effect theory 173, 175–6
  marginalization 63
  mortality 83, 199–200
  price sensitivity 132
  social class 63, 202
  social costs 183–4
  social justice 143, 145–9
  socioeconomic development 193–200
  tourism 195–6
  unemployment 64, 166–7, 173–4, 175
alcohol dehydrogenase 2 (*ALDH2*) 85, 105
ALICE RAP v, 3, 130, 131
alkali mixing 18
alkaloids 20, 21
alveolar macrophages 79
Alzheimer's disease 27, 87
America
  adolescent substance use 119
  amphetamine use 202
  cocaine use 103, 201
  historical drug use 17, 18
  native North Americans 19
  opioid use 201, 202
  prohibition 148
  see also United States
American Council on Science and Health 222
amphetamines
  burden of 103
  health effects 92–3
  socioeconomic development 201, 202
  use in US 29
AMSTAR 125
analgesics 27
Andes 17
anthelmintics 26–7
antibody response 79
antidepressants 201
antipsychotics 201

anxiety 121–2
anxiety-sensitivity 122
archaeological evidence of substance use
  16–20
Areca catechu (betel nut) 17, 18, 19, 26
arecoline 18, 26
Asia
  alcohol consumption 102, 196, 197
  amphetamine use 201
  gambling and Internet gaming 39
  injecting drug use 202
  tobacco consumption 99
'astroturf' organizations 223
attention, nicotine effects 27
attention deficit and hyperactivity disorder
  41, 121
attitudes
  automatic attitudes to substance use 131–3
  of health professionals to addiction 153
austerity measures 163–4
Australia
  Aborigines 17, 18
  alcohol-attributable mortality 199
  alcohol use and economic conditions 167
  economic recession and addictive
    behaviours 169, 170
  injecting drug use 202
  tobacco consumption 204
Austria
  government expenditure attributable to
    illicit drugs 185
  lobbying transparency 229
automatic attitudes 131–3
autonomy 60
availability 44
aversive learning 24

B
bacterial infection 26
banning substances 242
behavioural addictions 37, 39
  health effects 95–6
  see also specific behaviours
behavioural control problems 120
betel nut 17, 18, 19, 26
Better Life Index 58–9
binge-drinking 88, 89, 119, 120, 175, 198
binge-eating 39
bitter taste receptors 24
blood–brain barrier 24
brain development and damage 120, 131
Brazil
  alcohol consumption 199, 200
  tobacco consumption 205
British Nutrition Foundation 223
buccal route of administration 18
burden of addictive substances 78, 96–105,
  197–8

C
caffeine 27
Canada, adolescent substance use 119
cancer 80–1, 84–6, 105
cannabis
  adolescent use 119, 120
  analgesic effects 27
  anthelmintic effects 26
  automatic attitudes to 131
  burden of 103
  decriminalization in Portugal 91
  European policies 65
  European use 64
  harm ranking 190
  health effects 92–3
  socioeconomic development and use of
    201
  US users 29
  well-being and prohibition 64–6
capitalism 146–7
cardiovascular disease 81–2,
  87–8
Caribbean
  cocaine use 103
  injecting drug use 202
cassava 26
caterpillars 23, 26
Catha edulis (khat) 17, 18–19, 20
cathine 18
Central Asia
  alcohol consumption 102, 197
  injecting drug use 202
  tobacco consumption 99
Centre for Policy Studies 220
Change4Life 224
China
  alcohol consumption 196
  tobacco consumption 204
Chinese migrant workers 150
civic engagement 60
civil society
  corporate influence 222–4
  transparency 227–9
class justice 144
cleft lip 80
Climate Schools programme 126
coca 17, 18, 19, 20
Coca Cola 42
cocaine
  in Americas 103, 201
  crack 29, 43, 61–2, 150–1
  health effects 92–3
  pharmacology 19
  US consumption 29
cognitive behavioural therapy 126
cognitive enhancement 27
colonialism 194, 195
commercial interests 2, 43

Commission on the Measurement of
   Economic Performance and Social
   Progress (Stiglitz Commission) 55–6, 58
Committee on Publication Ethics (COPE) 226
commodification 44
communism 147
competence 60
conduct disorder 121, 122
conflicts of interest 221–2, 226–7, 230–1
contact hypothesis 153
contextual factors
   adolescent substance use 121
   social context of net-widening 42–5
continuum of behaviour 239–42
corporate capture 220
   civil society 222–4
   science 221–2
corruption 216–24, 226
cost of illness study 181
Cotesia congretate 22
crack cocaine 29, 43, 61–2, 150–1
crime 60, 216–24, 242
Croatia, government expenditure attributable
   to illicit drugs 185
cultural factors, automatic attitudes 131–3
CYP1A1 105
Cyprus, government expenditure attributable
   to illicit drugs 185
cytochrome P450 24
Czech Republic
   alcohol-attributable mortality 199
   government expenditure attributable to
      illicit drugs 185

D
dementia 27, 87
democracy 60
Democracy Institute 227
Denmark, government expenditure
   attributable to illicit drugs 185
dependence
   clinical criteria for 38
   as mental illness 154
depression 87, 121–2
derogation 2
deviance paradigm 152
diabetes mellitus 81, 86
*Diagnostic and Statistical Manual of Mental
   Disorders*
   DSM-IV 38, 171
   DSM-5 39, 171
digestive disease 88–9
disability-adjusted life years (DALYs) 78, 96,
   99–100, 102, 103, 197–8
discrimination 65, 152–3, 155
disinhibition 122
dissemination, evidence-based
   prevention 129–30

Donors Capital Fund 228
Donors Trust 228
dopamine system 15, 16, 40–1
dosage 43
drug hardening 43
drug use
   adolescents 119
   automatic attitudes to 131
   burden of 96, 98, 102–4
   counter-exploitation of neurotoxins 25–8
   ecological perspective 13, 20–4, 30
   economic conditions 168, 170
   evolutionary novelty 13, 16, 24–5
   foods 19–20
   health effects 90–5, 104
   hijack hypothesis 15–16, 28
   international drugs treaties 200
   paradox of drug reward 13–15
   punishment model 20–4
   routes of administration 18, 25
   social costs 184–6
   social justice 149–50
   societal perceptions of 61–2
   socioeconomic development 200–3
   socioeconomic status 202
drunkenness 131, 147, 193
Duboisia hopwoodii (pituri) 17, 18

E
Easterlin paradox 54
eastern Europe
   alcohol consumption 102, 148, 149, 197
   burden of drug use 103
   injecting drug use 202
   opioid use 201
   tobacco consumption 99
eating disorders 39
e-cigarettes 208
ecology 13, 20–4, 30
economic recession 161–76
   alcohol consumption 166–7, 169–70
   austerity measures 163–4
   drug use 168, 170
   gambling 171–2
   impact on addiction-related
      behaviours 165–72
   mechanisms of effect on addictive
      behaviours 172–6
   pro-cyclical versus counter-cyclical
      effects 165–6
   tobacco consumption 167–8, 170
   unemployment 162–3
Ecuador, archaeological evidence of coca use 17
education 60
enemy-reduced (-free) space 26
environment
   adolescent substance use 121
   well-being and 60

ephedrine 18–19
equality, productivity and 144
Erythroxylum coca (coca) 17, 18, 19, 20
Estonia
  alcohol-attributable mortality 199
  economic recession and addictive
    behaviours 167, 170
  government expenditure attributable to
    illicit drugs 185
ethanol 85–6, 89
Ethiopia, ancient use of khat 17
ethnicity 65–6
eudaimonic well-being 57
Europe
  addictive behaviours in last fifty years 3
  adolescent substance use 119
  adolescent substance use policy 123–4
  burden of addictive substances 99, 102,
    103, 197
  cannabis policy 65
  cannabis use 64
  cohort studies of risk factors for substance
    use 130
  economic crisis and alcohol
    consumption 167
  governance and well-being 68–72
  government expenditure attributable to
    illicit drugs 185, 186
  injecting drug use 202
  opioid use 201–2
  social costs of addiction 181–6
  social justice and alcohol consumption 148,
    149
  welfare state 144
European Alcohol and Health Forum 224
European Food Information Council
  (EUFIC) 223
European Food Safety Authority (EFSA)
  230
European Policy Forum 220
European Statistical System Committee
  (ESSC) 56
European Union (EU)
  economic recession 161, 162–4, 169
  GDP 145, 162
  GDP and alcohol dependence 184
  inequality 145
  life expectancy 145
  lobbying transparency 229
  quality of life indicators 58
  revolving door transparency 230, 231
  unemployment 162–3
evolution 5–6
evolutionary novelty 13, 16, 24–5
Exorista mella 23
externalities 2
externalizing behaviours 121,
  130–1

F
family, adolescent substance use 121
family-based therapy 126
fava beans 26
fertility 80
Finland
  alcohol-attributable mortality 199–200
  government expenditure attributable to
    illicit drugs 185
  temperance movement 147, 148
foetal exposure 80, 84
food
  as addictive substances 37, 39
  drugs as 19–20
  production 44
  see also sugar consumption
Foresight Project on Mental Capital and
  Wellbeing 55, 56
formal social control 45
Framework Convention on Tobacco Control
  (FCTC) 203
France, government expenditure attributable
  to illicit drugs 185
free markets 45
front groups 223
fructose 43
functional magnetic resonance imaging 40

G
gambling
  as an addiction 39
  dopamine system 40, 41
  economic recession 171–2
  engineering of 43
  harm 191
  health effects 95–6
  increasing accessibility of 44
  social control 45
  social costs 186, 242
gaming *see* Internet gaming/gambling
gender differences
  burden of addictive substances 99, 100, 102,
    103
  tobacco-related mortality 204
genetic issues
  cancer risks 85, 105
  predisposition to substance use 121
Germany
  economic recession and addictive
    behaviours 169
  government expenditure attributable to
    illicit drugs 185
Gini Index 145
Global Adult Tobacco Survey 204, 205
global health burden of addiction 78, 96–105,
  197–8
globalization 44, 45
Good Behaviour game 126

governance
  models for drugs policy 68–72
  partnerships 224
  theoretical perspectives 216
  well-being and 60, 68–72, 216, 231
Grammia incorrupta 23
Greece
  economic recession 164
  government expenditure attributable to
    illicit drugs 185
gross domestic product (GDP)
  alcohol consumption and 102, 196–7
  alcohol dependence in EU 184
  EU 145, 162
  well-being and 53–4
Gross National Happiness 58
GSTM1 105
GSTT1 105

H
habit-forming substances 37, 207
haemorrhagic stroke 88
harm
  adolescent substance use 120–3
  beyond the individual consumer 1–2,
    241
  comparative ratings 190–1
  health effects of addictive substances 78–96,
    100, 102, 104, 241
  inequalities 104–5
  policy-related 91, 95
  quality of life and material living conditions
    and 61–4
  see also social costs
harm reduction 62, 126
health and well-being 60
health burden of addiction 78, 96–105,
  197–8
health care budget cuts 163–4
health effects of addictive substances 78–96,
  100, 102, 104, 241
health insurance 152
health outcomes 203
health professionals
  attitudes to addiction 153
  knowledge of substance use 155
heart disease 81–2, 87–8
heavy use over time 240–1
hedonic balance 38
help-seeking behaviour 152
heroin 29
hijack hypothesis 15–16, 28
Hippocrates vi
historical accounts of substance use
  16–20
HIV 84
hopelessness 122
housing 59

Hungary
  alcohol-attributable mortality 199
  government expenditure attributable to
    illicit drugs 185
  lobbying transparency 229
hypertension 87–8
hypnotics 201

I
Iceland, economic recession and addictive
    behaviours 164, 168, 170
illicit drugs *see* drug use
IMAGEN 130
immune system 79, 83, 84
implicit attitudes 131–3
impulse-control disorders 42
impulsivity 120, 122, 130–1
income
  addictive behaviour and 166
  alcohol use 173, 175–6
  well-being and 54, 59
India
  alcohol consumption 199
  tobacco consumption 205
industrial production 43
Industrial Revolution 146, 194
inequality 144–5, 191–2
infectious diseases 26, 79, 83–4
informal social control 44
injecting drug use 25, 202
injuries, alcohol-related 89–90
innate immunity 79
Institute for Policy Research (IPR) 228–9
Institute of Economic Affairs (IEA) 223–4,
  227, 228
institutional corruption 218–20
insulin resistance 86
internalizing disorders 121–2
International Committee of Medical Journal
  Editors (ICMJE) 226
International Expert Working Group for a New
  Development Paradigm 56
International Life Sciences Institute (ILSI) 223
International Society of Addiction Journal
  Editors (ISAJE) 226, 227
Internet, regulated use 37
Internet gaming/gambling 39, 40, 41, 43, 44,
  45
intervention, adolescent substance use
  123–32
Ireland, government expenditure attributable
  to illicit drugs 185
ischaemic heart disease 88

J
Japan, cancer deaths 105
jobs 59 *see also* unemployment
journals, conflicts of interest 226–7

K
khat 17, 18–19, 20

L
labelling 63, 152
Lamu 196
Latin America, drug use 103, 202
Latinos 150, 151
laudanum 150
laws 62, 65, 150, 154, 217
leukocytes 79
LifeSkills Training 126
Lithuania
 government expenditure attributable to
  illicit drugs 185
 lobbying transparency 229
liver disease 88–9
lobbying 219–20
 transparency 229–30
Luxembourg, government expenditure
 attributable to illicit drugs 185

M
macrophages 79
malaria (*Plasmodium falciparum*) 26
malignant neoplasms 80–1, 84–6, 105
Malta, government expenditure attributable to
 illicit drugs 185
Manduca sexta 22
marginalization 62–3, 152, 192–3
market liberalization 45
Marxism 143–4
mass media campaigns 125
material living conditions 61–4
maternal exposures 80, 84
medicalization of addiction 153–4
memory, nicotine effects 27
mental health 27, 87, 121–3
mephedrone 217
mesolimbic dopamine system 15, 16, 40–1
methadone maintenance treatment 66, 67
Mexico, tobacco consumption 205
Micronesia, betel nut chewing 19
Middle East, injecting drug use 202
moral panic 61–2
mortality
 alcohol-related 83, 199–200
 tobacco-related 204
multitrophic interactions 22

N
nationalization 144
native North Americans 19
natural killer cells 79
neoliberalism 219–20
Nepal, alcohol consumption 200
Netherlands
 budget cuts 163–4

economic recession and addictive
 behaviours 169
lobbying transparency 229
net-widening of addiction 37–8, 41–5
neuroimaging 40
neuropsychiatric conditions 81, 87
neurotransmitters, plant compounds
 interfering with 14, 20–1
New Zealand, injecting drug use 202
Nicotiana attenuata 21
Nicotiana gossei 17
Nicotiana rustica 17, 18
Nicotiana tabacum 17, 18
nicotine
 African 'pygmy' exposure 30
 anthelmintic effects 26–7
 beneficial effects 22
 cognitive enhancer 27
 defensive functions 21
 multitrophic interactions 22
 physical health effects 208
 withdrawal 81
Nigeria
 drugs as foods 19
 tobacco consumption 205
norpseudoephedrine 18
North Africa, injecting drug use 202
North America
 burden of drug use 103
 injecting drug use 202
northeast Africa, ancient use of khat 17
Norway
 alcohol-related mortality 199
 economic recession and addictive
  behaviours 170
novelty, evolutionary 13, 16, 24–5
'nudging' 243

O
Oceania 200, 201, 202
Office of National Statistics 56, 58
opioids
 analgesic effects 27
 burden of 103
 health effects 92–3
 medicinal use 200
 socioeconomic development 201, 202
opioid substitution treatment 66–8
opium 150
oppression paradigm 152

P
pan-addiction model 39–41
pancreatitis 89
panic anxiety 122
parasitic disease 22–3, 25–7, 30–1, 79, 83–4
partnership governance 224
peer influence 121

perestroika 149
perinatal exposure 80, 84
permanent income hypothesis 172
personality-targeted interventions 128, 129
personality traits 122–3
pharmacophagy 22, 25–6
phenolics 20
pituri 17, 18
plants
    archaeological evidence of use 17
    counter-exploitation of neurotoxins 25–8
    defences 20–1
    domestication 25
    neurotransmitter effects 14, 20–1
Plasmodium falciparum 26
Platform on Diet Physical Activity and
        Health 224
Platyprepia virginalis 26
pneumonia 83–4
Poland
    alcohol and social justice 145–6, 148–9
    government expenditure attributable to
        illicit drugs 185
    lobbying transparency 229
policies
    adolescent substance use 123–4, 133–4
    capture 224–6
    comprehensive 70
    criminality 217
    European cannabis policy 65
    failure of top-down policies 29
    formal social control 45
    future developments 242–3
    governance models 68–72
    harm creation 91, 95
    harm reduction 62
    stigma-targeting 154, 155
    strategy-based 68–9
    structure-based 68, 69–70
    substance-based 69–70
    UK expenditure on drugs policy 64–5
    well-being and 55–6, 215
pornography 39, 40, 43, 44, 45
Portugal
    decriminalization of cannabis 91
    government expenditure attributable to
        illicit drugs 185
post-democracy 220
pregnancy 80, 84
prevention, adolescent substance use 123–32
Preventure Programme 128, 129
process addictions 37, 38–9
productivity, equality and 144
prohibition 2, 64–6, 91, 95, 148–50, 207, 217
propination 145
proximate biological explanations 24
Prussia, alcohol availability 146
psychiatric diagnoses 41

psychosocial interventions 126–32
psychosocial treatment 126
psychostimulants 201
psychotropic medications 201
public relations 219–20
pulmonary diseases 80
punishment model 20–4

Q
quality of life 58, 60, 61–4

R
racial differences in harm 104–5
realist review 167
regulation 2
reinforcement 13 *see also* reward
research issues 28–9, 30–1
Responsibility Deal 224
revolving door 225–6, 230–1
reward
    hijack hypothesis (reward model) 15–16, 28
    paradox of drug reward 13–15
    reward deficiency hypothesis 40–1
    sensitivity 122, 130, 131
role theory 175
Romania, government expenditure attributable
        to illicit drugs 185
routes of administration 18, 25
Russia
    alcohol consumption 102, 199
    class justice and social justice 144
    tobacco consumption 204

S
safety
    safety and disease approach 68
    well-being and 60
schizophrenia 27
school-based prevention programmes 125,
        126–7, 128
science
    corporate influence 221–2
    transparency 226–7
Science Media Centre 222
sedatives 201
selective prevention 127–8
self-inflicted injuries 89–90
self-medication 122, 175
self-stigma 152, 154
sensation-seeking 122, 131
skills development 125, 126, 127
Slovakia, government expenditure attributable
        to illicit drugs 185
Slovenia
    government expenditure attributable to
        illicit drugs 185
    lobbying transparency 229
snus 208

social control structures 44–5
social coordination 175
social costs 181–6
    alcohol addiction 183–4
    drug use 184–6
    gambling 186, 242
    tobacco dependence 184
social exclusion 4, 63, 151, 164–5
socialist movement 147–8
social justice 143–56
    alcohol access 143, 145–9
    drug prohibition 149–50
    historical background 143–4
    stigma 151–5
    well-being and 144–5
social networks 60, 91
social welfare expenditure 176
society
    net-widening effects 42–5
    norms 62, 121
    perception of drug use 61–2
    response to addiction 2
    well-being see well-being
socioeconomic development 189–208
    alcohol consumption 193–200
    definition 191
    drug use 200–3
    inequality 191–2
    patterns of use and problems
        196–206
    process 193–6
    tobacco consumption 203–6
socioeconomic status
    alcohol-related harms 63
    alcohol-related mortality 199–200
    drug use 202
    health outcomes 203
    marginalization and 193
    socioeconomic differentiation 191–2
    tobacco consumption 205
    treatment outcomes 152
soft drinks 42
Solidarity movement 148–9
South Asia, injecting drug use 202
South Korea
    alcohol consumption 196
    cancer deaths 105
Soviet Union, alcohol availability
        148, 149
Spain, economic recession and addictive
        behaviours 169
spices 26
State socialism 144
stereotyping 151, 155
Stiglitz Commission 55–6, 58
stigma 2, 62, 65, 91, 95, 151–5, 192–3
    self-stigma 152, 154
'stop and search' checks 65–6

strategy-based policy 68–9
stroke risk 88
structural discrimination 152–3, 155
structure-based policy 68, 69–70
subcultures 63
Sub-Saharan Africa, tobacco consumption
        99, 205
substance-based policy 69–70
sugar consumption 37, 39, 40–1, 42, 43, 44,
        45, 217
sugar substitutes 208
sustainable development 55
Sweden, alcohol-attributable mortality 199
symbolism 148–9
systems-based prevention 130–1

T
tannins 20
targeted prevention 127–8
TB 83
temperance movement 147, 148
Thailand
    alcohol consumption 196
    archaeological evidence of betel nut
        chewing 17
    tobacco consumption 205
THC 26
think-tanks 223, 227, 228–9
Timor, archaeological evidence of betel nut
        chewing 17
tobacco consumption
    burden of 96, 97, 99–100
    economic conditions 167–8, 170
    as food 19
    genetic differences in risk 105
    habit-forming substance 37
    health effects 79–82, 100
    historical use 17, 18
    mortality 204
    social costs 184
    socioeconomic development
        203–6
    US users 29, 205
tobacco hornworm (*Manduca sexta*) 22
tourism 195–6
trade agreements 45
tranquillizers 201
transparency 226–31
treatment of addiction
    adolescents 126
    availability 42
    marginalization 63
    opioid substitution treatment 66–8
    outcomes and social status 152
    in US 42
tritrophic interactions 22
tuberculosis 83
Turkey, tobacco consumption 205

U
ultimate biological explanations 24
'unelected' 216, 220
unemployment
    alcohol use 64, 166–7, 173–4, 175
    economic recession in EU 162–3
    gambling 171–2
    well-being and 59
UN General Assembly 56
United Arab Emirates, burden of drug use
    103
United Kingdom (UK)
    alcohol-attributable mortality 199
    domains of well-being 58
    gambling and the economic recession 171
    government expenditure attributable to
        illicit drugs 185
    government expenditure on drugs
        policy 64–5
    institutional corruption 219–20
    lobbying transparency 229
    minimum pricing of alcohol 224
    neoliberalism 219–20
    revolving door transparency 230
    'stop and search' checks 65–6
    well-being on policy agenda 55, 56
United States (US)
    addiction treatment 42
    alcohol-attributable mortality 199
    crack cocaine and social justice 150–1
    drug use 29, 30
    economic recession and addictive
        behaviours 169, 170
    gambling revenue 171, 172
    lobbying transparency 229, 230
    moral panic over crack cocaine 61–2
    racial differences in harm 104–5
    revolving door transparency 230
    tobacco consumption 29, 205

V
vascular dementia 87
Venezuela, alcohol consumption 196
violence 90
vodka production 146, 148
vulnerability to substance use 13, 122–3, 130

W
welfare state 144
well-being 4, 53–60
    defining 56–8
    domains (dimensions/components) 58–60
    dynamic model 56–7
    eudaimonic 57
    GDP and 53–4
    governance and 60, 68–72, 216, 231
    income and 54, 59
    living conditions and opioid substitution
        treatment 66–8
    measurement 57–8
    policy and 55–6, 215
    prohibition and 64–6
    social justice and 144–5
    two-way links with addiction 61–8
    well-being and relational management
        approach 68–9
Whitehall Wellbeing Working Group
    (W3G) 55
work–life balance 60
World Happiness Report 56
World Health Organization (WHO) 78
World Trade Organization 45

Y
years lived with disability 77–8
youth *see* adolescent substance use